Dairy Nutrition

Editor

ROBERT J. VAN SAUN

VETERINARY CLINICS OF NORTH AMERICA: FOOD ANIMAL PRACTICE

www.vetfood.theclinics.com

Consulting Editor
ROBERT A. SMITH

November 2014 • Volume 30 • Number 3

ELSEVIER

1600 John F. Kennedy Boulevard ● Suite 1800 ● Philadelphia, Pennsylvania, 19103-2899

http://www.vetfood.theclinics.com

VETERINARY CLINICS OF NORTH AMERICA: FOOD ANIMAL PRACTICE Volume 30, Number 3
November 2014 ISSN 0749-0720, ISBN-13: 978-0-323-32688-9

Editor: Patrick Manley
Developmental Editor: Yonah Korngold

Veterinary Clinics of North America: Food Animal Practice (ISSN 0749-0720) is published in March, July, and November by Elsevier Inc., 360 Park Avenue South, New York, NY 10010-1710. Subscription prices are $235.00 per year (domestic individuals), $326.00 per year (domestic institutions), $110.00 per year (domestic students/residents), $265.00 per year (Canadian individuals), $430.00 per year (Canadian institutions), $335.00 per year (international individuals), $430.00 per year (international institutions), and $165.00 per year (international and Canadian students/residents). To receive student/resident rate, orders must be accompanied by name of affiliated institution, date of term, and the signature of program/residency coordinator on institution letterhead. *Clinics* subscription prices. All prices are subject to change without notice. **POSTMASTER:** Send address changes to *Veterinary Clinics of North America: Food Animal Practice*, Elsevier Health Sciences Division, Subscription Customer Service, 3251 Riverport Lane, Maryland Heights, MO 63043. Customer Service (orders, claims, online, change of address): Elsevier Health Sciences Division, Subscription Customer Service, 3251 Riverport Lane, Maryland Heights, MO 63043. Tel: 1-800-654-2452 (U.S. and Canada); 314-447-8871 (ouside U.S. and Canada). Fax: 314-447-8029. E-mail: journalscustomerservice-usa@elsevier.com (for print support); journalsonlinesupport-usa@elsevier.com (for online support).

Reprints. For copies of 100 or more, of articles in this publication, please contact the Commercial Reprints Department, Elsevier Inc., 360 Park Avenue South, New York, NY 10010-1710. Tel.: 212-633-3874; Fax: 212-633-3820; E-mail: reprints@elsevier.com.

Veterinary Clinics of North America: Food Animal Practice is covered in *Current Contents/Agriculture, Biology and Environmental Sciences, MEDLINE/PubMed (Index Medicus),* and *Excerpta Medica.*

Contributors

CONSULTING EDITOR

ROBERT A. SMITH, DVM, MS
Diplomate, American Board of Veterinary Practitioners; Veterinary Research and
Consulting Services, LLC, Greeley, Colorado

EDITOR

ROBERT J. VAN SAUN, DVM, MS, PhD
Diplomate American College of Theriogenologists; Diplomate American College of
Veterinary Nutrition; Professor and Extension Veterinarian, Department of Veterinary and
Biomedical Sciences, College of Agricultural Sciences, Pennsylvania State University,
University Park, Pennsylvania

AUTHORS

MICHAEL S. ALLEN, PhD
University Distinguished Professor, Department of Animal Science, Michigan State
University, East Lansing, Michigan

HELEN M. GOLDER, BAgSci (Hons.)
SBScibus; Dairy Science Group, Faculty of Veterinary Science, The University of Sydney,
Camden, New South Wales, Australia

MARY BETH HALL, PhD
Research Animal Scientist, USDA-ARS, U.S. Dairy Forage Research Center, Madison,
Wisconsin

KEVIN J. HARVATINE, MSc, PhD
Assistant Professor of Nutritional Physiology, Department of Animal Sciences, Penn State
University, State College, Pennsylvania

ALEXANDER N. HRISTOV, MSc, PhD, PAS
Professor of Dairy Nutrition, Department of Animal Science, Pennsylvania State University,
University Park, Pennsylvania

THOMAS C. JENKINS, MSc, PhD
Professor Emeritus, Department of Animal and Veterinary Sciences, Clemson University,
Clemson, South Carolina

HÉLÈNE LAPIERRE, agr, MSc, PhD
Research Scientist, Dairy and Swine Research and Development Centre, Agriculture and
Agri-Food Canada, Sherbrooke, Québec, Canada

IAN J. LEAN, BVSc, DVSc, PhD, MANZCVS
SBScibus; Dairy Science Group, Faculty of Veterinary Science, The University of Sydney,
Camden, New South Wales, Australia

JAVIER MARTÍN-TERESO, PhD
Manager Ruminant Research Centre, Nutreco Research and Development, Boxmeer, The Netherlands

HOLGER MARTENS, VMD
Professor of Veterinary Medicine, Department of Veterinary Physiology, School of Veterinary Medicine, Free University of Berlin, Berlin, Germany

DAN F. McFARLAND, MS
Agricultural Engineering Educator, Penn State Extension York County, York, Pennsylvania

THOMAS J. OELBERG, PhD
Diamond V, New Ulm, Minnesota

GARRETT R. OETZEL, DVM, MS
Diplomate American College of Veterinary Nutrition (Honorary); Professor, Food Animal Production Medicine Section, Department of Medical Sciences, School of Veterinary Medicine, University of Wisconsin-Madison, Madison, Wisconsin

ROBERT A. PATTON, MS, PhD, PAS
President and Nutritionist, Nittany Dairy Nutrition Incorporated, Mifflinburg, Pennsylvania

PAOLA PIANTONI, Veterinaria, MS
PhD Candidate, Department of Animal Science, Michigan State University, East Lansing, Michigan

WILLIAM J. SEGLAR, DVM, PAS
Senior Nutritionist/Veterinarian, Global Nutritional Sciences, Global Forages Division, DuPont-Pioneer, Johnston, Iowa

RANDY D. SHAVER, PhD, PAS
American College of Animal Science-Nutrition; Professor and Extension Dairy Nutritionist, Department of Dairy Science, University of Wisconsin, Madison, Wisconsin

CHARLES J. SNIFFEN, PhD
Dairy Consultant and President, Fencrest, LLC, Holderness, New Hampshire

WILLIAM STONE, DVM, PhD
Diamond V, Auburn, New York

WILLIAM S. SWECKER Jr, DVM, PhD
Diplomate American College of Veterinary Nutrition; Professor, Department of Large Animal Clinical Sciences, Virginia-Maryland Regional College of Veterinary Medicine, Virginia Tech, Blacksburg, Virginia

JOHN T. TYSON, MS
Agricultural Engineering Educator, Penn State Extension Mifflin County, Lewistown, Pennsylvania

ROBERT J. VAN SAUN, DVM, MS, PhD
Diplomate American College of Theriogenologists; Diplomate American College of Veterinary Nutrition; Professor and Extension Veterinarian, Department of Veterinary and Biomedical Sciences, College of Agricultural Sciences, Pennsylvania State University, University Park, Pennsylvania

Contents

Veterinarians serving dairy clients can provide systematic investigations of nutritional problems. The foundation of a nutritional investigation is a careful evaluation of the diet being consumed by the cows. This information is supplemented by herd health and production records, evaluation of the cows (particularly locomotion and body condition scoring), and biological tests. All data collected during a herd investigation contain inherent error. Diagnostic conclusions from the herd investigation are most plausible when information collected from different sources all indicates similar conclusions.

VETERINARY CLINICS OF NORTH AMERICA: FOOD ANIMAL PRACTICE

RELATED INTEREST

Veterinary Clinics of North America: Small Animal Practice
July 2014 (Vol. 44, Issue 4)
Clinical Nutrition
Dottie Laflamme and Debra L. Zoran, *Editors*

THE CLINICS ARE NOW AVAILABLE ONLINE!
Access your subscription at:
www.theclinics.com

Preface

Dairy Nutrition

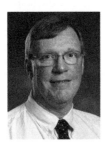

Robert J. Van Saun, DVM, MS, DACT, DACVN, PhD
Editor

It has been 23 years since the last *Veterinary Clinics of North America: Food Animal Practice* issue devoted to dairy cattle nutrition was published. Drs Thomas Herdt and Charles Sniffen were the editors for that issue in 1991. I am much honored to have been asked to be the guest editor for this issue given both previous editors were my mentors during my graduate education in dairy cattle nutrition. I owe much to both of these scientists relative to my professional development. This situation of student and mentor lineage and time period between issues may reflect on the small population of dairy nutrition veterinarians and underscores the need for veterinarians to work closely with dairy nutritionists. With feed costs accounting for more than half of total milk production costs and the well-documented critical role of nutrition in animal health and reproductive performance, it is essential that veterinarians and animal scientists work together to support and enhance dairy farm profitability and sustainability through nutritional avenues. Over the course of my veterinary education and practice career, there has been greater veterinary interest in becoming more familiar with application and monitoring of dairy cattle nutritional programs. The intent of this issue was to provide foundational information addressing current dairy cow feeding practices integrated with methods to assess adequacy of the nutritional program.

The previous *Veterinary Clinics of North America: Food Animal Practice* dairy nutrition issue covered calf, heifer, and dry cow feeding programs as well as various lactating cow nutrient requirements, grouping strategies, bovine somatotropin use, nutrition-reproduction interactions, nutritional monitoring, and nutritional consulting; essentially the full continuum of dairy nutrition. Much has changed over the past 23 years in improving our theoretical and applied understanding of how to feed dairy cows for health and performance. During this time, the National Research Council (NRC) had just released a sixth edition of Nutrient Requirements of Dairy Cattle (1989) and published a seventh edition in 2001. An indication of the expanding scope of dairy cow nutrition is reflected in the size of the NRC reports going from 157 to 381

Vet Clin Food Anim 30 (2014) xi–xii
http://dx.doi.org/10.1016/j.cvfa.2014.08.004
vetfood.theclinics.com

pages between 1989 and 2001. A new committee is being convened to generate the next edition, but the end product is still a few years from completion.

There are always new research and practical approaches to feeding cows that continue to refine our practices between NRC publications. It was quite a challenge, considering the current scope of dairy nutrition topics and new developments, to identify appropriate themes for this issue. I am extremely grateful to the American Association of Bovine Practitioners (AABP) membership in guiding my decision process in developing the topical material for this issue. In response to an e-mail request for suggested topics, I received an outstanding number of recommendations that were mostly incorporated into this issue. It is unfortunate I was not able to incorporate all suggestions, but some recent *Veterinary Clinics of North America: Food Animal Practice* issues have addressed dairy heifer management (March, 2008), transition cow management (November, 2004), and metabolic diseases (June, 2013).

In response to AABP member suggestions, articles for this issue are grouped to address nutritional basics (feed analysis, ensiled forage management), nutrient feeding practices (carbohydrates, proteins, lipids, macrominerals, and microminerals), and diagnostic practices (TMR audits, nonnutritional factors influencing nutrition, herd nutritional diagnostic investigations). Most articles have multiple authors to promote the animal science and veterinary perspectives on the given topics. Authors were challenged to provide a balance between current mechanistic modeling approach to nutritional practices and recommendations for clinical assessment or monitoring practices. Articles on rumen feeding management and transition cow nutritional management integrate information provided in many of the other articles and address the two most critical aspects of dairy nutrition for veterinarians. It is evident that there is no single best method for feeding dairy cows. As one might expect, all authors do not necessarily agree on the interpretation of available data and translation of this into methods for nutritional management. However, there is a consistent pattern to their recommendations, which is emphasized by all of the authors. No matter what approach is taken in formulating dairy cow diets, careful monitoring of cow performance is the best reflection of her nutritional adequacy. This places the veterinarian interested in dairy nutrition in a critical management role of being the unbiased monitoring agent of the nutrition program. One does not always have to be involved with nutritional formulations in being an important component of the dairy nutritional program.

Finally, I would like to thank those individuals who accepted my invitation and served as independent reviewers of the articles. It is through their efforts that the information provided is of the highest quality. This issue would not be the quality document that it is without the dedicated efforts of all of the authors. I am greatly indebted to these individuals for their efforts and willingness to be contributors to this issue. All authors are highly respected nationally and internationally. This issue provides an international perspective on the most current dairy cattle nutritional practices and recommendations appropriate for dairy veterinarians to become an integral part of their client's nutrition program.

Robert J. Van Saun, DVM, MS, DACT, DACVN, PhD
Department of Veterinary and Biomedical Sciences
College of Agricultural Sciences
Pennsylvania State University
115 W.L. Henning Building
University Park, PA 16802-3500, USA

E-mail address:
rjv10@psu.edu

Feed Analyses and Their Interpretation

Mary Beth Hall, PhD

KEYWORDS

- Feed analysis • Carbohydrates • Proteins • Fats • Minerals • Digestion
- Composition

KEY POINTS

- Assays differ in their accuracy and precision. For analytical values to be most useful, select analyses with needed accuracy and apply results within the bounds of assay precision.
- Crucial to the relevance of compositional values to the feed of interest, it is the user's responsibility to obtain a representative subsample for analysis and, in conjunction with the analytical laboratory, verify that the values are realistic.
- Carbohydrates can be analyzed as water-soluble, starch, and fiber fractions that relate to their ruminal and digestive fates.
- The most common methods for separating feed protein into fractions related to rates of ruminal degradation are based on differences in protein solubility.
- In vitro fermentability assays for carbohydrates are useful for describing relative differences among feedstuffs.
- Compositional and digestibility analyses should be used within diet formulation systems that are calibrated to the values generated by the specific analyses. Different assays used to measure a given feed characteristic may differ in their results.
- A number of needed assays, such as bioavailability or ruminal availability of nutrients and ruminal rates of protein fermentation, do not yet have definitive, commercially available methods for use in the field.

FACTORS AFFECTING USE OF FEED ANALYSES

Before we discuss feed analyses proper, it is critical that the user understands the impact of various factors on how to appropriately interpret and use the analytical values. Some key elements to consider are the type of assay, accuracy, precision, agreement between sample and what is actually fed, and use of rolling averages.

Type of assay used matters because sample or assay characteristics may change how results are interpreted, and accepted or rejected. Two general types of feed

Disclosures: None.
USDA-ARS, U.S. Dairy Forage Research Center, 1925 Linden Drive West, Madison, WI 53706, USA
E-mail address: MaryBeth.Hall@ARS.USDA.GOV

Vet Clin Food Anim 30 (2014) 487–505
http://dx.doi.org/10.1016/j.cvfa.2014.07.001   vetfood.theclinics.com

assay are chemical (sometimes called "wet chemistry") and near infrared (NIR) reflectance spectroscopy.

Chemical Analysis

Chemical analysis encompasses the traditional analyses performed in the laboratory, such as gravimetric (by weight), spectrophotometric (by detection of color change), chromatographic (separation of analytes in columns or on paper), and spectroscopic (absorption of wavelengths) analyses. Within chemical analyses, assay types can be subdivided into those that measure empirical fractions or specific analytes. An empirical assay is one in which the assay itself defines the fraction being measured, such as neutral detergent fiber (NDF), water-soluble carbohydrates (WSC), soluble protein, and ether extract. These assays tend to be colorimetric or gravimetric, and, typically, there is no analytical standard available that represents a "pure" compound. It is essential that an empirical assay be run exactly as the agreed-on protocol describes (ie, official methods of Association of Analytic Chemists [AOAC]), or the assay does not measure what it was intended to measure. In contrast, assays that measure analytes detect specific, identifiable compounds, such as minerals, carbohydrates, amino acids, or fatty acids. The purified analytes themselves are used as standards to measure and possibly verify that the analyte of interest is what was measured. These assays may be colorimetric with chemistry that is specific for a given compound (nitrogen, glucose), chromatographic (gas chromatography, high-performance liquid chromatography [HPLC]), or spectroscopic (atomic absorption or inductively coupled plasma optical emissions spectrometry). Both types of assays may use "standards," particularly in colorimetric, chromatographic, or spectroscopic assays. A "standard" is the purified, known material or solutions made from it that is used in an assay and against which all sample results are compared so as to calculate their composition. For example, solutions with known concentrations of purified compounds providing known amounts of specific elements are used as standards in mineral analyses, whereas solutions with differing concentrations of purified sucrose are used to make standard curves for the phenol-sulfuric acid assay to detect soluble carbohydrates.

Near Infrared Spectroscopy Analysis

NIR involves shining near-infrared light on ground feed samples, detection of the reflected light, and determination of composition based on the correlation of the detected spectra with calibrations made to chemical analysis data. NIR should be performed only on feed samples for which adequate calibrations are available. Typically, that allows reliable analysis of individual feeds, but the reliability or accuracy may decline with the degree to which the sample deviates from the samples included in the database on which the NIR calibrations were developed, such as with uncommon feeds or mixed samples, such as total mixed rations (TMR). The organic portions of feeds are detected by NIR, but minerals are not. Although mineral content may be correlated with other feed components, a chemical method should be used to obtain accurate mineral content information. NIR may be more repeatable, but cannot be more accurate than chemical analyses because it includes both the variability of the chemical analyses on which it is based as well as that within its calibrations. NIR is useful, requires less time, and is typically less expensive than are chemical analyses, but chemical analyses are preferred when highest accuracy is required.

Analysis Interpretation

In addition to the quality control practiced by analytical laboratories, it is up to the user to apply critical thought to evaluation of results. Do the results look realistic? If not, how do

I determine (1) if the analysis is correct or (2) what was the basis for the strange result? It is the user's responsibility to have information that describes sample collection, source, and handling that were in their control so that they are in a better position to work with the analytical laboratory to understand the results, or need for reanalysis or resampling.

Accuracy

Describes whether or not an analysis measures what it is intended to measure. Does an assay measure the intended fraction, or do other compounds interfere and increase or decrease the result? Generally, analyses for analytes should be reliable if performed properly with appropriate standards. Results of empirical assays may represent different components in different samples and have different sources of interference. This does not reduce the accuracy of the assay, per se, but the meaning of the result could differ among samples. For example, WSC represents the water-soluble carbo-hydrates extractable from feeds. However, the carbohydrate composition of WSC differs among forages (eg, sucrose may predominate in WSC from legumes, whereas fructans may be the main component in cool season grasses). Soil contamination inflates NDF values that are not on an ash-free basis because, although biogenic silica is soluble in neutral detergent, soil and rock are less so.

Certain sample types cannot be accurately analyzed with certain methods. For example, NDF analysis was developed to be applied to forage and feed samples. When applied to sporocarps (fungi), samples become slimy, do not filter, and do not give acceptable results.[1] The glucose oxidase–peroxidase assay cannot be used to measure glucose in fermentation media because the reducing conditions of the media interfere with the reaction (M. B. Hall, PhD, unpublished observation, 2009). An assay designed to detect starch contamination in meat cannot be used on liver products, because the glycogen that naturally occurs in liver will be erroneously detected as a contaminant.[2] In recognition of the issue of compatibility of assay and sample type, the official methods of the AOAC include mention of sample types that should not be analyzed with a given method because the results will not accurately describe what the method is intended to measure.

Precision

Precision addresses variability in analytical values and limits of detection of assays. In all analytical methods, there is some degree of variation even in properly determined analytical values. This is normal and can be due to the chemistry of the method, or the slight variations contributed by subsampling in the laboratory, weighing, pipetting, transferring samples, filtering, and so on. The analytical variation does differ by assay and can differ by sample type within assay; it is smaller for values determined in a single laboratory as compared with values determined across multiple laboratories. Variability related to an assay is separate from that introduced by variation among subsamples obtained from the original source feed. Limit of detection describes the smallest concentration that can be reliably measured with an assay.

Analytical Variation

So, what does analytical variation look like? It means that a properly run assay produces a range of results for a given sample. An example: the average standard deviation (SD) in NDF analyses performed with sodium sulfite and amylase, on a with-ash basis run in a single laboratory is 0.48%, which is rather small.[3] The 95% probability limits describing the range where properly performed analytical results will fall is calculated as 2 × the SD × 2.8. So the range around the mean into which NDF analyses will fall is 2 × 0.48% × 2.8 = 2.69%, or the mean ± 1.3% units. That means that analytical values determined on a 40% NDF alfalfa silage will fall between 41.3% and 38.7% NDF. If we were analyzing for fiber in a feed with only 2% NDF, the analytical variation does not necessarily decrease. So, using the same 0.48% SD of the NDF analysis, the values for this sample would fall between 0.7% and 3.7% NDF on a DM basis. For a 30-hour NDF digestibility (NDFD) assay, the analytical variability is greater: within a single laboratory there is a 95% probability that results will fall within ±5.1 percentage units around the mean.[4]

The analytical precision of an assay sets bounds for how precisely the results should be applied. For instance, for the 30-hour NDFD values determined multiple times by multiple laboratories, forages that were 5 percentage units or closer to each other could not be declared as different.[4] It would make sense that expression of such values should not go beyond the right of the decimal, as that suggests greater precision than the assay supports. Issues regarding precision have implications for how we compare and value feedstuffs and how we apply the information to use and develop ration formulation software.

In addition, how well the subsample sent to the laboratory represents the composition of a feed source affects the accuracy of how well the results describe the original feedstuff, and variation in repeated analyses of the feed source. The variation in subsample results has potential to be greater than the analytical variability. Subsample variability can be affected by the sampling methods used and how variable the feed source is. Appropriate subsampling is the only way to help ensure that the analytical results accurately reflect the feeds actually being fed to the animals.

FEED SAMPLING

Obtaining representative subsamples of feeds is a crucial first step in obtaining useful feed analyses. Feeds such as hays and silages may vary by bale or layer in the silo. Feed samples such as corn silage or mixed feeds can readily separate if particles vary in density or size. The goal is to obtain samples that accurately represent the feeds the animals are receiving. The more variable a given feed, the more samples may need to be taken over time to adequately describe the average. It is recommended to wait on sampling if an adverse weather event like a severe rainstorm changes or damages a feed so that it does not represent what the herd normally receives.

Individual Feed Sampling

The diverse forms of feed each require a separate approach for proper sampling. The most comprehensive information on properly sampling feeds is available from the American Association of Feed Control Officials, and for forages from the National Forage Testing Association. Hay from multiple bales must be cored, perpendicular to the end or round side of the bale; grab samples do not give an accurate cross section. Submission of 20 cores is recommended. Silage may be best sampled into a 5-gallon bucket over the course of a feeding as it is being run from an upright silo, or from a feeding's worth of material defaced from a bunk silo and mixed. Rather than hand-picking material from the silo face, the sample will contain what the cows will be fed, and the person sampling does not risk life and limb to silo unloaders and bunk silo avalanches. The silage can be put into a large plastic trash bag and tumbled/not shaken by hand to mix to avoid separation before subsampling. Concentrates can be sampled from commodity sheds or bins, with note taken as to any apparent nonuniformity within or among loads. Any time you take a chopped or ground sample by hand, put your hand or sampling tool underneath the sample and pick up to avoid losing fine material. Liquids, such as molasses or whey, should be agitated before sampling so as to capture typical amounts of solids and liquid. Pastures may be sampled by collecting 15 to 20 samples hand clipped at the height they will be grazed from a paddock that is about to be grazed.

Total Mixed Ration Sampling

Properly sampling TMR is a challenge. Analyzing individual feeds and verifying that they are properly weighed and mixed is preferable. Total mixed rations are complex samples, typically containing particles of differing sizes and densities that can be prone to separation. If the TMR was not adequately mixed, the composition of the material may change from start to finish of unloading from the mixer. Grab samples are often not adequate because the feed may not be homogeneous in the feed bunk. One approach to sampling TMR is to take samples from 3 sections of the feed bunk just after the material has been unloaded and before the cows have access to the feed. Remove entire vertical sections of TMR at the beginning, middle, and far end of the bunk. This will help to prevent separation and ensure that a representative sample was taken. Mixing these large samples to further subsample them to send them off for analysis is a challenge. Putting the sample on a large sheet of plastic and mixing it by pulling up a corner of the plastic so that the feed is rolled over on itself will mix it, and should be repeated 3 times from each corner of the plastic (a total of 12 rolls). Split the final pile into 4 quadrants, take one quadrant and quarter it again, and take a quarter to send for analysis.

Rolling Averages

Taking multiple samples of a feed over time is a common way to monitor feeds fed continuously out of a large stock, such as silage or a commodity from an individual supplier. Unless there is indication that there is a new, gross change in composition or quality of the feed (eg, obvious visual change), use a rolling average of the 3 most recent analyses.[5] This will avoid making changes in the rations when the changes in analyses actually reflect sampling and analytical variation. If there is an obvious or known change in the feed, restart the rolling average using feed analyses from the new feed.

DRY MATTER

Dry matter (DM) concentration is the simplest and most central of feed analyses. Feed consists of 2 fractions: DM and matter lost on drying. Because diets are most commonly formulated on a DM basis, accurate determination of DM sets the foundation for use of any other compositional results. Use of current DM analyses of moist feeds allows adjustment of feed mixes to ensure that the desired proportions of feeds are delivered to the cow. DM concentrations in feedstuffs are commonly determined in the laboratory in forced-air ovens at 55°, 60°, 105°, or 135°C. On the farm, DM can be determined using a Koster tester, microwave, or, more recently, stationary or equipment-mounted NIR sensors. In the non-NIR methods, DM is determined as the weight of the dried sample divided by the weight of the initial sample. Accurate DM determination requires that the sample be completely dry, but that no losses due to browning, charring, or spilling of sample occur, as these will result in losses in DM.

- For more information on determining dry matters on farm go to: Measuring dry matter content of feeds at http://www.caes.uga.edu/publications/pubDetail.cfm?pk_id=7730

DMs of moist feeds should be determined at least weekly, preferably 3 times per week, or when unusual change is noted. High-moisture feedstuffs, such as silages, can be variable in DM content and should be monitored. DM content within a silo will vary with the moisture content of the original material and with water movement, and compression. For example, DM content of alfalfa silage varied vertically from 34.6% at 50 cm from the bunk floor to 26.7% at 2.3 m in a bunk silo.[6] Such variation is typically more of an issue with perennial crops, such as alfalfa, than with others, such as corn silage. Precipitation events can grossly decrease DM concentrations of unsheltered feeds and this should be taken into account when feeding, or else considerably less DM will be provided from the affected feeds if they are fed on a wet weight basis without correction for the additional water.

CARBOHYDRATES

Carbohydrates provide 70% to 80% of diet DM in dairy cattle diets. Current analyses partition them into fractions related to their digestion or fermentation characteristics, based on our current understandings (**Fig. 1, Table 1**).[7] To begin with, carbohydrates are partitioned into fiber and nonfiber. Neutral detergent fiber (NDF) represents "fiber" that is digestible only by rumen microbes and typically ferments more slowly than other carbohydrates. In comparison, nonfiber carbohydrates (NFC) are assumed to be 98% digestible, may ferment more rapidly than fiber in the rumen, and some are digestible in the small intestine.[8] The array of carbohydrates, associated analyses that are commonly commercially available, and digestion characteristics are shown in **Table 1**.

Nonfiber Carbohydrates

For many feeds, NFC calculated by difference gives a not unreasonable starting estimate of the NFC content of feeds. One weakness of NFC estimated by difference is that errors associated with each of the individual assays used to calculate it will be pooled in this fraction. Additionally, compounds that are not measured as NDF, crude protein, ether extract or ash, and that are not carbohydrates will fall by default into this fraction. For example, fermentation acids in silage, such as lactic acid, are included in NFC, but do not provide as much energy to rumen microbes as carbohydrates do.[9] Calculated NFC grossly overestimates NFC in cane molasses, because 10% of the DM is composed of browning reaction products, which are not detected by the

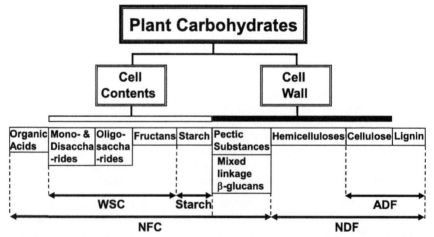

Fig. 1. Scheme of analysis for plant carbohydrates for use in ration formulation. Organic acids and lignin are not carbohydrates. (*From* Hall MB, Eastridge ML. Carbohydrate and fat: considerations for energy and more. The Professional Animal Scientist 2014;30:140–9.)

component analyses used to calculate NFC.[10] For molasses, total sugars as invert, which encompasses the glucose, fructose, and sucrose content reported by molasses manufacturers, should be used to describe molasses NFC content for diet formulation.

Sugars

"Sugars" has been used to denote rapidly fermenting soluble carbohydrates in cell contents. As determined with current analyses, this fraction consists of more than glucose, fructose, sucrose, and lactose that are traditionally termed "sugars"; it also includes oligosaccharides and fructans from cool-season grasses. Grouping this assortment of carbohydrates together can be justified because they appear to be treated similarly by rumen microbes. They all can be fermented to lactate, they may be converted to stored glycogen by microbes (confirmed for all but stachyose; possibly to a lesser extent with lactose), and seem to differ mostly by rate of fermentation.

Both water-soluble carbohydrates (WSC) and 80% ethanol-soluble carbohydrates (ESC) have been used to measure the "sugar" fraction. However, WSC is preferable to ESC because it completely extracts fructans, whereas ESC only partially extracts them. Efforts had been made to use WSC minus ESC to estimate the amount of long-chain fructans in grasses, but results were mixed and this approach is not recommended. The problem is that the assays use 2 different methods to measure carbohydrate, which do not give equivalent values for a given carbohydrate (see further discussion later in this article). Additionally, water or 80% ethanol may extract different blends of carbohydrates. This creates challenges for accurately measuring or comparing the amounts of extracted carbohydrate when a single type of carbohydrate is used as the standard for the assays. The issue is the degree to which the single carbohydrate does or does not serve as an appropriate standard for the different blends of carbohydrate. ESC is typically measured with the phenol-sulfuric acid assay (PSA),[11] whereas WSC is often measured with a reducing sugar assay (RSA) after acid hydrolysis; RSA is designed to measure monosaccharides, so longer-chain carbohydrates must be hydrolyzed for analysis. Both lactose and maltose are underestimated by RSA due to incomplete or no hydrolysis with the conditions normally used to hydrolyze sucrose in feedstuffs.[12] Proteins and noncarbohydrate reducing substances can interfere with and inflate values from RSA.

The PSA and RSA results for WSC in feedstuffs can differ, even when the 2 assays are using essentially the same carbohydrate as a standard.[12] Sucrose (glucose and fructose bonded together) and 50:50 glucose:fructose are commonly used for PSA and RSA standards, respectively, because it is a WSC that commonly predominates in plant materials. Using these standards, both assays give the same analytical value for measurement of sucrose. However, using those same standards, the 2 assays give different values when used to measure nonsucrose carbohydrates extracted from feeds, with RSA typically overestimating amounts of carbohydrates containing fructose (like fructan) and PSA underestimating them. Ideally, a carbohydrate that represents the predominant carbohydrate in feed samples should be used as the standard, but this is typically not feasible considering the diverse profile of carbohydrates that are found together in individual feeds. Recent work indicates that use of PSA with a sucrose standard gives WSC values for feeds closest to those found with high-performance ion chromatography (M. B. Hall, PhD, unpublished observations, 2013).

Starch

Starch is a polysaccharide component of NFC that predominates in diets that include grain crop silages or grain supplementation, as it is primarily a carbohydrate of plant

Table 1
Carbohydrate fractions, methods of analysis, components, and digestion characteristics

Fraction	Method	Components	Digestion Characteristics
Nonfiber carbohydrates	By difference calculation as: 100 − (CP + NDF + EE + ash), on a DM basis. The CP in NDF may be subtracted from the NDF value to avoid subtracting it in both CP and NDF; less of an issue if sodium sulfite is used in the NDF analysis.	Non-NDF carbohydrates, and compounds not measured by or errors in the CP, NDF, EE, and ash assays	Assumed to be 98% digestible in the total tract, variable as to small intestinal digestibility.
Organic acids from fermentation	Water extraction. HPLC.	Products of carbohydrate fermentation in silage: acetate, propionate, butyrate, lactate, etc.	Supply little energy to support microbial growth in the rumen, but are usable by the cow.
ESC	Extract with 80% ethanol, detection with PSA. Colorimetric.	Monosaccharides (glucose, fructose), disaccharides (sucrose), oligosaccharides (stachyose, raffinose, short-chain fructans)	Readily fermented by rumen microbes; likely soluble in the rumen. ESC may be converted to microbial glycogen by ruminal bacteria and protozoa. Monosaccharides are digestible in the small intestine.
WSCs	Extract with water, detect with PSA, or with RSA after acid hydrolysis. PSA gives closer agreement with HPIC than does RSA. RSA gives incomplete detection of lactose and maltose. Colorimetric.	Same carbohydrates as found in ESC, plus longer chain fructans, and lactose	Same as for ESC, except that there may be limited conversion of lactose to glycogen. Fructans are not digestible in the small intestine.
TSAI	Dilute molasses with water, detection most commonly by HPIC.	Glucose, fructose, sucrose	Same as for ESC, except available to small intestinal digestion if sucrose is hydrolyzed.

Starch	Gelatinize sample, hydrolyze with amyloglucosidase with or without use of heat-stable, α-amylase, detect released glucose. 0.9 × enzymatically released glucose = starch. Colorimetric or HPLC.	Starch, glycogen, maltooligosaccharides; all α-1, 4–α-1, 6-linked glucose carbohydrates	Digestible by microbes or small intestinal enzymes. Digestibility greatly influenced by particle size and protein matrix in which the starch is embedded.
NDF	Extract with boiling neutral detergent, soak/rinse residue with boiling water and then acetone. Most commonly, heat-stable, α-amylase is added to remove starch, and sodium sulfite to remove protein. Gravimetric.	Neutral detergent fiber; hemicellulose, cellulose, lignin, neutral detergent-insoluble CP; with or without ash	Digestible only by microbes.
ADF	Extract with boiling acid detergent, soak/rinse residue with boiling water and then acetone. Gravimetric.	Acid detergent fiber; cellulose, lignin, acid detergent-insoluble CP; with or without ash	Digestible only by microbes.
Sulfuric acid lignin	Digest acid detergent residue with 72% sulfuric acid, soak/rinse residue with boiling water and then acetone. Gravimetric.	Lignin, cutin	Indigestible. Used to estimate indigestible NDF.
Crude fiber	Samples extracted sequentially in hot acid and hot alkali. Gravimetric.	Variable	Does not accurately describe a nutritionally relevant fraction.

Abbreviations: ADF, acid detergent fiber; CP, crude protein as nitrogen × 6.25; DM, dry matter; EE, ether extract; ESC, ethanol-soluble carbohydrate; HPIC, high-performance ion chromatography; HPLC, high performance liquid chromatography; NDF, neutral detergent fiber; PSA, phenol-sulfuric acid assay; RSA, reducing sugar assay; TSAI, total sugars as invert; WSC, water-soluble carbohydrate.

seeds and some tubers (eg, potatoes, cassava). Starch is entirely composed of glucose covalently bound with α-1, 4-linkages with α-1, 6-linked branches. This differs from cellulose, another homoglucan, which has only β-1, 4-linkages. The most common, commercially available starch assays for individual or mixed feeds rely on the specificity of enzymes, typically heat-stable α-amylase and amyloglucosidase (glucoamylase), to hydrolyze only the linkages in starch to release glucose, which is then measured with glucose-specific assays (eg, glucose oxidase–peroxidase assay, HPLC). There may also be free glucose in the sample that should not be allocated to starch content. Starch content is calculated as ([free + enzymatically released glucose] – [free glucose]) × 0.9. The 0.9 factor accounts for the weight of water removed for each covalent bond made between glucose molecules. Historically, sucrose has been a common interference that can inflate values in starch analyses. This occurs when run conditions or enzyme preparations have the side activity of hydrolyzing sucrose to release glucose and fructose; the glucose is detected as being associated with starch.[13] Evaluating enzymes and run conditions and using those that avoid sucrose hydrolysis can guard against this interference.

Fiber Measures

"Fiber" most commonly refers to hemicellulose, cellulose, and lignin, which comprise the cell wall and give forage its distinctive digestive and physical effects. It is partitioned into NDF, acid detergent fiber (ADF), and lignin. Analysis of NDF varies in whether heat-stable, α-amylase or sodium sulfite is added.[3] Amylase removes starch and sulfite breaks disulfide linkages to remove protein. Thus, their combined use gives NDF values that are more hemicellulose, cellulose, and lignin, and less-contaminating material. The only advisable reason not to use sodium sulfite is to produce residue on which neutral detergent-insoluble nitrogen (NDIN or neutral detergent fiber crude protein [NDFCP], both expressed as crude protein with N × 6.25) can be measured. Subtraction of NDFCP from the NDF value is appropriate only when both assays are run using the same reagents.

Acid detergent fiber is composed of cellulose, lignin, and acid detergent-insoluble nitrogen (ADIN or acid detergent fiber crude protein [ADFCP], both expressed as crude protein with N × 6.25). ADIN has been used to estimate undigestible or heat-damaged protein in feeds. However, at least some portion of heat-damaged proteins may be digestible and used by the animal.[14]

Ash contamination

Ash, which is the mineral in feedstuffs that remains after incinerating a sample, is important to the discussion of fiber because of its potential to inflate values. Common variants of NDF and ADF analyses report results on a with-ash or ash-free basis. Ash in feed samples comes from minerals in plant cells, added minerals, from soil contamination, or from biogenic silica that naturally covers plant cells. Biogenic silica is a common component of grasses. "Ash-free" requires that the residue remaining after extraction with neutral or acid detergents be incinerated and the residual ash subtracted so that it is not counted as part of the fiber. "With-ash" leaves that mineral as part of the fiber and so inflates the fiber value and estimates of potentially fermentable cell wall. Most commercial analyses give fiber values on a with-ash basis; it improves turnaround time on samples and is often a low value. Soil contamination can inflate both NDF and ADF analyses because neither will completely solubilize it. An ash analysis of a feed sample with heavy soil contamination also will show unusually high ash values (approximately 5% of dry matter more than average values for a feed). If the high ash content is specific to the subsample, the best solution is to send in a different, uncontaminated sample. If the feed source itself is high in ash, running the fiber measures on an ash-free basis is the best way to determine what carbohydrate is present. Biogenic silica is soluble in neutral detergent, but is quantitatively recovered in the residue with acid detergent.[15] To get an accurate assessment of carbohydrate in ADF in this situation, ADF should be determined on an ash-free basis, or by running a sample sequentially through the NDF and then ADF analyses.

Lignin

Lignin is an indigestible polyphenolic compound that is covalently linked to other components in plant cell walls. It typically increases with increasing plant maturity and reduces the digestibility of the cell wall carbohydrates with which it is associated. The extent of digestibility of NDF has been estimated as $0.75 \times (NDFn - L) \times (1 - [L/NDFn]^{0.667})$, where NDFn is NDF minus the crude protein in NDF, and L is sulfuric acid lignin.[8] Lignin $\times$ 2.4 has also been used to estimate the portion of NDF made indigestible by its association with lignin.[16] Neither of the lignin-related estimates may be the most accurate approach to determining indigestible fiber as compared with fiber remaining after extensive in vitro or in situ fermentation; research in this area is ongoing.

Crude fiber

Although crude fiber is used in labeling of feeds, it does not accurately represent the fermentable or indigestible fiber fraction. In fact, crude fiber varies by feed in the extent to which hemicellulose, cellulose, and lignin are solubilized and not included in crude fiber.[15] Crude fiber is not an appropriate measure to use to describe the nutritional value of feeds.

Neutral Detergent-Soluble Fiber

Neutral detergent-soluble fiber (NDSF) is part of NFC because these carbohydrates are soluble in neutral detergent, but they are not digestible by mammalian enzymes. NDSF content of feeds has been calculated by difference to estimate carbohydrates, such as pectic substances and mixed linkage β-glucans. Originally the fraction was defined as (ethanol-insoluble residue [EIR] – crude protein [CP] in EIR) – (NDF – NDFCP) – starch.[17] With the understanding that short-chain fructans are soluble in 80% ethanol and some portion of the long-chain fructans are not, NDSF includes long-chain fructans (primarily in cool-season grasses), pectic substances, and the mixed linkage β-glucans and other carbohydrates of similar solubility. This fraction has the same issue as does NFC: errors within the individual assays become a part of the estimation of NDSF.

Carbohydrate Composition

Commercial laboratory Web sites and National Research Council publications[8] can be the best sources of carbohydrate composition values on feedstuffs. It is important to recognize that composition of feeds can vary by region and by growing season. In the case of by-product feedstuffs, changes in processing methods over time can result in changes in composition, making historical values unrepresentative of what is presently available. For example, starch contents of hominy feed declined as the value of starch for other purposes (eg, biofuel production) increased. Common sources of different carbohydrates are as follows:

- Sugars: include monosaccharides: glucose, fructose, simple sugars; and disaccharides: sucrose, lactose. Fresh forages, sugar beet or citrus pulps, molasses, and bakery products. Residual monosaccharides up to 9% of DM can be found in silages, particularly those above 30% DM (M. B. Hall, PhD, unpublished observation, 2005). Lactose is found only in milk-derived products, such as milk, whey, whey permeate, and milk replacer.

- Oligosaccharides: maltooligosaccharides, galacto-oligosaccharides. Maltooligosaccharides are breakdown products of starch and are found in bakery products. Galacto-oligosaccharides, such as stachyose and raffinose, are found in soybeans, canola, and sugar beets.
- Fructans (fructosans). The short-chain (oligosaccharide) and long-chain (polysaccharide) fructans consist of chains of fructose typically with a glucose molecule at one end. They are found in cool-season grasses. Commercially available inulin is derived from chicory.
- Neutral detergent soluble fiber: pectic substances, mixed linkage β-glucans, fructans. Pectic substances are found in legume forages, citrus and beet pulps; mixed linkage β-glucans are found in small grains.
- Starch: found in silage and grain from corn, sorghum, millet, rice, and small grains, and products produced from grain (eg, bakery waste, wheat middlings, hominy feed), as well as in tubers, such as potatoes. Many nongrain forages will contain low levels of starch (<2% of DM).
- Neutral and acid detergent fibers. In legume, grass, and grain forages, and in plant-based byproduct feeds. Not found in animal-derived products except as contaminating plant material or an analytical artifact.

PROTEIN

CP is useful in ruminant nutrition because, although the cow requires amino acids (AAs) to meet requirements, ruminal microbes can use nonprotein N to synthesize AAs, given adequate energy and carbon skeletons. The mass of CP is estimated as nitrogen (N) × 6.25, which denotes that N makes up 1/16 of the mass of protein. The 6.25 factor is acceptable for corn grain, and is commonly applied to forages, but other feeds may have other factors (eg, milk protein = 6.38; wheat protein = 5.7). In ruminant nutrition, the application of CP factors other than 6.25 is done to calculate the mass taken up by protein for calculations of NFC or efficiency of N utilization by the animal; the N content itself is what is important for diet formulation.

All CP sources are not nutritionally equal. Some are more rapidly used in the rumen (soluble peptides, ammonia), some are more slowly used (N associated with NDF), and some may be indigestible (N associated with lignin).[16] Protein fractions have largely been separated on the basis of solubility (**Table 2**)[18]; however, solubility or specific fractions may or may not accurately describe the digestibility of N in all feeds. There are soluble N fractions in heat-damaged feeds that can be indigestible,[19] and N in ADF fractions of heat-treated feeds that are digestible.[14] AA analyses are available from specialized laboratories, but these do not parse out ruminally degradable and undegradable AA fractions of feeds. Compared with carbohydrates, proteins have lacked common, commercially available in vitro ruminal digestibility assays, due in large part to the challenge of separating microbial protein from feed protein. Results with enzymatic methods to estimate ruminal protein degradability have varied with how well they agreed with measures of ruminal in situ protein degradation.[20] The 2001 Dairy NRC provides a table of information on protein fractions in feeds, ruminal rate of protein degradation, and AA composition of ruminally undegradable protein for a variety of feedstuffs.[8]

FATS

Ether extract (EE) has been used to measure fats in feeds, but the nutritional relevance of the measure is questionable. Ether or similar solvents extract not only the

Table 2
Protein fractions, methods of analysis, components, and digestion characteristics

Fraction	Method	Components	Digestion Characteristics
CP	Analysis of sample for N content, typically through Kjeldahl analysis (colorimetric titration) or Dumas combustion analysis. CP = N × 6.25.	True protein, amino acids, ammonia, nucleic acids, all molecules containing nitrogen	Digestibility is variable and dependent on the characteristics of the components.
Ammonia	Water extraction and titration or use of a specific electrode.	Ammonia	Usable by rumen microbes. Rapidly used.
Soluble protein	Extract with buffer to solubilize proteins. CP in residue is measured. Soluble protein as % of CP = 1 − (Residual CP/ Original CP) × 100	True protein, peptides, nonprotein nitrogen	Potentially very rapidly used in the rumen.
Nonprotein nitrogen (NPN)	Water-extracted N is precipitated with tungstic acid or trichloroacetic acid to remove larger protein molecules. Residual feed and precipitate is analyzed for N. NPN as % of CP = 1 − (Residual CP/Original CP) × 100	Amino acids, short peptides, ammonia, nucleic acids, etc.	Usable by rumen microbes. Potentially very rapidly used in the rumen.
NDIN; NDFCP	Extract with boiling neutral detergent, soak/rinse with boiling water and then acetone. Most commonly, heat-stable, α-amylase is added to remove starch; sodium sulfite is not used. Residue analyzed for CP as N × 6.25.	Proteins associated with cell wall or tannins, and heat-damaged proteins	Minus ADFCP approximates a slowly degraded protein pool.
ADIN; ADFCP	Extract with boiling acid detergent, soak/rinse with boiling water and then acetone. Residue analyzed for CP as N × 6.25.	Proteins associated with lignin or tannins, and heat-damaged proteins	Estimated to be indigestible in forages. Some heat damaged proteins in ADIN are digestible and can be used.[14]

Abbreviations: ADFCP, acid detergent fiber crude protein; ADIN, acid detergent-insoluble nitrogen; CP, crude protein; N, nitrogen; NDFCP, neutral detergent fiber crude protein; NDIN, neutral detergent-insoluble nitrogen; NPN, nonprotein nitrogen.

nutritionally available fatty acids, triglycerides, and so forth, but also pigments, waxes, cutin, and other indigestible materials of the correct solubility. The degree to which EE is useful for nutritional purposes depends on the proportion of indigestible material in it. The value of EE as a percentage of DM minus 1 has been used for diets to estimate the amount of fatty acids in EE, but accuracy of this value depends on how closely 1% of DM represents the non–fatty acid fraction of EE.[21] Feedstuffs can be directly analyzed for fatty acid content.[22] Such analysis is more nutritionally relevant, but is also more expensive. Fatty acid analysis with identification of individual fatty acids can be used to examine the levels of potentially biologically active fatty acids present in feeds.

Sample handling can affect analysis for fats. Triglycerides can break down to release glycerol and fatty acids, and fatty acids are reactive. As anyone who has seasoned a cast iron frying pan with shortening can attest, fats can be converted chemically to a material that reacts more like fiber and in which case the original fat is no longer detectable. Ground plant materials should not be stored for an extended period or else fats may react and become undetectable. Use of an acid hydrolysis step during analysis for fats can help to release some bound fats and fatty acids in triglycerides.[22]

Description of EE, fatty acid, and other analyses are listed in **Table 3**.

DIGESTIBILITY AND RATE ASSAYS

Ruminal digestibility or fermentation rates of feed fractions are most commonly measured in vitro in anaerobic fermentations with rumen inoculum. These measures have been used to provide information with which to compare fermentability of feeds and so their relative energy contributions, as well as being used as numeric values in diet formulation programs. When a feedstuff is fermented in vitro, there is an initial lag phase where little or no disappearance of the substrate is noted, and then the fraction steadily disappears as it is fermented. Finally, a plateau is reached where no more of

Table 3
Other feed fractions and analyses

Fraction	Method	Components	Digestion Characteristics
EE	Extract sample with ether or hexane and determine EE as loss of weight. An acid hydrolysis may be used to increase extraction. Gravimetric.	Triglycerides, fatty acids, waxes, cutin, pigments	Digestibility is variable and dependent on the characteristics of the components.
Fatty acids	Feed is extracted with hexane or ether. Extract is hydrolyzed to release fatty acids. HPLC.	Fatty acids	Digestible/absorbable in the small intestine.
Minerals	Incinerate sample, solubilize ash, measure by atomic absorption, inductively coupled plasma spectrometry, etc.	Individual elements	Variable. No indication of bioavailability.
Ash	Incinerate sample at 500° to 600°C for 2 h or a constant weight. Gravimetric.	Minerals, carbonates	Variable.

Abbreviations: EE, ether extract; HPLC, high-performance liquid chromatography.

the fraction disappears, as it has entirely disappeared or has reached its maximal extent of digestion (**Fig. 2**). Samples can be harvested at different points during the fermentation to measure remaining substrate and evaluate how much of the fraction of interest has fermented by that time.

Rate of Fermentation

Rates of fermentation (kd) describe the disappearance of a fraction in a feed per unit of time, and are usually expressed as exponential rates. Rates apply only to the potentially digestible portion of a fraction; the unfermentable portion has a rate of zero. Rates are also calculated only during the actively fermenting period, excluding the lag phase. The length of the lag is affected by availability of substrate, temperature, how the inoculum was handled (aeration, chilling, exposure to nonreducing conditions), whether the inoculum donor had been fed feeds containing the substrates being fermented, and so forth. Particle size of the sample has potential to alter fermentation, with more finely ground material being more available to fermentation and reducing the effect of physical form. Fermentation rates have generally been calculated using multiple time points to describe the pattern of substrate disappearance.

Neutral Detergent Fiber Digestibility

Digestibility of NDF (NDFD) describes the energy available from NDF. NDFD as a percentage of sample NDF is calculated as 1 − (residual NDF/initial NDF) × 100. Most commonly, 1-mm ground, dry samples are fermented for 24, 30, or 48 hours. The

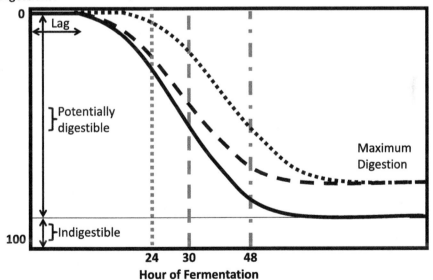

Fig. 2. Examples of patterns of NDF digestion over time. The dotted line has the longest lag time, the solid line has the greatest extent of NDF digestion. The dotted and dashed lines have the same rates of fermentation, but would analyze differently because of differences in the length of the lag phase. Measures at earlier hours are more sensitive to differences in rates, but variation in the data is greater there, too. Lag time, potentially digestible fraction, and indigestible fraction are shown for the solid line example. (*Modified from* Hall MB. Forage digestibility: how to deal with something that makes or breaks rations. In: Proceedings of the Penn State Dairy Nutrition Workshop. Grantville (PA): 2013. p. 29–32.)

48-hour measurement is that used in the 2001 Dairy NRC for calculating fiber digestibility, in lieu of calculating it as a function of lignin.[8] The 24-hour and 30-hour time points are more sensitive to detecting differences in rates rather than extents of fermentation, as they are generally located in the more actively fermenting portion of the fermentation (see **Fig. 2**). Longer, 240-hour fermentations are used to describe the indigestible NDF fraction, or, conversely, amount of potentially digestible NDF, a value that is needed for calculation of NDF kd. An alternate approach that has been used for estimating indigestible NDF is to use the value of lignin percentage of feed DM $\times$ 2.4.[16]

NDFD is a very useful, but not extremely precise measure. It can provide directional comparisons of the energy provided by fiber in different feedstuffs. In a ring test in which 10 laboratories repeatedly analyzed 14 alfalfa, corn forage, or grass samples for 30-hour NDFD, the laboratories were largely able to consistently rank samples similarly within fermentation runs.[4] However, the variability of the numeric NDFD values was such that if samples were not more than 5% units of NDFD apart, statistically, they were not designated as different. The precision of the NDFD measures were such that in a given laboratory for a specific sample, measured analytical values had a 95% probability of falling within ±5.1% units of the mean; the value was ±6.7% across analyses performed in different laboratories. When you consider that NDFD is measured from stacked assays (original sample NDF, in vitro fermentation, NDF on fermentation residue), each with their own variability, the variation is not surprising. NDFD is certainly useful for comparing feeds for energy content, but it should not be used with greater precision than the assay supports.

Different methods are used to measure NDFD. In the ring test, 6 of 8 laboratories that used some variant of the Goering and Van Soest[23] method gave similar results, regardless of whether filter bags, Erlenmeyer flasks, or sealed, shaken tubes were used in the fermentation.[4] The 2001 Dairy NRC 48-hour NDFD is based on the Goering and Van Soest system.[8] Another system that uses preincubated inoculum gave NDFD values that were approximately 60% of the Goering and Van Soest values.[24] Values from the 2 fermentation methods are not interchangeable. Values from any method should be used only in diet formulation or evaluation programs that are calibrated to use results from that specific method.

Starch Digestibility

Measurement of in vitro starch digestibility (StarchD) has been evolving. Currently, a single time point of 7 hours is commonly used with moderately coarsely ground samples. The coarser grind is used so that physical characteristics of the grain can show their effects with in vitro analysis; particle size and protein matrix of grains affect availability of starch granules for fermentation by rumen microbes. Compositional assays associated with StarchD that describe the impact of the protein matrix are prolamin in dry corn[25] (as prolamin increases, StarchD decreases) and ammonia in high-moisture corn[26] (as ammonia increases, StarchD increases). Enzymatic analyses have been used to describe StarchD in terms of extent of release of glucose from starchy feeds in a specific time period to assess degree of processing and starch availability.[27] Not surprisingly, enzymatic degradation and glucose release are also correlated with particle size.[28] Both in vitro and compositional assays give directional differences among samples that are useful to consider in ration formulation. At this time, the relationship between StarchD and in vivo digestion has not been established.

Gas Production

Gas production measurement is another way to monitor fermentation of feedstuffs. Feeds are fermented with mixed rumen microbes in sealed vessels and the pressure or volume of gas produced directly from fermentation (CO_2, CH_4) or from neutralization of fermentation acids by buffers in the media is measured over time.[29] Gas pressure or amount of gas produced is measured continuously or at periodic intervals. The resultant curves are approximately the inverse of substrate disappearance curves (gas increases as substrate disappears over time). Measured gas production does not describe fermentation of specific fractions in feeds, as the gas produced from one or another feed component cannot be isolated. "Curve peeling" may be applied to the curves to separate gas generated from fermentation of slow and fast pools that presumably depict relatively rapidly (WSC, starch, soluble fiber) and slowly (starch, NDF) fermenting carbohydrates.[30] Rates of fermentation can be calculated from the gas curves, but, again, the rates cannot be ascribed to specific carbohydrates. Gas production is related to amount of carbohydrate fermented, although the yield of gas per unit of carbohydrate fermented may not be identical among fractions.[31]

MEASURES FOR WHICH WE HAVE NO COMMONLY AVAILABLE FEED ANALYSES

There are a number of measures for which we presently have no commonly available, definitive commercial analyses:

- Plant organic acids
- Nonfructan soluble fiber
- Fructans
- Bioavailability of minerals
- Ruminal protein degradability or undegradability
- Rates of carbohydrate fermentation, except for starch and NDF
- Rates of protein fermentation and use by rumen microbes

What we need are analyses that are shown to reflect responses in the animal and to which ration formulation programs can be calibrated. These will need to be tested and our systems of analysis changed as better approaches become available.

REFERENCES

1. Hanson AM, Hall MB, Porter LM, et al. Composition and nutritional characteristics of fungi consumed by *Callimico goeldii* in Pando, Bolivia. Int J Primatol 2006. http://dx.doi.org/10.1007/s10764-005-9014-z.
2. AOAC. Method 958.06. In: Horwitz W, editor. Official methods of analysis. 18th edition. Gaithersburg (MD): AOAC INTERNATIONAL; 2005.
3. Mertens DR. Gravimetric determination of amylase-treated neutral detergent fiber in feeds with refluxing in beakers or crucibles: collaborative study. J AOAC Int 2002;85:1217–40.
4. Hall MB, Mertens DR. A ring test of in vitro neutral detergent fiber digestibility: analytical variability and sample ranking. J Dairy Sci 2012;95:1992–2003.
5. Weiss WP, Shoemaker D, McBeth L, et al. Within farm variation in nutrient composition of feeds. In: Proceedings of the Tri-State Dairy Nutrition Conference. Fort Wayne (IN): 2012. p. 103–17.
6. Muck RE, Huhnke RL. Oxygen infiltration from horizontal silo unloading practices. Trans ASAE 1995;38:23–31.
7. Hall MB, Eastridge ML. Carbohydrate and fat: considerations for energy and more. The Professional Animal Scientist 2014;30:140–9.
8. National Research Council (NRC). Nutrient requirement of dairy cattle. 7th edition. Washington, DC: National Academy of Science; 2001.

9. Russell JB, Wallace RJ. Energy yielding and consuming reactions. In: Hobson PN, editor. The rumen microbial ecosystem. Barking (United Kingdom): Elsevier; 1988. p. 185–215.

10. Binkley WW, Wolfram ML. Composition of cane juice and cane final molasses. Scientific Research Report Series No. 15. In: Hudson CS, Wolfrom ML, editors. Advances in carbohydrate chemistry, vol. VIII. New York: Academic Press, Inc; 1953. p. 291–314.

11. Dubois MK, Gilles A, Hamilton JK, et al. Colorimetric method for determination of sugars and related substances. Anal Chem 1956;28:350–6.

12. Hall MB. Efficacy of reducing sugar and phenol-sulfuric acid assays for analysis of soluble carbohydrates in feedstuffs. Anim Feed Sci Technol 2013;185:94–100.

13. Hall MB, Jennings JP, Lewis BA, et al. Evaluation of starch analysis methods for feed samples. J Sci Food Agric 2001;81:17–21.

14. Machacek KJ, Kononoff PJ. The relationship between acid detergent insoluble nitrogen and nitrogen digestibility in lactating dairy cattle. The Professional Animal Scientist 2009;25:701–8.

15. Van Soest PJ. Nutritional ecology of the ruminant. 2nd edition. Ithaca (NY): Cornell University Press; 2009.

16. Sniffen CJ, O'Connor JD, Van Soest PJ, et al. A net carbohydrate and protein system for evaluating cattle diets: II. Carbohydrate and protein availability. J Anim Sci 1992;70:3562–77.

17. Hall MB, Hoover WH, Jennings JP, et al. A method for partitioning neutral detergent-soluble carbohydrates. J Sci Food Agric 1999;79:2079–86.

18. Licitra G, Hernandez TM, Van Soest PJ. Standardization of procedures for nitrogen fractionation of ruminant feeds. Anim Feed Sci Technol 1996;57:347–58.

19. Van Soest PJ, Mason VC. The influence of the Maillard reaction upon the nutritive value of fibrous feeds. Anim Feed Sci Technol 1991;32:45–53.

20. Stern MD, Bach A, Calsamiglia S. Techniques for measuring nutrient digestion in ruminants. J Anim Sci 1997;75:2256–76.

21. Allen MS. Effects of diet on short-term regulation of feed intake by lactating dairy cattle. J Dairy Sci 2000;83:1598–624.

22. Sukhija PS, Palmquist DL. Rapid method for determination of total fatty acid content and composition of feedstuffs and feces. J Agric Food Chem 1988;36: 1202–6.

23. Goering HK, Van Soest PJ. Agriculture handbook no. 379: forage fiber analyses: apparatus, reagents, procedures, and some applications. Washington, DC: USDA-ARS; 1970.

24. Goeser JP, Combs DK. An alternative method to assess 24-h ruminal in vitro neutral detergent fiber digestibility. J Dairy Sci 2009;92:3833–41.

25. Larson J, Hoffman PC. Technical note: a method to quantify prolamin proteins in corn that are negatively related to starch digestibility in ruminants. J Dairy Sci 2008;91:4834–9.

26. Hoffman PC, Mertens DR, Larson J, et al. A query for effective mean particle size in dry and high moisture corns. J Dairy Sci 2012;95:3467–77.

27. Xiong Y, Bartle SJ, Preston RL. Improved enzymatic method to measure processing effects and starch availability in sorghum grain. J Anim Sci 1990;68:3861–70.

28. Blasel HM, Hoffman PC, Shaver RD. Degree of starch access: an enzymatic method to determine starch degradation potential of corn grain and corn silage. Anim Feed Sci Technol 2006;128:96–107.

29. Beuvink JM, Spoelstra SF. Interactions between substrate, fermentation end-products, buffering systems and gas production upon fermentation of different

carbohydrates by mixed rumen microoganisms in vitro. Appl Microbiol Biotechnol 1992;33:852–9.

30. Schofield P, Pitt RE, Pell AN. Kinetics of fiber digestion from in vitro gas production. J Anim Sci 1994;72:2980–91.

31. Hall MB, Pell AN, Chase LE. Characteristics of neutral detergent-soluble carbohydrate fermentation by mixed ruminal microbes. Anim Feed Sci Technol 1998; 70:23–39.

Management and Assessment of Ensiled Forages and High-Moisture Grain

William J. Seglar, DVM, PAS[a],*, Randy D. Shaver, PhD, PAS[b]

KEYWORDS

- Silage quality • Forage quality • Ensiled forage • Forage and grain crops
- Nutritional value • Fermentation • Digestibility • Evaluation

KEY POINTS

- Forage crop options affect dairy cow performance and health.
- Environmental growing conditions, more than seed genetic selection, determines the final forage quality fed to dairy cattle.
- Forage digestibility is influenced by growing conditions and length of time in silo storage.
- Harvest and ensiling management determines success of forage fermentation process and silage feeding value.
- On-farm tests and forage laboratory samples are available for determining forage quality of ensiled forages and grains.

FORAGE AND GRAIN CROPS ENSILED FOR DAIRY PRODUCTION

The diversity of geographies and growing environments dictate the types of ensiled forages that are used for dairy production. Feed cost represents the largest single expenditure on most livestock operations. The production of high-quality silages can help reduce the cost associated with feeding concentrates and supplements. For dairy producers, whole-plant corn, high-moisture corn, alfalfa, cereal, and a variety of grass species are the silages of most economic significance.

SPECIFIC FORAGE CROP HYBRIDS AND VARIETIES AND IMPACT OF THE GROWING ENVIRONMENT
Forage Production Considerations

- Decisions on forage product options based on genetic nutritional traits are important; however, environmental and management factors have the greatest influence on forage quality.

Disclosures: none.
[a] Global Nutritional Sciences, Global Forages division, DuPont-Pioneer, Northwest 62nd Avenue, Johnston, IA 50131, USA; [b] Department of Dairy Science, University of Wisconsin, 1675 Observatory Drive, Madison, WI 53706, USA
* Corresponding author.
E-mail address: bill.seglar@pioneer.com

- Corn silage quality at time of harvest is primarily influenced by harvest maturity, kernel processing (PROC), theoretical length of chop, and length of storage time in silos.
- Corn offers a diversity of feeding options, which include corn silage, high-moisture shelled corn, high-moisture ear corn (HMEC), snaplage (SNAP), dry corn (DC), and stalklage.
- Legume, grass, and cereal forage quality is contingent on stage of maturity at time of harvest and wilting time to achieve proper dry matter (DM) content at time of ensiling the crop.
- Temperature and moisture are 2 environmental variables during plant growth that highly influence forage quality of corn, legumes, grass, and cereal forage crops.

Forage categories

Plants are classified as C3 and C4 carbohydrate producers, and the primary difference is within plant cells in which photosynthesis for carbon fixation events occur. C3 plants are cooler season crops that have a longer growing season and higher water demands (**Table 1**). In contrast, C4 plants are warm season crops that are water efficient and drought tolerant. **Table 2** compares water usage requirements for several C3 with C4 crops; alfalfa is a C3 crop that has the highest water demand, whereas C4 sorghum crops use about one-third of the water required by alfalfa.[1]

Crop scientists monitor growth rates with calculators based on ambient temperature where using corn for example, growth starts at 7.2°C, maximizes at 22–30° C range, and ceases at 46°C. A Growing Degree Unit (GDU) calculation is used in the United States that is based on a linear relationship of growth to temperatures in the 10–30°C range. The GDU formula along with an example for corn is shown in **Table 3**. Using alfalfa in contrast, this crop starts growing at 5°C compared to corn at 10°C. Using the calculation for alfalfa and same daytime and night time temperature inputs as showing in the table, there would be 15.0 GDU accumulated for that day.[2]

Corn utilization as ensiled forage or grain

Corn is the predominant cereal crop grown throughout the world, because compared with all cereal crops, corn is unique in its ability to outyield the other crops on a ton/acre and nutrients/acre basis.[2] Corn growth and development are typically categorized by a staging system that divides plant development into vegetative (before flowering) and reproductive grain development (after flowering) stages. The reproductive stages are key growth periods for capturing crop harvest opportunities intended for (1) whole-plant corn silage (WPCS), (2) high moisture ear corn (HMEC) or snaplage (SNAP), high-moisture shelled corn (HMSC), and (4) dry corn (DC).

Table 1	
Characteristics of cool and warm season grasses	
Cool Season Grasses (C3)	**Warm Season Grasses (C4)**
Optimal growth at cooler temperature (70°F)	Optimal growth at higher temperature (95°F)
More digestible and higher in crude protein	Less digestible and lower in crude protein
Longer growing season	More drought tolerant
Higher water demands	More efficient at using water

Data from Teutsch C. Using mixtures of summer forages for improved forage yields in dry conditions. J Anim Sci 2013;91(E-Suppl 2)/J Dairy Sci 96(E-Suppl 1):406. [abstract 358].

Table 2
Water use in forage crops

| Crop | Water Used | | Reference |
	kg H$_2$O/kg DM	% of Alfalfa	
Alfalfa (C3)	844	100	Bennett & Doss, 1963[63]
Bromegrass (C3)	828	98	Martin et al, 1976[64]
Wheat (C3)	505	60	Martin et al, 1976[64]
Orchardgrass (C3)	418	50	Bennett & Doss, 1963[63]
Sudangrass (C4)	380	45	Martin et al, 1976[64]
Corn (C4)	372	44	Martin et al, 1976[64]
Sorghum (C4)	271	32	Martin et al, 1976[64]

Data from Teutsch C. Using mixtures of summer forages for improved forage yields in dry conditions. J Anim Sci 2013;91(E-Suppl 2)/J Dairy Sci 96(E-Suppl 1):406. [abstract 358].

The reproductive maturity of corn is assessed by plant moisture, as shown in **Table 4**. WPCS is based on whole-plant moisture content, whereas high-moisture and dry grains are based on kernel moisture content.

During corn grain development, corn maturity for WPCS falls with a 63% to 68% whole-plant moisture range. Corn grain reaches blacklayer, or becomes physiologically mature, at about kernel 33% moisture, which is suitable for ensiling as HMEC or SNAP. Usually the corn and cob mix is 6% points higher than measured kernel moisture. At a post blacklayer stage or 25% to 32% kernel moisture, the grain is suitable for ensiling HMSC, and at less than 15% moisture, the corn is suitable for dry grain storage.

Corn silage WPCS contributes greatly to supplying the energy, starch, and forage neutral detergent fiber (NDF) needs of high-producing dairy cows, reducing purchased feed costs from expensive grain and byproduct supplements, and generating milk revenue for dairy producers. It is coveted as a forage source for ruminants around the world, because of its agronomic yield potential and energy value relative to other forage crops. The energy value of WPCS is related primarily to the content and digestibility of starch.[3] Starch content is related to grain versus stover yields or the proportion of grain in whole-plant DM, which can range from 0% to 45% and is largely dependent on the hybrid, agronomic practices, crop stressors (eg, drought, early frost) and stage of maturity at harvest, resulting in WPCS starch concentrations that average 30% but range from 0% to 45% (DM basis). Depending on starch content and thus energy value, WPCS can be targeted to a wide range of livestock groups. Energy-dense WPCS is required for high-producing dairy cows or growing beef cattle, whereas low-energy (<65% total digestible nutrients) WPCS is best for low-producing and dry dairy cattle, dairy replacement heifers, or beef brood cows.

Table 3
GDU calculations for corn and alfalfa

Crop	Calculation	Example	GDU
Corn	[(Daily maximum temperature + daily minimum temperature)/2] − 10	[(30°C+10°C)/2] − 10	10.0
Alfalfa	[(Daily maximum temperature + daily minimum temperature)/2] − 5	[(30°C+10°C)/2] − 5	15.0

Table 4		
Corn harvest opportunities for corn silage and grain		
Corn Use	**% Moisture[a,b]**	**Plant Part Moisture**
Corn silage	63–68	Whole plant
HMEC/SNAP	26–33	Kernel
	32–39	HMEC/SNAP product
High-moisture corn (HMC)	25–32	Kernel
DC grain (shelled corn)	<15	Kernel

[a] % Moisture is used by crop producers, whereas cattle producers use % DM terminology.
[b] % DM = 100 − % moisture.

Moderately cool and dry growing conditions improve WPCS nutritional quality, and slight moisture stress stimulates seed (grain) production. Cool temperatures (especially at night) seem to inhibit secondary cell wall development, which can negatively affect fiber digestibility. The lack of adequate moisture is the single most limiting factor for corn growth.

Growing conditions affect WPCS nutritive values before and after silking differently, as indicated in the following:

- Between plant emergence and tassel stage may increase NDF digestibility (NDFD) but results in shorter plants and less silage tonnage
- During tasseling and silking results in the great yield reduction
- Kernel development stage does not affect NDFD but can reduce grain fill (starch content) and yield

In general, dry conditions during the vegetative stages of plant growth enhance fiber digestibility (NDFD). Higher than normal temperatures tend to moderate the positive effect that low moisture has on improving NDFD. Wetter than normal conditions during vegetative growth, although they improve whole-plant yield (taller plants), tend to reduce fiber digestibility.

The digestibility of starch in WPCS is influenced primarily by PROC, stage of maturity at harvest, and length of time undergoing fermentation in the silo before feeding; total tract starch digestibility can vary by about 20% units.[4] Ruminal digestibility of NDF affects DM intake (DMI) and milk production by dairy cows and can vary for WPCS by up to 20% units, depending primarily on lignin content and corn hybrid type.[5,6] Other than brown midrib (BMR) hybrids, the genetic variation in NDFD among corn hybrids is minimal. **Fig. 1** summarizes the factors that influence the nutritive value of corn silage.

Hybrids Ferraretto and Shaver[4] performed a meta-analysis to determine the impact of WPCS hybrid type on intake, digestion, and milk production by dairy cows. The dataset comprised 139 treatment means from 45 peer-reviewed journal articles from 1990 to 2013. Hybrid categories were those selected for stalk (conventional, dual purpose, or isogenic vs BMR vs leafy) or grain (conventional, yellow dent vs nutridense vs high oil vs waxy) characteristics or those that were genetically modified compared with their isogenic counterparts. All hybrids were harvested as WPCS and fed as the primary forage component in rations for lactating dairy cows. Intakes of DM and milk yield were 1.1 and 1.4 kg/d per cow greater, respectively, for BMR than the conventional hybrid. Lactation performance was similar for leafy compared with the control. Fiber digestibility was greatest, whereas starch digestibility was lowest, for BMR. The only effects observed for hybrids selected for grain characteristics and harvested as WPCS

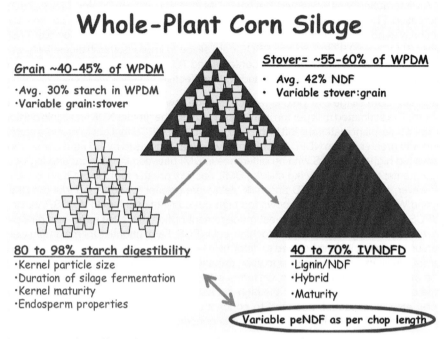

Whole-Plant Corn Silage

<u>Grain ~40-45% of WPDM</u>

•Avg. 30% starch in WPDM
•Variable grain:stover

<u>Stover= ~55-60% of WPDM</u>

• Avg. 42% NDF
• Variable stover:grain

<u>80 to 98% starch digestibility</u>

•Kernel particle size
•Duration of silage fermentation
•Kernel maturity
•Endosperm properties

<u>40 to 70% IVNDFD</u>

•Lignin/NDF
•Hybrid
•Maturity

Variable peNDF as per chop length

Fig. 1. Factors that affect whole-plant corn silage. (*Courtesy of* Joe Lauer, PhD, UW Madison Agronomy Department.)

were reduced milk fat and protein concentrations for the high-oil treatment compared with control and other treatments. Lactation performance was unaffected by feeding genetically modified corn hybrids harvested as WPCS compared with isogenic controls. Choosing hybrids based on yield and agronomic traits for WPCS production is important, because these factors drive the nutritional quality of the forage.

Maturity, cut length, and kernel processing: Ferraretto and Shaver[7] performed a meta-analysis to determine the impact of dry matter (DM) content, kernel processing (PROC) and theoretical length of cut (TLOC) of WPCS on intake, digestion and milk production by dairy cows. The dataset was comprised of 106 treatment means from 24 peer-reviewed journal articles from 2000 to 2011. Categories for DM content at silo removal and PROC and TLOC at harvest were: ≤ 28% very low DM (VLDM), >28% to 32% low DM (LDM), >32% to 36% medium DM (MDM), >36% to 40% high DM (HDM), and >40% very high DM (VHDM) DM; 1 to 3 or 4 to 8 mm roll clearance or unprocessed; 0.48 to 0.64, 0.93 to 1.11, 1.27 to 1.59, 1.90 to 1.95, 2.54 to 2.86, and ≥ 3.20 cm TLOC.

Milk yield was decreased by 2 kg/d per cow for VHDM. Fat-corrected milk (FCM) yield decreased as DM content increased. Total tract digestibility of dietary starch (TTSD) was reduced for VHDM compared with HDM and LDM. Processing (1–3 mm) increased TTSD compared with 4 to 8 mm PROC and unprocessed corn silage. Milk yield tended to be 1.8 kg/cow/d greater, on average, for PROC (1–3 mm) and unprocessed WPCS than 4 to 8 mm PROC. The TLOC of WPCS had minimal impact on any of the parameters evaluated. Starch digestibility and lactation performance were reduced for dairy cows fed diets containing corn silage with greater than 40% DM or WPCS with insufficient PROC.

An interaction was observed between DM content and PROC for TTSD. PROC increased TTSD for diets containing corn silage with 32% to 40% DM. Also, an interaction was observed between TLOC and PROC for TTSD. PROC increased diet TTSD when TLOC was 0.93 to 2.86 cm. PROC corn silage to improve starch digestibility was effective across a wide range of DM contents and TLOC but did not overcome adverse effects of VHDM content on TTSD and was ineffective at very long TLOC.

High cut Corn silage DM yield is reduced as the row-crop head is raised from 15 to 45 cm. The estimated milk per ton increases, because the greater NDF and lignin portion of the whole-plant material is left in the field, resulting in WPCS that contains more starch and with greater in vitro NDFD.[8] Actual milk yield was increased by 1.5 kg/d per cow for cows fed high-cut WPCS with no difference in DMI between the low-cut and high-cut treatments; feed efficiency (kg milk/kg DMI) was 3% greater for high cut than low cut. However, both in vitro NDFD and milk yield were greater for cows fed low-cut BMR hybrid WPCS compared with cows fed high-cut conventional hybrid WPCS.[9] Varying WPCS height of cutting is a harvest management option, because estimated milk per acre is reduced by only 1% to 3% for high-cut WPCS. Farm priorities for maximum yield versus higher quality can be used to determine height of cutting guidelines for individual farms, which may vary from year to year, depending on the yield and quality of the crop and existing on-farm inventories. On farms with erodible land, more beneficial crop residue can be left in the field with the high-cut harvest without sacrificing much milk per acre. Also, because nitrates tend to concentrate in the bottom portion of the stalk, raising the crop-head helps minimize nitrate concerns in drought years.

Silage fermentation/starch digestibility Highly vitreous corn types contain greater concentrations of prolamin proteins than floury or opaque corn types in DC.[10] This factor affects extent of rumen digestion with feeding of DC grain, whereas the prolamin/starch relationship has a lower impact on WPCS, HMEC, or high-moisture corn (HMC). Starch granules in the corn endosperm are surrounded by hydrophobic prolamin proteins, which are slowly degraded.[11] Hoffman and colleagues[12] reported that ensiling high-moisture corn for 240 days reduced zein protein subunits that cross-link starch granules and suggested that the starch-protein matrix was degraded by proteolytic activity over an extended ensiling period. This finding could explain reports of greater ruminal in situ starch degradability for HMSC with greater moisture contents and duration of silage fermentation compared with feeding DC.[13] Newbold and colleagues[14] reported ruminal in situ starch and crude protein (CP) degradabilities (ie, soluble protein) increased for WPCS as the length of silage storage time increased. Increased WPCS in vitro starch digestibility with greater length of silage storage time has also been reported by others.[15]

The Larson and Hoffman[10] turbidity assay determination of total zein protein content did not detect a reduction in zein protein subunits over the ensiling period for HMC, as measured by high-performance liquid chromatography (HPLC).[12] However, ammonia content increased, as HPLC zein protein subunits decreased in HMC. Ammonia nitrogen has been suggested in combination with mean particle size (MPS) for modeling the effects of corn maturity, moisture content, and length of silage fermentation time on ruminal and total tract starch digestibilities and rate of ruminal starch degradation for high-moisture corn at feed-out.[16] Young and colleagues[17] reported that the addition of protease enzymes and greater length of the ensiling period increased ammonia nitrogen content and ruminal in vitro starch digestibility in WPCS.

Shredlage Shredlage (SHRD) is corn silage harvested with a self-propelled forage harvester (SPFH) fitted with aftermarket cross-grooved processing rolls that run at a greater speed differential than conventional processing rolls (**Fig. 2**). With some

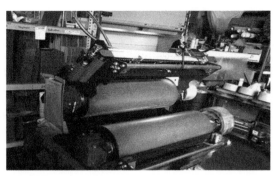

Fig. 2. SHRD processor. (*Courtesy of* Shredlage, LLC, with permission. Available at: http://www.shredlage.com/.)

SPFH brands and models, the TLOC can be set longer up to 26 to 30 mm compared with commonly used 17-mm to 19-mm TLOC. Compared with conventional-processed corn silage (CPCS) harvested with the SPFH set at 19 mm TLOC, the most obvious difference for corn SHRD harvested with the SPFH set for a longer TLOC is a greater proportion of coarse stover particles in SHRD. When fed in rations for lactating dairy cows, this factor can increase the physically effective NDF (peNDF) content of the ration, which is important for proper rumen function, cow health, and milk fat content. An important aspect of the corn SHRD concept is that excellent PROC may be achieved, even with a longer TLOC, allowing for high starch digestibility. Furthermore, the cross-grooved rolls with greater speed differential used for producing corn SHRD may cause greater damage to the coarse stover particles and allow for greater digestibility of the fiber.

A feeding trial conducted by Ferraretto and Shaver[7] with lactating cows was conducted at the University of Wisconsin-Madison to compare corn SHRD (SHRD; 30 mm TLOC) with CPCS (19 mm TLOC). The proportion of coarse stover particles was greater for SHRD than CPCS for samples collected during feed-out from the silo bags throughout the feeding trial (32% vs 6% as-fed particles retained on the coarse or 19-mm screen of the Penn State Particle Separator).[18] PROC scores on feed-out samples averaged 75% for SHRD and 60% for CPCS. The SHRD and CPCS were similar in DM (34%) and starch (36%) contents, pH (3.6), and silo bag packing density (17 lb DM per ft^3).[19] Midlactation cows were used in the 10-week continuous-lactation experiment with respective treatment total mixed ration (TMR) containing 50% (DM basis) from either SHRD or CPCS. Averaged over the treatment period, DMI and FCM yield tended to be greater by 0.7 and 1.1 kg/d per cow, respectively, for SHRD than CPCS. Total tract dietary starch and NDFDs were greater for cows fed SHRD than cows fed CPCS. Measurements of weigh-backs during the trial did not show feed sorting for either treatment.

More research is needed to determine the variables (eg, TLOC, maturity, roller mill engineering) that influence processing goals by SHRD and CPCS. Furthermore, further research is needed regarding fiber digestibility in SHRD and CPCS with longer TLOC and its relative peNDF compared with hay crop silage, whole cottonseed, and chopped hay or straw, to allow for better decisions on how best to use WPCS processing options in dairy cattle diets.

High-moisture corn Corn harvested as grain can be ensiled and fed as HMSC or HMEC. Harvest is carried out with a combine, which dictates that dry-down in the field should be about 30% kernel moisture before harvest.[20] For HMEC harvest, combines are adjusted to retain only a portion of the cob, which that ends up in the combine bin with the grain. The proportion of cob in HMEC can vary, and therefore, starch and fiber concentrations are variable in HMEC, and feed analysis for these 2 nutrients is required during feed-out. Furthermore, the cob contains approximately 6% more moisture than the kernel, which means moisture content of the HMEC product is greater than HMSC harvested at the same kernel moisture.[21] Frequent analysis for the moisture content of HMSC and HMEC is required during silo feed-out.

HMSC and HMEC needs to be rolled before ensiling into most storage systems, except for oxygen-limiting seal systems, in which whole grain is stored and rolled or ground during the unloading process. Typically high-moisture corn is coarse-rolled before ensiling to about 1500 μ MPS for HMSC.

SNAP SNAP is another option for harvesting HMEC. SNAP is harvested using an SPFH fitted with a corn combine head. Use of an SPFH for production of SNAP allows the corn harvest to be initiated earlier (33% kernel moisture) and proceed more rapidly, with PROC performed immediately during the harvest process by way of the SPFH on-board roller mill rather than later at the silo as with HMSC or HMEC.[22,23]

Nutritionists may be concerned about reduced energy content of SNAP, because it comprises kernels, cob, husk, and shank from the ear and possibly some leaf material from above the ear, which serve to dilute its starch content with fiber compared with HMSC or ground dry shelled corn. Starch and fiber concentrations can be highly variable in SNAP, and feed analysis for these 2 nutrients is required during feed-out. Similar to HMEC, the nonkernel portion of SNAP contains more moisture than the kernel, which means that the moisture content of SNAP is greater than HMSC harvested at the same kernel moisture by several few percentage units, and frequent analysis for the moisture content of SNAP during feed-out is required.

Compared with DC, harvest of corn as SNAP with its increased moisture content may increase rate and extent of ruminal starch digestibility[22,23] through breakdown of the less formed starch-protein matrix in the kernel endosperm during the ensiling process.[12,16] This factor could contribute to reduced milk fat content[24,25] when SNAP is fed to lactating dairy cows.[26] On the other hand, harvest of SNAP that is too dry reduces the digestibility of the cob or fiber fraction and can reduce the digestibility of the starch fraction if the kernels are not processed properly, thereby reducing the energy value of SNAP. Because of concerns over low-energy content or high ruminal starch digestibility, SNAP is often fed in combination with ground dry shelled corn rather than alone as the sole source of grain in dairy cattle diets. Similar concerns over high ruminal starch digestibility can arise for both HMSC and HMEC with high moisture contents at ensiling, fine processing, and a long length of silo fermentation time before feeding.[12,16,24,25]

Stalklage The stalk residue remaining after corn grain harvest can be ensiled successfully if it is adequate in moisture content and chopped and packed properly. Greater than 45% moisture content is recommended for good stalklage preservation, which is dependent on speed of harvest and field dry-down conditions, which are highly variable from field to field and year to year. The use of an acid-based forage additive is advised when ensiling at less than 55% moisture content. However, when performed properly, corn stalklage can provide an excellent feed ingredient for inclusion in rations for dry dairy cattle, dairy replacement heifers, or beef brood cows, because of its high NDF content and low energy value. It is recommended that corn stalklage be fine chopped with the chopper set for a 4-mm to 6-mm TLOC to improve silo packing density, augment silage fermentation, and minimize sorting in the feed-bunk.

Legume silages
Alfalfa Legume crops have deep tap root systems, which go as far as 20 to 30 ft into the earth. Therefore, much of the high water demand for alfalfa comes from subsoil levels unattainable by other crops. This situation offsets the drought tolerance of alfalfa in that often this crop has normal growth patterns during water deprivation, when cereal crops show signs of drought stress.

Alfalfa is a perennial legume crop, which typically has multiple harvest cuttings during the growing season.[27] Legume forages provide their highest nutritive quality during early vegetative growth; however, this factor is offset by substantially lower DM yields. Typically, alfalfa is harvested at initiation of the reproductive flowering stage of growth to produce the most nutritive leaf/stem ratio to produce the most nutritive value on a per acre basis. Advanced crop maturity results in lowered leaf/stem ratios, and thus, cell wall concentrations increase. Because the stems are less digestible, NDFD tends to be decreased with advanced stages of maturity. Because there is more indigestible NDF, voluntary intakes are restricted because of rumen fill limitations. The maturity effects on digestion and intakes are listed as follows:

- Cell wall concentrations increase and cell contents decrease
- Cell wall digestibility decreases
  - Lowered NDFD
  - Grass lignification occurs faster (2 times) than legumes (20%).
- Voluntary intake decline because of rumen fill limitations and increases in NDF cell wall concentrations.

Although temperature and water deficiency are the biggest environmental factors influencing alfalfa yields, solar radiation and day lengths are other influencers of yield and quality.[28] Growing conditions that promote the highest alfalfa quality are long day lengths, cool nights, and moderately dry weather. Warm, wet weather tends to produce the poorest-quality alfalfa. Cool, wet growing conditions produce high-quality alfalfa, as a result of low NDF and low lignification. Light promotes carbohydrate production (every 1-hour increase in day length can increase digestibility by about 0.2% units).

Alfalfa silage, with its higher contents of protein, pectin, and macrominerals and minimal starch content, complements corn silage to form the forage base of many dairy cattle rations. High-quality alfalfa silage is produced by cutting the first cutting stand at a late-bud stage of maturity (and approximately 30 days thereafter) with a swather and windrowing the crop in the field, and wilting down to % moisture ranges based on silo structures, as shown in **Table 5**. Alfalfa should be chopped at 6 to 12 mm TLOC before ensiling the crop.

Table 5
% Moisture when ensiling alfalfa into various storage structures

Silo Structure	% Moisture[a,b]
Horizontal bunker/pile	55–65
Horizontal bagged	55–65
Upright stave	55–68
Upright sealed	45–55
Balage (round bale silage)	45–55

[a] % Moisture is used by crop producers, whereas cattle producers use % DM terminology.
[b] % DM = 100 − % moisture.

Alfalfa harvest at the late-bud stage of maturity allows for lower NDF (38%–42%) and acid detergent fiber (ADF; 28%–32%) concentrations and higher CP (20%–22%) content, energy value, intake potential, and milk production than harvesting alfalfa at early to full bloom maturity stages.[29] Relative feed value (RFV) is an index of quality based on NDF and ADF concentrations as predictors of hay crop forage intake potential and energy value, respectively.[30] RFV is commonly available on commercial forage test reports and used routinely in comparisons of hay crop silage quality. Alfalfa silage with RFV 150 or greater is the quality targeted for high-producing dairy cows. However, the RFV estimates do not account for differences in NDFD that may exist among hay crop silages. Measurement of ruminal in vitro NDFD is incorporated into the calculation of a revised RFV or relative forage quality (RFQ), where forage energy value is estimated using summative equations and DMI potential is estimated using NDF and NDFD (**Fig. 3**).[31]

The use of NDFD measurements in forage evaluation schemes detects variation in forage quality not detected in schemes based solely on fiber concentrations (ie, grasses and alfalfa-grass mixtures that have lower lignin contents and thus higher NDFD than alfalfa). Although alfalfa silage is high in CP relative to most other silages, an issue for dairy cattle nutritionists with alfalfa silage is the high soluble protein concentration, which results in high ruminal degradability of the protein.

Harvesting alfalfa silage at the correct maturity stage and DM content under good ensiling practices including the use of silage inoculants to decrease pH rapidly is important for controlling ruminal protein degradability. Laying alfalfa swaths (4 m cut width) in wide windrows (2.4–2.7 m wide) reduced drying times in the field to the desired DM content for ensiling compared with narrow windrows (1.2–1.5 m wide), which reduces the potential for rain damage and field losses during wilting.[32]

Red clover The CP, NDF, ADF, and macromineral concentrations of high-quality red clover and alfalfa silages are reasonably similar.[33] However, the ruminal degradability of protein in red clover silage (65%–75% of CP) is lower than for alfalfa silage (75%–85% of CP), because polyphenol oxidases in red clover inhibit plant proteases and proteolysis during silage fermentation. In a summary of feeding trials, DMI was consistently reduced for cows fed red clover silage compared with alfalfa silage, whereas milk production was either similar or reduced only slightly for red clover silage. The specific reasons for the DMI reduction caused by the feeding of red clover

Relative Feed Value (RFV)

$$RFV = \frac{\%DDM \times \% DMI}{1.29}$$

$$\%DDM = 88.9 - (0.779 \times \% ADF)$$

$$\% DMI = 120/\% NDF$$

Relative Forage Quality(RFQ)

$$RFQ = DMI, (\% \text{ of } BW \times TDN, \% \text{ of } DM)$$

For alfalfa, clover, and legume/grass mixtures

$$DMI = 120/NDF + (NDFD-45) \times 0.374 /1350 \times 100$$

$$TDN = (NFC \times .98) + (CP \times .93) + (FA \times .97 \times 2.25) + (NDFn \times (NDFD/100)) - 7$$

Fig. 3. RFV and RFQ calculations. ADF, Acid Detergent Fiber; BW, Body Weight; CP, Crude Protein; DDM, Digestible Dry Matter; DMI, Dry Matter Intake; FA, Fatty Acids; NDF, Neutral Detergent Fiber; NDFD, Neutral Detergent Fiber Digestion; NDFn, Neutral Detergent Fiber Non-available; NFC, Non-Fiber Carbohydrate; TDN, Total Digestible Nutrients.

silage have not been elucidated. Cows pass black loose manure when fed red clover silage; however, no plausible mechanism that explains the black feces and laxative effect in cows has been agreed. For the highest quality and milk production potential, harvest red clover silage at late bud to early bloom maturity. Harvest DM, TLOC, and ensiling guidelines for red clover silage are similar to alfalfa silage.

Soybean Severe drought-stressed or early frost–damaged soybean fields can be harvested as silage.[34] However, yields are usually low, at only 1 to 2 tons forage DM per acre. The CP, NDF, ADF, and macromineral concentrations of soybean and alfalfa silages are similar. Harvest DM and ensiling guidelines for soybean silage are similar to alfalfa silage, except that a finer TLOC of 6 to 9 mm is recommended for soybean silage. Soybean silage is generally limited to 15% to 20% of ration DM. Visual maturity indicators for soybean silage include: (1) completion of seed fill within pods and (2) lower leaves turning yellow. A more mature crop produces higher fat content, which depresses fermentation quality. Harvest at an earlier stage of maturity results in lower harvest losses (because of less seed loss) but has greater silage palatability.

Grass silages

Grass silage is generally higher in NDF content and NDFD and lower in CP and lignin contents than alfalfa silage at similar stages of harvest maturity (ie, early cut vs late cut). Environmental conditions usually dictate whether the haycrop grown for silage production is predominantly grass or predominantly legume. For the highest-quality grass silage for lactating dairy cows, harvest should be at the late boot stage of maturity. Harvest DM, TLOC, and ensiling guidelines for grass silage are similar to alfalfa silage. Harvest of grass silage at the heading stage of maturity increases yield per acre and NDF content but reduces CP content and energy value, thereby improving it as forage for replacement heifers and dry cows. **Table 6** provides growth stages of grass crops.[35]

However, grasses along with alfalfa can luxury consume potassium from the soil and be high enough in potassium to cause subclinical or clinical milk fever related to high dietary cation-anion difference (DCAD) (see to article by Hall elsewhere in this issue). Haycrop silage to be fed to dry cows should be analyzed for potassium and DCAD, with rations formulated accordingly for DCAD, by dilution with corn silage or anionic salt inclusion in the diet, or both.

Varieties Ryegrass tends to be lower in NDF and higher in NDFD than other grass varieties, but Italian ryegrass is an annual and thus most suitable for emergency forage situations. Perennial ryegrasses are subject to major winterkill issues in northern climates, and ryegrass can be more difficult to chop and handle through the ensiling

Table 6	
Notable growth stages of grass crops	
Stage of Maturity	**Definition of Maturity Stage**
Boot	Grain head or spike found near top of plant inside the flag leaf sheath
Head	Grain head fully emerges from flag leaf sheath
Flower	Grain head anthers emerge and shed pollen
Milk	Grain kernels develop and fill with white, milky liquid
Soft dough	Grain kernels well formed and have rubbery dough consistency to touch

Data from Collar C, Aksland C. Harvest stage effects on yield and quality of winter forage. In: 31st California Alfalfa Symposium. Davis (CA): University of California Cooperative Extension, University of California; December 11–13, 2001.

process. New York researchers[35] have found the newer endophyte-free tall fescue varieties to be winter tolerant and high yielding, with high quality and milk production potential compared with other grass varieties. Old tall fescue varieties that contain an endophytic fungus that causes silage palatability issues should be avoided. Timothy tends to be higher in NDF content and lower in CP content and energy value than other common grass varieties, including orchardgrass and smooth brome grass.

Legume-grass mixtures In some major dairy regions, it is common to plant legume-grass mixtures on pure stands, resulting in silage nutrient composition intermediate between legumes and grasses depending on seeding rates and stand densities of each. Benefits to mixing 30% to 40% grass with alfalfa compared with 100% alfalfa seeding include improved yield in the seeding year, improved yield in later years if alfalfa stands are reduced by winterkill, wider harvest window for second and later cuttings, faster field wilting to desired moisture content for ensiling, and greater resistance to traffic damage from tractors and farm implements.[36] Seeding mixtures with alfalfa should be either endophyte-free tall fescue or orchardgrass, but not timothy or smooth bromegrass, which tend to produce most of their yield in the spring or first cutting and have a maturity progression that is too fast relative to the alfalfa. More frequent analysis of forage nutrient composition is recommended for legume-grass mixtures than pure stands, because quality variation may be more highly variable during feed-out of these silages.

Noncorn cereal silages

Varieties Cereal crops such as barley, oats, wheat, rye, triticale (wheat × rye cross), and forage sorghum can be harvested, stored, and fed as whole-plant silage. Winter wheat and rye are the common winter cover crops that are harvested in the spring as cereal silage in northern climates. Spring planted oats or oats and peas harvested in the early summer as silage are also common in northern climates. For the highest quality (highest CP and NDFD and lowest NDF) for lactating dairy cows, harvest should be when the cereal crop is in the late boot stage of maturity. Later harvest, in the flowering stage, can be performed to increase yield per acre and improve its quality parameters (ie, higher NDF and lower CP concentrations) for lower producing cows, replacement heifers, and dry cows.[37]

Forage sorghum, sudangrass, and sorghum-sudangrass hybrid for silage These silages are generally lower in yield per acre and quality (higher NDF content and lower starch content and energy value) than corn silage. Therefore, they usually are found in northern climates only during drought years as an emergency forage source and in southern regions, where agronomic conditions favor sorghum over corn production. Forage sorghums are monitored for maturity by visual examination of the head and are harvested at the middough stage on kernel maturity, with whole-plant DM, TLOC, PROC, and ensiling guidelines similar to those provided for corn silage. For the highest-quality silage for lactating dairy cows, sudangrass or the hybrid should be harvested at 4 feet of growth and field wilted to less than 70% moisture before ensiling. Harvesting later, taller increases yield per acre but decreases quality, which may be appropriate for replacement heifers and dry cows. BMR varieties are available commercially that have been shown to increase DMI and milk production in dairy cows compared with conventional varieties.[38]

Cereal crop forages

Cereal crop forages are annual crops; during plant growth, those forages have a vegetative growth stage followed by a reproductive stage that produces seed or a starch-rich grain source. Most of these crops have 1 harvest period, although several sorghum-sudan varieties can have several harvest cuttings during the growing season. The nutritional value of cereal grains changes throughout the growing stages of the crop. The vegetative stage grows by leaf emergence, followed by stem development, and then, further leaf development until the crop enters the reproductive stage. **Fig. 4** shows the growth phases of cereal forages.

The digestibility and protein content of leaves and stems decline as the plant proceeds through heading, flowering, and grain development. Digestibility of the head decreases through milk stage and then rebounds as grain fills with highly digestible starch and protein. This rebound is an important aspect of small grain forages, which distinguishes them from those forage grasses and legumes for which seed weight never becomes a significant portion of the forage crop.

Varieties of small grains that have high grain yield and grain/stem ratios are the most likely to have the biggest rebound in digestibility as the plant reaches maturity. Small grains at the boot stage of maturity typically are higher in protein content and NDFD than those harvested at the soft dough stage, whereas those at soft dough have higher yield and concentration of nonfiber carbohydrates. Protein and digestibility of boot and soft dough stage forages compare favorably with benchmark values for alfalfa and corn silage.[39]

In the central and western Canadian provinces, whole-plant barley silage usually replaces corn silage as predominant forage feed. In that situation, harvest is carried out in the soft dough stage of grain development to increase its starch content and energy value. Harvest DM, TLOC, and ensiling guidelines for cereal silages are similar to alfalfa and grass silages. The foregoing discussion with regard to potassium and DCAD for grass silage applies to cereal silage also.

High-Moisture Ensiled Cereal Grains

Both barley and wheat have been harvested, stored, and fed this way, but barley is the most common. The best moisture content for harvest of high-moisture ensiled barely is 25% to 35% grain moisture, with 30% moisture optimum. When moisture content decreases lower than 25%, the crop should be left for harvest as dry barley. A coarse

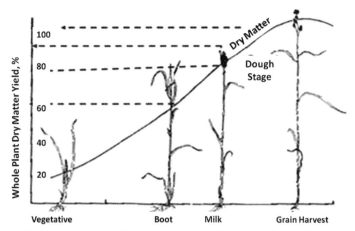

Fig. 4. Growth phases of cereal silages. (*Courtesy of* Steve Barnhart, PhD, Department of Agronomy, Integrated Crop Management News and Iowa State University Extension. Available at: http://www.extension.iastate.edu/CropNews/2011/0621barnhart.htm.)

roll for high-moisture barley is recommended to enhance packing and silo fermentation. Because the rate and extent of ruminal starch digestibility are inherently greater for barley than corn starch, fine grinding is discouraged, and high-moisture barley may need to be fed with DC or barley to minimize adverse effects on rumen function and milk fat content.

Sorghum varieties are a group of cereal forages commonly grown in water-deficient areas, such as the Southwestern United States, because of their lower water demands. Forage sorghum does respond well to timely irrigation, and maximum forage yields can usually be obtained with 12 to 16 in of irrigation water. Corn grown under the same environments requires approximately 26 in of irrigation water to achieve maximum silage yield potential.[40]

SILAGE STORAGE
Silage Production Considerations

- An efficient fermentation process in the silo produces silages that are well preserved, highly palatable, and rich in nutrient content for feeding dairy cattle.
- Silage best management practices and use of quality forage additives drive fermentation efficiencies for minimizing silage inventory losses and producing highly nutritious forages.
- Problem silages may exist when ensiling the crop at low DM contents, which may result in clostridial spoilage, whereas ensiling the crop at high DM contents increases the risk of aerobic instability.
- Catastrophic weather, such as hail, drought, floods, and early frost, affect forage quality and management decision on the harvest and storage of stressed crops.
- Nitrate and prussic acid content is increased with grass-based crops such as corn and cereal crops but are of minimal concern with legume and grass crops.

The Fermentation Process

Silage fermentation can be simplified for discussion purposes into the 3 phases shown in **Fig. 5**. Silages experience aerobic conditions during harvest and filling, followed quickly by anaerobic conditions that initiate bacterial growth for production of silage acids and pH decline, and back to aerobic conditions during feed-out, with potential effects of yeast, mold, and *Bacillus* spoilage microbes.[41,42]

DM loss (shrink) begins with plant cell respiration and aerobic microflora using carbohydrate sources (primarily sugar), thereby producing water, heat, and carbon

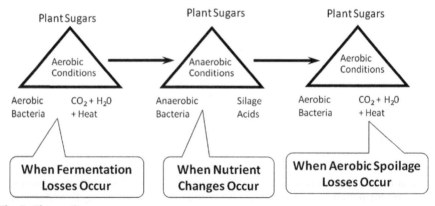

Fig. 5. The ensiling process.

dioxide. It is this carbon, lost to the atmosphere, that causes shrink loss. Wilting time and speed of harvest affect the extent of aerobic field losses. These processes continue until oxygen is depleted within the silage mass. Plant moisture and compaction play a role in reducing the length of the aerobic phase in the storage structure by reducing silage porosity. The reexposure of silage to aerobic conditions can be divided into 2 areas: (1) top and side exposure and (2) face exposure during feedout. Silage additives should be used when all forage harvest and ensiling management recommended practices for producing high-quality silage have been met or when high-risk damaged forages must be harvested. Additives are classified as (1) bacterial, (2) enzyme, (3) acid, and (4) nutrient, of which the most common in North America are the bacterial inoculant and acid products. Good silage can be made better through the proper use of well-researched silage additives; however, these additives do not make poor silage good.[43]

The *Pioneer Silage Zone Manual*[44] gives further details regarding environmental factors that influence the fermentation process regarding substrate utilization, end products produced, and forage shrink (DM) losses.

Silage Storage Systems

Silage storage requires physical structures where the forage can be delivered and packed tightly for air exclusion. The decision on the type of storage system for ensiled forage is based on several factors: (1) type of silage, (2) herd size, (3) available labor, (4) capital investment, (5) access to equipment service, (6) feeding management, and (7) flexibility for future needs.[45] The rate at which silage needs to be fed is the primary factor in determining the size of the silo. **Table 7** shows suggested harvest moisture percentage goals and ranges for expected DM percentage storage losses.

Horizontal and vertical storage structures are the 2 broad classifications of silo types. Horizontal silos in the form of bunker-walled and silage-pile structures are more likely to exist in larger dairy operations, because of large capacity requirements along with needing to maximize efficiencies of labor and power resources. These silos best can be filled and fed out with properly sized conventional farm equipment and require less energy to move silages into TMR mixers.

Plastic-bagged silos provide one of the most flexible systems for silage storage, in that with dairy expansion, increased storage capacity can be met simply by filling more silage bags. Capital investment cost is not an issue other than investment in a bagging machine. Another feature of bagged silage is the ability to segregate and

Table 7		
Storage system harvest moisture ranges and expected DM losses		
Structure	**% Moisture[a,b] at Harvest**	**% DM Losses at Feed-Out**
Pile system	60–68	16–40
Bunker system	60–68	12–25
Concrete stave	60–65	7–15
Oxygen limiting	55–65	5–15
Bagged	60–65	7–15
Balage	40–60	10–25

[a] % Moisture is used by crop producers, whereas cattle producers use % DM (DM) terminology.
[b] % DM = 100 − % moisture.
Data from Harrison JH, Fransen S. Silage management in North America. Field guide for hay and silage management in North America. National Feed Ingredients Assn; 1991. p. 33–49.

identify crops based on hybrid/variety types, harvest maturities, and environmental factors.

Balage is an alternative plastic storage system that involves ensiling low DM round bales with ensiling moisture percentages ranging from 40% to 60%. The ensiling moisture range is lower than other silage storage systems, which are in the 60% to 68% moisture range. The hay baling machine must be designed to create tightly packed bales and then wrapped with several layers of plastic for driving optimal fermentation and storage life.[46]

Vertical structures are typically referred to as tower silos and exist as cement or stave top unloading or sealed bottom unloading structures. The latter structure is designed with 1-way air and gas vents along with an air bag in the silo to maintain an oxygen-free environment. Both types require greater mechanization during filling and feed-out, although they require less area for construction, and have a smaller exposed surface area of silage compared with horizontal silos. DM losses typically are 7% to 15% for stave and 5% to 10% for sealed structures. Silo filling and feed-out limitations dictate the size of the dairy operation in which it is feasible to store ensiled forages in vertical storage systems.

Harvesting and Ensiling Management

Harvest management, maturity, wilting, and crop processing practices were discussed within the crops section and are tightly linked with ensiling management. Preharvest weather-related catastrophes such as floods, droughts, wind, hail, and early frosts jeopardize the dairy producers' goal of producing the highest-quality forages needed to maximize dairy production. Such weather events cause silage inventory issues as a result of yield losses and reduction of silage quality.

Immature corn silage because of effects of hail, frost, or drought

Reduced grain development in immature corn decreases WPCS starch concentration at time of harvest. The crop may range from earless silage, in which there is no starch, to a minimal 5% to 6% unit starch reduction. Immature WPCS generally has higher stover soluble sugar contents, which needs to be considered by nutritionists. NDFD may be higher in WPCS harvested from mild drought-stressed and heat-stressed growth environments. Knowing the starch and sugar concentrations and NDFD in immature WPCS is essential for balancing rations.[47]

Weather-damaged corn crops may appear to be dry, and producers may want to harvest and ensile as WPCS immediately. However, immature corn can maintain high moisture contents in the stalks; therefore, it is imperative to monitor dry-down rates to harvest at the desired whole-plant DM contents.

Managing flood-damaged corn for silage Floods can contaminate crops with large amounts of organic debris, resulting in high levels of yeast, mold, and *Bacillus* spores that enter the silo with the crop. The prevention of aerobic instability requires critical attention to ideal ensiling management practices such as packing, sealing, and maintaining proper feed-out rates. A bacterial inoculant is indicated, because naturally occurring lactic acid–producing bacteria are washed off the crop from flood waters. Monitoring the silage at feed-out for mycotoxins and ash levels is advised so that feeding management can be altered with the inclusion of flood damages WPCS. The following reference checklist when harvesting flooded forage crops includes,

- Closely monitor harvest DM content
- Segregate flooded forages into separate silos
- Target least affected fields for silage

- Harvest above silt line if possible
- Inoculate with a well research-proven bacterial inoculant
- Screen for mycotoxins
- Monitor ash levels to determine severity of flood damage
- May increase likelihood of Listeriosis and heavy metal cases in cattle

Harvesting and feeding weather-impaired alfalfa Nutritional effects of weather delays during harvest, such as rain, can directly influence nutritional value of the alfalfa crop. NDFD is primarily determined by harvest maturity, leaf retention, and environmental conditions. Exposure to rain or delayed wilting in the field can increase respiration losses, leach out water-soluble carbohydrates, and increase leaf loss. Wet conditions usually delay harvest, causing advanced maturity, which increases fiber NDF content and reduces digestibility and intake potential.

Drought conditions generally decrease alfalfa yields, but quality usually remains high because of the increased leaf/stem ratio. Short but leafy plants increase the protein content of the crop. Plants with fine stems show lower NDF content with higher digestibility. However, drought plus extremely high temperatures usually reduces NDFD, as a result of increased lignification.[28]

Factors That Affect Silage Quality

The storage structure must be filled as rapidly as possible to diminish time spent in the initial aerobic ensiling phase of the fermentation process. A balance needs to exist with rate of forage delivery compared with adequate packing of the forage in silo. If forages are delivered to the silo site too fast, packing tractors may not have sufficient time to adequately eliminate air from the crop.

Bunker silos should be filled from back to front rather than from bottom to top; the progressive wedge method shown in **Fig. 6** prevents disruption of previously ensiled forage. Bunker and pile structures need adequate packing for exclusion of oxygen from the silage mass for achieving a fast and desirable anaerobic fermentation.

Packing ensures the elimination of oxygen, thus minimizing aerobic activity and maximizing anaerobic fermentation. **Table 8** shows the top 10 with R^2 greater than

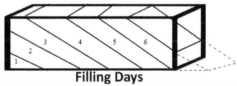

Filling Days

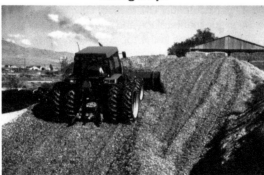

Fig. 6. Progressive wedge filling technique.

Table 8
Top 10 correlation factors with silage density

Factor	Correlation
Initial layer thickness	−0.279
Average packing tractor weight	0.262
Average wheel load	0.2224
DM content	0.209
Total weight of packing tractor(s)	0.200
Tire condition (1 = new, 3 = bald)	0.195
Average particle size	0.194
Packing time, min/ton (as fed)	0.162
Speed of packing (1 = >8 km/h, 4 = <1.6 km/h	0.147
Number of packing tractors	0.146
Wheels per packing tractor	0.126

Data from Muck RE, Moser LE, Pitt RE. Post-harvest factors affecting ensiling. In: Buxton DR, Muck RE, Harrison JH, editors. Silage science and technology. Madison (WI): American Society of Agronomy, Crop Science Society of America, Soil Science of America; 2003. p. 251–304.

10 out of 18 factors that are correlated with desirable packing densities for minimizing nutrient and DM losses and enhance stability at feed-out. The main factors with R^2 0.20 or greater that affect packing include: (1) initial layer thickness, (2) average packing tractor weight, (3) average wheel load, (4) DM content of the crop, and (5) total weight of packing tractors.[48]

Modern high-capacity forage harvesters make it critical that there exist enough packing tractors with adequate weight to achieve good compaction. A good rule of thumb is to have 800 lbs of packing tractor for each ton per hour of harvest or filling capacity. For example, if the filling rate is 100 ton per hour, 80,000 lbs of pack tractor would be needed.[49]

The bunker and pile structure needs to be properly sealed; plastic tarp is usually used to cover the entire bunker surface, and a net of tires holds the tarp in place. Silage covers minimize surface molding and reduce nonvisual silage DM losses. Uncovered silos can have air penetration up to 4 feet below the silo surface, where oxygen becomes available for aerobic fermentation. The respiratory microbes use oxygen and water-soluble carbohydrates to produce heat, water, and carbon dioxide. Research shows that DM losses were 33% greater in the top 4 ft of the silo compared with silage losses below the 4-ft section.[50] Silo covering yields a 4:1 return on investment by eliminating 33% of potential DM losses. Oxygen barrier film products have been introduced to the silage marketplace and show promise in further mitigating surface mold and reducing DM losses in the top 3 to 4 ft of horizontal silos.[51]

Silage Quality Issues

Silage feeding issues are a result of not following strict silage management practices, resulting in less than ideal fermentations. Two general classes of silage quality issues are (1) aerobically unstable or (2) clostridial (secondary fermentation) silages. Usually ensiling the crop at lower than 60% moisture provides silage environments conducive to aerobic instability in contrast to greater than 70% moisture, which produces an environment contributing to clostridial fermentation issues.[52]

Aerobic instability can be identified by poor bunklife (hot forages or rations), less total energy availability, production of molds, animal intake and production problems, and mycotoxin issues. Soilborne yeast, mold, and *Bacillus* spores are the causative spoilage microbes that are incorporated along with crops during harvest. They are always present within ensiled crops and propagate when oxygen is introduced into the ensiled environment. Aerobic activity of spoilage microbes results from ensiling crops with less than recommended moisture contents, less than adequate compaction, without covering, or with slow feed-out rates. These conditions permit air penetration or entrapment in the silage, thus permitting the sporulation of aerobic spoilage microbes, which produce heating and palatability problems.

Aerobic instability caused by soilborne *Bacillus* activity generates great amounts of heat in silage. The first result of thermophilic *Bacillus* activity is the Malliard reaction, which is the binding of protein to fiber and is known as bound protein and quantified as acid detergent insoluble nitrogen (ADIN). Aerobically unstable forages and grains caused by *Bacillus* may: (1) appear dry and fluffy, (2) feel hot, (3) have a tobacco smell, and (4) appear brown/black. Refer to the article on feed analysis elsewhere in this issue for further information.

Clostridial secondary fermentation presents as green, slimy, unpalatable silage. DM losses often exceed 50%. Forages ensiled at greater than 70% moisture may undergo a different type of fermentation. Instead of lactic acid-producing bacteria predominating, large populations of *Clostridia* bacteria may grow in the silage. It is important therefore that haycrop silages are not harvested at 70% or more moisture to minimize the risk of clostridial spoilage in the silo, causing high butyric acid, ammonia, and amine concentrations and therefore issues with reduced DMI and lactation performance by lactating cows and ketosis in transition cows. These anaerobic bacteria can: (1) degrade lactate and amino acids, (2) produce butyric acid from lactic acid, (3) result in silages with pH greater than 4.5, and (4) cause unpalatable sour silage.

Butyric acid can reduce DMI and has the potential to predispose ruminants to ketosis. Recommendations are to limit daily intake of butyric acid to 50 g or less for dry cows and 75 g or less for fresh cows. Levels exceeding 150 g/d pose a high risk for ketosis for dry cows and at any stage of lactation when daily butyric acid intake exceeds 250 g. **Table 9** shows butyric acid silage feeding thresholds for early lactation cows.[53] For example, a dry cow consuming as little as 3 lb alfalfa

Table 9
Butyric acid silage feeding thresholds for fresh cows

% Butyric Acid in Silage (DM Basis)	mg/lb	50 g/cow/d	150 g/cow/d	250 g/cow/d
0.50	2.3	22.0	66.1	110.1
1.00	4.5	11.0	33.0	55.1
1.50	6.8	7.3	22.0	36.7
2.00	9.1	5.5	16.5	27.5
2.50	11.4	4.4	13.2	22.0
3.00	13.6	3.7	11.0	18.4
3.50	15.9	3.1	9.4	15.7
4.00	18.2	2.8	8.3	13.8
4.50	20.4	2.4	7.3	12.2
5.00	22.7	2.2	6.6	11.0

Data from Oetzel GR. Herd-level ketosis: diagnosis and risk factors. Auburn (AL): American Association of Bovine Practitioners; 2007. p. 67–91.

silage/d with 1.0% butyric acid would be ingesting 66 g, which exceeds the 50-g butyric acid threshold limit.

Increased ammonia nitrogen concentrations, expressed as a percentage of total nitrogen, result from clostridial bacteria through the proteolytic breakdown of protein into ammonia and other nitrogenous end products such as amines and amides that research indicates cause depressed cattle intake and silage palatability issues. Therefore, the measured ammonia nitrogen value in fermentation reports provides an indicator for the presence of the other nitrogenous end products that may result in feeding issues. Ammonia nitrogen, % of total nitrogen values should be less than 10% for corn and cereal and less than 15% for grass/legume silages.[54]

Forage Toxins

Nitrate poisoning in forages

Nitrate analysis is advised if the crop was stressed during the growing season or if high nitrate was present during tests that were performed to determine nitrate levels at harvest. Under normal growth conditions, there is little nitrate buildup in the plant even although the roots of the plant are absorbing large amounts of nitrate, because the stem and leaves normally convert nitrate to protein about as fast as it is absorbed by the roots. Under adverse weather events, such as droughts, frosts, or hail damage, this balance can be disrupted such that that the roots accumulate nitrates faster than the plant can convert nitrates to protein. The nitrate-to-protein cycle in a plant is dependent on 3 factors: (1) adequate water, (2) energy from sunlight, and (3) temperatures conducive to rapid chemical reactions.

If any one of these factors is inadequate, the root continues to absorb nitrate at the same rate and stores it unchanged in the stalk and lower parts of the leaves. When this situation develops, nitrate accumulates. Nitrates may also accumulate in plants from excessive nitrogen fertilization, for example, on fields where a large amount of manure have been applied. Some plants are more likely to accumulate nitrate that others. Crops capable of high levels of nitrate accumulation under adverse conditions include corn, small grains, sudangrass, and sorghum. Legumes are not subject to nitrate issues. If conditions exist for high nitrate levels, samples should be submitted to forage laboratories for nitrate analysis. If high levels are present, lifting the chopper head (eg, 18–20 in for corn and sorghum forages) minimizes the amount of high-nitrate forage brought into the silo.[55]

Feeding high-nitrate forages fed to cattle may induce symptomatic labored breathing, because they interfere with the ability of the blood to carry oxygen. Because of nitrate reduction during the ensiling process, nitrates may be reduced by as much as 50%; therefore, toxic levels of nitrate coming in with the crop may feed out within tolerable plant concentrations. **Table 10** provides recommended safe feeding levels for silages with increased nitrate levels.

Prussic acid poisoning in forages

Prussic acid poisoning primarily occurs in sorghum and sorghum-sudangrass crops that are growing rapidly under early frost, drought, or heat stress conditions. Dhurrin is a compound produced in sorghum and sudangrass plants that is degraded by cattle to release prussic acid (hydrogen cyanide).

High levels of nitrogen fertilizer or manure increase the likelihood of prussic acid poisoning, which is indicated by dark green color in plant growth. Most prussic acid is lost during the hay curing process because of dissipation of the gas into the atmosphere; however, reduction of prussic acid by the ensiling is minimal, because of the high packing densities that exist in silages.[56] Harvesting sorghum-sudangrass silages

Table 10 Nitrate levels in forages for cattle		
Nitrate Ion (%)	**Nitrate Nitrogen (ppm)**	**Recommendations**
0.0–0.44	<1000	Safe to feed under all conditions
0.44–0.66	1000–1500	Safe to feed to nonpregnant animals. Limit use for pregnant animals to 50% of total ration on a DM basis
0.66–0.88	1500–2000	Safely fed if limited to 50% of the total DM ration
0.88–1.54	2000–3500	Feeds should be limited to 35%–40% of the total DM in the ration. Feeds >2000 ppm nitrate nitrogen should not be fed to pregnant animals
1.54–1.76	3500–4000	Feeds should be limited to 25% of total DM in the ration. Do not feed to pregnant animals
>1.76	>4000	Feeds containing these levels are potentially toxic. Do not feed

Adapted from Sniffen CJ, Chase LE. Nitrates in dairy rations. Department of Animal Science, Cornell University Ithica, NY; 1981.

at a higher chop height helps decrease dhurrin concentrations in the crop by leaving rapidly growing tillers in the field.

SILAGE FEED-OUT
Silage Feeding Considerations

- Silage evaluations during feed-out can be performed by collecting on-site observations and measurements that help dairy clients feed higher and more consistent quality silages.
- Proper silage sampling techniques and using silage fermentation analytical services help identify silage feed-out issues.
- Frequent monitoring NDF and starch digestibilities of silages permits fine-tuning of dairy rations that provide the dairy animal with nutritional requirements for optimal production, health, and fertility.

Feed-out management requires that: (1) a proper amount is removed daily and (2) a clean silo face is maintained, with no loose silage present for extended periods. Losses resulting from slow removal account for up to 50% of DM loss and in the form of plant sugars, not fiber. Aerobic organisms consume water-soluble carbohydrate, thus reducing the energy content of the forage. Silage defacers have been introduced to the North American silage marketplace in recent years and have been proved to maintain aerobic stability during feed-out.[57]

Silo Safety

Making silage quality assessments during feed-out requires approaching horizontal silos for making observations and collecting silage samples. Many horizontal silos are built too high to be safe. In **Fig. 7**, the silo face is 4 times the height of the vehicle, meaning that the face is approximately 32 ft high. A silage overhang, as shown in the image, breaking loose and falling 32 feet could cause injury or even death. Anytime the silo face seems compromised, it is wise to have unloader equipment collect representative silage and bring it into a safe location for making observations and collecting samples.

- ◆ **Many silos are built too high to be safe**
  - • **Cause feedout challenges**
  - • **Risk avalanches**
- ◆ **Machinery at silo sites can be dangerous**

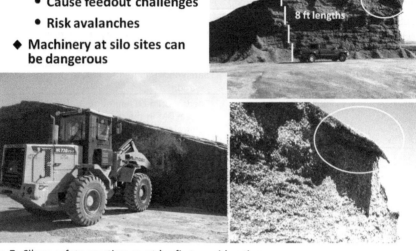

Fig. 7. Silage safety practices must be first consideration.

Silo gas is another danger when working around silos during silo filling and up to 3 weeks after ensiling. Tower silos are especially dangerous. This is the period when nitrates are reduced into lethal silo gas when they combine with organic silage acids to form nitrous oxide. The nitrous oxide decomposes to water and a mixture of nitrogen oxides, including nitrogen oxide, dioxide, and trioxide. These forms of nitrogen are volatilized as a brownish gas in the atmosphere. This gas is heavier than air and lethal to humans and livestock. It is advisable to run the silo blowers for at least 15 minutes before entering recently filled silos. **Fig. 8** summarizes silo gas talking points.

Sample collection

The sample intended for nutritional analysis must be as representative as possible of the entire silo face being fed out. Refer to the article on feed analysis elsewhere in this issue for further information.

Do not sample problem silage as removed from a TMR mixer or an upright silo unloader chute so as not to mask the trouble spots with normal silage. Silage problems often exist in focal areas of the silo, and therefore, samples must be collected in those unique areas of the silo. It helps to have comparative samples from both problem and

- • Silo gas forms after filling and persists 2-3 weeks
- • VENTILATE! Run blowers 15-20 minutes before entering silo
- • Keep workers, children and livestock clear of area
- • Beware of bleach-like odors and following colors
  - › nitric oxide   → colorless
  - › nitrogen dioxide   → red-brown
  - › nitrogen tetraoxide → yellow

Fig. 8. Silo gas talking points.

normal silage to help troubleshoot the relative extent of the problem. Likewise, in the case of aerobic instability, when heating occurs at the face of the silo, it is often advisable to collect the silo face hot sample and then another deep sample 2 to 3 feet behind the face for using as a baseline comparison.

Silage evaluations are often a result of dairy cattle observations such as inconsistent manure in pens or presence of corn grain in the manure. The veterinarian providing nutritional consultation services should develop a protocol that transitions from dairy cow observations to monitoring of the feed delivery system, which often points to making evaluations of the silages being fed in the diet. Refer to the article on TMR evaluation elsewhere in this issue for further details regarding feed delivery systems.

The list of subjective observations to make before approaching the silo face include evaluating: (1) face management, (2) changes in packing density, (3) feed-out rate, (4) whether silage is removed evenly across the entire face daily, (5) demarcation lines, and (6) inconsistent pockets or channels that may show up as color variations, pack differences, or obvious spoilage areas. While collecting this information, evaluate the integrity of the silo for safety to determine if approaching the silo face is advisable.

On-site testing equipment can provide instantaneous and economical objective data compared with submitting samples for laboratory analysis. However, both are often used during silage evaluations so that on-site assessments can be validated with laboratory data. **Table 11** compares on-site evaluations with laboratory analysis.

Silage pH observations can be collected with litmus paper or a pocket pH meter to probe silage at different focal locations to determine if the pH is uniform or if pockets of clostridial growth or aerobic instability are the reasons for increased pH. An economical way of conducting a silo site pH test is with the use of pH litmus paper, which usually costs around $5.00/roll; approximately 100 tests can be run per roll.

Silage pH testing with litmus paper involves placing 1 to 2 oz of equal parts silage and water into a container and then using a stir stick to mix for at least 1 minute. Then, tear off a strip of pH litmus paper and dip it into the silage solution. Next, compare the color of the litmus strip with the color chart on the container, as shown in **Fig. 9**. Legume silages such as alfalfa and clover always have a higher terminal pH in the 4.0 to 4.5 range compared with grass and corn silages with a 3.7 to 4.2 range. The differences are caused by differences in DM content and buffering capacity for these crops.

Table 11
On-site silage evaluations compared with laboratory analysis

On-Site Testing	Sampling/Laboratory Tests
Immediate answers	Provides quantitative data
More economical	May take days for results
Permits client face-time	Involves laboratory and shipping expenses
A professional offering	
Evaluation Tools	Laboratory Tests
pH testers	Nutritional
Thermometers	Digestibility
Density Probe	Fermentation
PROC cup	Spoilage microbes
Penn State Particle Separator	Mycotoxins

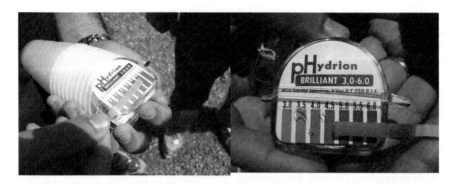

Preserved Silage-silo center   **Unstable Silage-silo edge**

Fig. 9. Example of pH determination from silage in 2 locations.

Temperature monitoring equipment is used for gathering data that help determine consistency of the silage fermentation. Often, temperature data complement pH information, and using aerobic instability from yeast as an example, the unstable silage is a result of yeast consuming lactic acid for substrate, which causes pH to increase and generation of heat. As discussed in the biology of fermentation, respiratory activities of spoilage microbes create carbon dioxide and water, which accounts for DM losses but also generation of heat. Therefore, collection of data at various locations in the silo helps support your discussion with management regarding the losses that occur when aerobic activity is permitted to occur during the feed-out phase. The ideal ensiling temperature is within 15°F of ambient temperatures at time of harvest and filling of the silo. Temperatures in excess of the 15°F limit indicate either (1) inefficient front-end fermentation or (2) excessive spoilage microbe activity during silage feed-out. Temperatures that approach or exceed 130°F to 140°F indicate *Bacillus* spoilage activity, causing increased ADIN in laboratory reports.

Two types of thermometers are recommended: (1) a 3-ft compost temperature probe and (2) a noncontact thermometer; both of which are $100 investments. Temperature probes permit recording temperature data from 1.5 to 2 ft behind the silo face, which should be an aerobically stable area of the silage mass. The deeper readings are compared with data collected from the noncontact thermometer on the silo face.

Internal temperature is not an absolute value but rather is based on what the ambient temperature was at time of harvest. This information can be obtained from farm management and the value does not need to be exact, but it is to be hoped that an approximate temperature during silage harvest can be recalled and shared for making silage evaluation assessments. If this temperature is within 15°F of ambient harvest temperatures, the fermentation process is considered normal and should be considered as the baseline temperature.

Once a baseline temperature has been established, use the noncontact thermometer by positioning about 20 to 30 ft away from the silo face and aim the thermometer at the desired silo face location for data collection. Pull back the trigger and the face temperature appears on the display. The reading is instantaneous, so that many face temperatures across and up and down the face can be collected and recorded quickly. Ideally, face temperatures should be collected several hours after silage has been removed from the face so that if aerobic instability exists, it may be quantified with the temperature readings.

Compare the various face temperatures with the internal temperature, as shown in **Fig. 10**. The goal for stable silage is to have the face temperature be the same or lower than that of the internal temperature. Similar temperatures mean that the silage is stable, whereas if the face temperature is lower, that indicates heat dissipation off the silo face. This finding is perfectly normal and is more apparent during months when ambient air temperatures are cold. If the surface temperature is greater than 15°F higher than the internal baseline temperature, then it may be concluded that aerobic instability exists during silage feed-out.

Silage density probes provide a report card assessment regarding how well the forage was packed at silo filling time. Data are reported in pounds of silage (DM or as-fed basis) per ft³. **Fig. 11** shows sources where density probes can be purchased along with an electric cordless or gas-powered drill and a gram scale needed for the analysis.

The test is performed by coring into the silo face to the advised depth, which results in a sample that is contained within a predefined geometric cubic area. Then, the sample is removed with a wooden tamper and weighed on a gram scale. Once the weight data are recorded, the DM content of the silage has to be determined, which usually exists on forage analysis reports that have been run. Otherwise, a Koster tester or microwave oven is needed to perform a DM determination. Once the grams and DM are recorded, refer to a conversion chart, which can be found and printed off from the Dairy One Web site http://dairyone.com/analytical-services/feed-and-forage/master-forage-probe/dcsingle/, and use it to determine the silage density in DM lb/ft³. Some consultants and silage articles in farm publications may refer to "as-fed" silage densities, so it is always important to clarify if the densities collected are on a DM or as-fed basis.

Corn silage should be in the 14 to 16 DM lb/ft³ range, whereas grass and alfalfa silage should be in the 16 to 18 DM lb/ft³ range. Sharing these results with farm managers during silo feed-out provides a report card for determining if proper packing tractor weights existed during silo filling.

If the silo face is unsafe to approach, an alternative option for silage density assessment is to download a spreadsheet calculator from the Internet, from which average

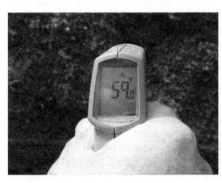

◆ This silage has 67° F. **internal temperature**

◆ History indicates 60-65° harvest temps

◆ **Face temp is 59° F.**

◆ 67° - 59° = 8° temp difference

◆ **Conclusion:**

  – This silage is stable

  – Internal heat is dissipating off face

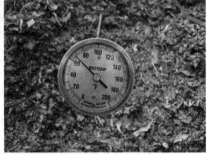

Fig. 10. Usefulness of the noncontact thermometer with temperature probe data.

- Assesses how well silage is packed
- Reported in lbs/ft.[3]
- Use density calculator
- Need a scale
  - (~ $30.00 at Walmart)
- Probe cost ~$150.00
  - Dairy-1 sells a density probe

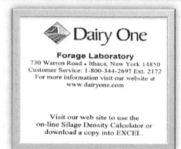

Think Safety....
do not probe bunkers with dangerous overhangs or obviously poor compaction

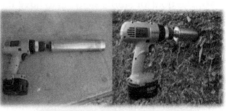

Refer to the UW calculator:
http://www.uwex.edu/ces/crops/uwforage/storage.htm
Safer way to go

Dairy One

Forage Laboratory
730 Warren Road • Ithaca, New York 14850
Customer Service: 1-800-344-2697 Ext. 2172
For more information visit our website at
www.dairyone.com

Visit our web site to use the
on-line Silage Density Calculator or
download a copy into EXCEL.

Fig. 11. Silage density determination.

packing densities can be determined based on removal rates and lb silage removed in that time frame. One such resource can be found in the University of Wisconsin's Forage Extension Web site: http://www.uwex.edu/ces/crops/uwforage/storage.htm.

The kernel processing cup and Penn State Particle Separator permit physical assessments that can be made at the silo to determine the availability of nutrients from the silage for digestion. Assessment of the degree of WPCS processing for kernel damage is 1 such test. Perhaps the most overlooked aspect of assessing corn silage at the bunker is attention to physical damage of the corn kernels. A (32-oz) beverage cup can be used as an on-farm method to quantify kernel damage. Fill the cup to the rim, spread the silage out on a flat surface, and pick out any half or whole kernel pieces. If the sample contains more than 3 or more of these whole or half kernel pieces, have a laboratory PROC test conducted to help in potentially discounting the energy value of the silage.[44]

However, often, the on-site assessment is validated by collecting samples and sending into commercial laboratories to obtain a more exact quantification of the degree of processing of the silage. The 32-oz beverage cup test is meant to stimulate discussions with chopping crews during harvest regarding degree of PROC, whereas the laboratory test is a direct quantification of how successful PROC was at harvest. A PROC score was developed at the US Dairy Forage Research Center, which involves sending a corn silage sample to a commercial feed testing laboratory, where it is dried, sieved through a series of wire mesh sieves of varying sizes, starch analyses performed, and the proportion of the starch in the sample that is retained or has passed through a 4.75-mm sieve is determined.[19] The finer starch or the starch that passes through this sieve is more highly digestible in the cow. **Table 12** provides guidelines for laboratory PROC evaluations.

Determination of chop length for effective fiber and contribution to rumen health is another physical nutritional assessment opportunity. The Penn State Particle Separator is an excellent way to make sure that proper chop lengths are being achieved during harvest. However, it is better to monitor particle size of forages being ensiled

Table 12
US Dairy Forage Research Center guidelines for PROC evaluations

% Starch in WPCS Passing Through the 4.75-mm Sieve	PROC Score
>70	Excellent
50–70	Adequate
<50	Poor

Data from Ferreira G, Mertens DR. Chemical and physical characteristics of corn silages and their effects on in vitro disappearance. J Dairy Sci 2005;88:4414–25.

at time of harvest to advise the chopper operator of needed changes rather than being hampered by what exists at feed-out. The Penn State Particle Separator comprises either 2 (19.0 and 8.0 mm)[58] or 3 (19.0, 8.0, and 1.18 mm)[18] sieves plus the bottom pan. Guidelines provided by Penn State Extension[59] are listed for corn and hay crop silages in **Table 13**.

DC and HMSC particle size is determined by using forage and grain laboratory services in which submitted grain samples are sieved through an official American Society of Agricultural Engineers (ASAE) 13-screen and collection pan stack system using the Tyler RoTap sieve shaker. The average particle size of material retained on a screen is calculated as the geometric mean of the diameter openings in 2 adjacent sieves in the stack. Once this calculation is performed for each screen, a MPS reported in μ is determined along with a standard deviation determination.[60] Field experience indicates that 1500 μ MPS is suitable for HMSC compared with 800 μ MPS for DC.

A field-based sieving system was tested by Baker and Herrman,[60] which used a short 5-sieve and collection pan system on the farm and determined that similar results were produced when compared with the official ASAE procedure. Another field study by Nuzback and colleagues[61] used a series of 4 sieves and collection pan, which was validated by making sampling comparisons against the ASAE sieve system. The study produced high correlations at $R^2 = 0.99$ for DC and 0.97 for HMSC.

Laboratory analysis of ensiled forages and grains is of value for quantification of silage quality and identification of silage feeding issues. Those analyses include: (1) nutritional and digestibility profiles, (2) silage fermentation profiles, and (3) spoilage microbial enumeration and identification. Performing all the tests can result in high laboratory expense; therefore, judiciously determine which questions need to be answered when selecting test offerings. For instance, if nitrate is the only concern,

Table 13
Corn silage and haylage particle silage recommendations

Screen	Particle Size (mm)	Corn Silage	Haylage
		% As Fed on Sieve or Pan	
Upper sieve	19.0	3–8	10–20
Middle sieve	8.0	45–65	45–75
Lower sieve	1.18	20–30	30–40
Bottom pan	<1.18	<10	<10

Data from Heinrichs J. Penn State Particle Separator. DSE 2013–186. Available at: http://www.extension.psu.edu/animals/dairy/health/nutrition/forages/forage-quality-physical/separator. Accessed November 7, 2013.

then the only additional test would be specific for determination of nitrate concentrations.

Nutritional measurements are discussed in the article on feed analysis elsewhere in this issue.

Digestibility measurements for NDF and starch provide value in silage reports when determining how digestibilities differ based on various ensiled crops and how long they were ensiled in the storage structure. Details on forage digestibility measurements can be found in the article on feed analysis elsewhere in this issue.

Silage fermentation profile analyses are available for evaluating silage quality on farms through commercial forage testing laboratories. Analyses commonly included in silage fermentation reports are pH, lactic, acetic, propionic and butyric acids, ammonia, and ethanol. Results from a fermentation profile analysis can determine whether an excellent, average, or poor fermentation has occurred. In most cases, the fermentation that a crop undergoes can be explained by various crop factors, such as moisture content, buffering capacity, and sugar content. However, management factors such as silo packing speed, silage pack density, type of additive used, chop length, silo management during storage, and silo management during feed-out can affect fermentation reports. **Table 14** provides the normal ranges for fermentation end products.[62] Lower DM legume and grass silages should have less than 0.5% butyric acid concentrations; a goal should always be to have no butyric acid present in silages.

Aerobic microbial assessments that determine yeast, mold, and *Bacillus* population counts are expressed in colony-forming units per gram of feedstuff (cfu/g). Aerobic microorganisms require oxygen from air penetration, thereby indicating aerobic instability. Aerobic microbial cfu counts less than 100,000 are desirable for each of the spoilage microbes (yeast, mold, and *Bacillus*).

1. Yeast: uses lactic acid as substrate in the presence of oxygen, thereby causing the increase of pH. DM losses occur from the production of carbon dioxide, water, and heat. Yeast activity precedes mold growth. Poor face management and observations of heating at the face are usually explained by high yeast counts.
2. Mold: when lactic acid concentrations are diminished by yeast and the pH increases higher than 4.5, the silage environment becomes conducive to mold

Table 14
Typical concentration of common fermentation end products in various corn, legume, and grass silages

End Product	Legume Silage (30%–40%)[a]	Legume Silage (45%–55%)[a]	Grass Silage (30%–35%)[a]	Corn Silage (30%–40%)[a]	HM Corn (70%–75%)[a]
pH	4.3–4.7	4.7–5.0	4.3–4.7	3.7–4.2	4.0–4.5
Lactic acid (%)	7–8	2–4	6–10	4–7	0.5–2.0
Acetic acid (%)	2–3	0.5–2.0	1–3	1–3	<0.5
Propionic acid (%)	<0.5	<0.1	<0.1	<0.1	<0.1
Butyric acid (%)	<0.5	0	<0.5	0	0
Ethanol (%)	0.2–1.0	0.5	0.5–1.0	0.5–1.0	0.5–1.0
Ammonia-N (% of CP)	10–15	<12	8–12	<10	—

[a] % DM of silage.

Data from Kung L, Shaver R. Interpretation and use of silage fermentation analysis reports. 2000. Available at: http://www.uwex.edu/ces/crops/uwforage/fermentaion.html. Accessed August 22, 2013.

growth. This situation results in musty, hot, energy-depleted, and unpalatable silage. Often, using laboratories that can accurately identify the storage mold helps determine likelihood of mycotoxins present that are not screened for by commercial laboratory offerings. An example is *Penicillium roquefortii*, which is the most common spoilage mold in silage and produces patulin and PR toxin.

3. *Bacillus*: fields may be highly contaminated with soilborne spores from this aerobe at harvest. *Bacillus* is highly thermophilic in the presence of oxygen and is primarily responsible for high bound protein (ADIN) values in silages. See bound protein description in article on feed analysis elsewhere in this issue.

Advised Silage Analysis Equipment and Where to Access

Silage Density Probe (The Master Forage Probe from Dairy One, Ithica, NY)
  http://dairyone.com/analytical-services/feed-and-forage/master-forage-probe/
Heavy-duty (high torque) 18-V cordless drill for silage density probe
  Available through hardware store retailers
NASCO' S3-Sieve Forage Particle Separator (Model C24682N) (NASCO, Fort Atkinson, WI)
  http://www.enasco.com/product/C24682N
Battery-operated, digital gram scale
  Available through hardware or kitchenware store retailers
pH strips (1 pack of 12 strips range of pH 3–7 with 0.5 increments)
  Available through veterinary equipment suppliers
36 inch REOtemp compost (windrow) temperature probe (with 5/16 inch shaft) (Biocontrol Network, Brentwood, TN)
  http://www.biconet.com/compost/thermometer.html
MiniTemp Noncontact Thermometer with Laser Sighting (Model B01376N) (NASCO, Fort Atkinson, WI)
  http://www.enasco.com/action/solr/select?q=MiniTemp+Non+Contact+Thermometer&x=11&y=14
Koster Hay/Haylage/Silage/High Moisture Grain Moisture Tester (Model C08633N) (NASCO, Fort Atkinson, WI)
  http://www.enasco.com/action/solr/select?q=Koster+Tester&x=10&y=11

REFERENCES

1. Teutsch C. Using mixtures of summer forages for improved forage yields in dry conditions. J Anim Sci 2013;91(E-Suppl 2)/J Dairy Sci 96(E-Suppl 1):406. [abstract 358].

2. Benson GO, Pearce RB. Corn perspective and culture. In: Watson SA, Ramstad PE, editors. Corn: chemistry and technology. St. Paul (MN): American Association of Cereal Chemists; 1994. p. 1–12.

3. Schwab EC, Shaver RD, Lauer JG, et al. Estimating silage energy value and milk yield to rank corn hybrids. J Anim Feed Sci Technol 2003;109:1–18.

4. Ferraretto LF, Shaver RD. Meta-analysis: effect of corn silage harvest practices on intake, digestion, and milk production by dairy cows. Prof Anim Sci 2012;28:141–9.

5. Oba M, Allen MS. Evaluation of the importance of the digestibility of neutral detergent fiber from forage: effects on dry matter intake and milk yield of dairy cows. J Dairy Sci 1999;82:589–96.

6. Jung H, Lauer J. Corn silage fiber digestibility: key points, historical trends, and future opportunities. In: Proc. 72nd MN Nutr. Conf. Owatonna (MN): 2011. p. 30–44.

7. Ferraretto LF, Shaver RD. Effect of corn shredlage on lactation performance and total tract starch digestibility by dairy cows. Prof Anim Sci 2012;28:639–47.
8. Neylon JM, Kung L Jr. Effects of cutting height and maturity on the nutritive value of corn silage for lactating cows. J Dairy Sci 2003;86:2163–9.
9. Kung L Jr, Moulder BM, Mulrooney CM, et al. The effect of silage cutting height on the nutritive value of a normal corn silage hybrid compared with brown midrib corn silage fed to lactating cows. J Dairy Sci 2008;91:1451–7.
10. Larson J, Hoffman PC. Technical note: a method to quantify prolamin proteins in corn that are negatively related to starch digestibility in ruminants. J Dairy Sci 2008;91:4834–9.
11. McAllister TA, Phillippe RC, Rode LM, et al. Effect of the protein matrix on the digestion of cereal grains by ruminal microorganisms. J Anim Sci 1993;71:205–12.
12. Hoffman PC, Esser NM, Shaver RD, et al. Influence of ensiling time and inoculation on alteration of the starch-protein matrix in high moisture corn. J Dairy Sci 2011;94:2465–74.
13. Benton JR, Klopfenstein T, Erickson GE. Effects of corn moisture and length of ensiling on dry matter digestibility and rumen degradable protein. Nebraska Beef Cattle Reports. Lincoln (NE): University of Nebraska Animal Science Dept; 2005. p. 31–3.
14. Newbold JR, Lewis EA, Lavrijssen J, et al. Effect of storage time on ruminal starch degradability in corn silage. J Dairy Sci 2006;84(Suppl 1):T94 (abst).
15. Der Bedrosian MC, Nestor KE, Kung L Jr. The effects of hybrid, maturity, and length of storage on the composition and nutritive value of corn silage. J Dairy Sci 2012;95:5115–26.
16. Hoffman PC, Mertens DR, Larson J, et al. A query for effective mean particle size of dry and high moisture corns. J Dairy Sci 2012;95:3467–77.
17. Young KM, Lim JM, Der Bedrosian MC, et al. Effect of exogenous protease enzymes on the fermentation and nutritive value of corn silage. J Dairy Sci 2012; 95:6687–94.
18. Kononoff PJ, Heinrichs AJ, Buckmaster DR. Modification of the Penn State forage and total mixed ration particle separator and the effects of moisture content on its measurements. J Dairy Sci 2003;86:1858–63.
19. Ferreira G, Mertens DR. Chemical and physical characteristics of corn silages and their effects on in vitro disappearance. J Dairy Sci 2005;88:4414–25.
20. Mader T, Erickson G. Feeding high moisture corn. Lincoln (NE): University of Nebraska – Lincoln Ext. Serv. Publ; 2006. G100.
21. Soderlund SD, Uhrig J, Curran B, et al. Influence of maturity on the yield and nutritional quality of four pioneer corn hybrids harvested as high moisture ear corn. Johnston (IA): Nutritional Insights, DuPont Pioneer; 2006.
22. Mahanna B. Renewed interest in snaplage displayed. Feedstuffs 2008;80(50): 12–3.
23. Lardy G, Anderson V. Harvesting and feeding corn as earlage. Fargo (ND): North Dakota State Univ. Ext. Serv. Publ; 2010. AS-1490.
24. Oba M, Allen MS. Effects of corn grain conservation method on feeding behavior and productivity of lactating dairy cows at two dietary starch concentrations. J Dairy Sci 2003;86:174–83.
25. Ferraretto LF, Crump PM, Shaver RD. Impact of cereal grain type and corn harvest and processing methods on intake, digestion and milk production by dairy cows through a meta-analysis. J Dairy Sci 2013;96:533–50.
26. Akins MS, Shaver RD. Effect of corn snaplage on lactation performance by dairy cows. Prof Anim Sci 2014;30(1):86–92.

27. Barnes DK, Sheaffer CC. Forages legumes and grasses. In: Barnes RF, Miller DA, Nelson JC, editors. Forages: an introduction to grassland agriculture, vol. I, 5th edition. Ames (IA): Iowa State University Press; 1995. p. 205–61.

28. Van Soest PJ. Environment and forage quality. Proceedings of the Pioneer Hi-Bred Pre-Conference Symposium of the Cornell Nutrition Conference. Rochester (NY): 1996. p. 1–9.

29. Nelson WF, Satter LD. Effect of stage of maturity and method of preservation of alfalfa on production by lactating dairy cows. J Dairy Sci 1990;73: 1800–11.

30. Rohweder DA, Barnes RE, Jorgensen N. Proposed hay grading standards based on laboratory analysis for evaluating quality. J Anim Sci 1978;47: 747–59.

31. Undersander DJ, Moore JE. Relative forage quality, vol. 4. Madison (WI): University of Wisconsin Extension Focus on Forage Series; 2002. No. 5. Available at: http://www.uwex.edu/ces/crops/uwforage/RFQvsRFV.htm.

32. Kung L Jr, Stough EC, McDonell EE, et al. The effect of wide swathing on wilting times and nutritive value of alfalfa haylage. J Dairy Sci 2010;93:1770–3.

33. Hoffman PC, Broderick GA. Red clover forages for lactating dairy cows. Madison (WI): University of Wisconsin Extension Focus on Forage; 2001. 3:11. Available at: www.uwex.edu/ces/crops/uwforage/RedCloverCows.pdf. Accessed November 6, 2013.

34. Undersander D, Jarek K, Anderson T, et al. A guide to making soybean silage. Forage and Grazinglands 2007. http://dx.doi.org/10.1094/FG-2007-0119-01-MG.

35. Cherney JH, Cherney JR. Grass for dairy cows. Proc MN Forage Day. 2009. Available at: www.extension.umn.edu/agriculture/forages/pdfs/grass_for_dairy_cows_21009.pdf. Accessed November 16, 2013.

36. Undersander D. Alfalfa grass mixtures. Proc. WI Crop Mgmt. Conf. Madison (WI): 2012. 51:88–90.

37. Barnhart S. Oats for forage. Ames (IA): Iowa State University Extension and Outreach; 2011. Available at: http://www.extension.iastate.edu/CropNews/2011/0621barnhart.htm. Accessed January 13, 2014.

38. Oliver AL, Grant RJ, Pedersen JF, et al. Comparison of brown midrib-6 and -18 forage sorghum with conventional sorghum and corn silage in diets of lactating dairy cows. J Dairy Sci 2004;87:637–44.

39. Collar C, Aksland C. Harvest stage effects on yield and quality of winter forage. In 31st California Alfalfa Symposium. Davis (CA): University of California Cooperative Extension, University of California; December 11-13, 2001.

40. Bean B, Marsalis M. Corn and sorghum silage production considerations. Proc High Plains Dairy Conf. Amarillo (TX): 2012. p. 1–7.

41. McDonald P. The biochemistry of silage. Wiley, Chalcombe, Cambridge University Press, Cambridge, UK; 1991. p. 48, 13 Highwoods Drive, Marlow Bottom, Bucks SL7 3PU.

42. Seglar WJ. Silage fermentation. Compendium's food animal medicine & management. 1997. p. 65–68.

43. Mahanna WC. Silage fermentation and additive use in North America. NFIA Proc. 1991.

44. Mahanna WC, Seglar WJ, Dennis S. Pioneer Silage Zone Manual. Johnston (IA): DuPont Pioneer Global Forages; 2012. 6900 N.W. 62nd Ave. 50131.

45. Harrison JH, Fransen S. Silage management in North America. In: Field guide for hay and silage management in North America. Arlington (VA): National Feed Ingredients Association; 1991. p. 33–49.

46. Weiss B, Underwood J. Round bale silage. Columbus (OH): Ohio State University Extension Publ; 1995. AGF01095. Available at: http://ohioline.osu.edu/agf-fact/0010.html.

47. Mahanna WC. Lessons learned from feeding the 1993 and 1994 corn crops. 4-States Applied Nutrition Conf Proc. Madison (WI): University of Wisconsin Extension; 1995.

48. Muck RE, Moser LE, Pitt RE. Post-harvest factors affecting ensiling. In: Buxton DR, Muck RE, Harrison JH, editors. Silage science and technology. Madison (WI): American Society of Agronomy, Crop Science Society of America, Soil Science of America; 2003. p. 251–304.

49. Ruppel KA, Pitt RE, Chase LE, et al. Bunker silo management and its relationship to forage preservation on dairy farms. J Dairy Sci 1995;78:141–53.

50. Bolsen KK, Dickerson JT, Brent BE, et al. Rate and extent of top spoilage in horizontal silos. J Dairy Sci 1993;76:2940–62.

51. Borreani G, Tabacco E, Cavallarini L. A new oxygen barrier film reduces aerobic deterioration in farm-scale corn silage. J Dairy Sci 2007;90:4701–6.

52. Seglar WJ. Ruminant disorders associated with pathogens found within ensiled forages. Proc. to the American Assn. of Bovine Practitioners Conf. Auburn (AL): 1999. p. 61–70.

53. Oetzel GR. Herd-level ketosis: diagnosis and risk factors. Proc to the American Assn of Bovine Practitioners Conf. Auburn (AL): 2007. p. 67–91.

54. Bergen WG. Protein conservation in silage management. West Des Moines (IA): Silage Management, National Feed Ingredient Association; 1984. p. 113.

55. Undersander D, Combs D, Howard T, et al. Nitrate poisoning in cattle, sheep and goats. UW Extension; 2001.

56. Busk PK, Moller BL. Dhurrin synthesis in sorghum is regulated at the transcriptional level and induced by nitrogen fertilization in older plants. Plant Physiol 2002;129:1222–31. Available at: http://www.plantphysiol.org/content/129/3/1222.full.pdf+html. Accessed January 13, 2014.

57. Holmes BJ. Bunker Silo Facers – Worth the Investment? 2003. Available at: http://fyi.uwex.edu/forage/files/2014/01/FacerFOF.pdf. Accessed August 26, 2014.

58. Lammers BP, Buckmaster DR, Heinrichs AJ. A simplified method for the analysis of particle sizes of forage and total mixed rations. J Dairy Sci 1996;79:922–92.

59. Heinrichs J. Penn State Particle Separator. DSE 2013-186. 2013. Available at: http://www.extension.psu.edu/animals/dairy/health/nutrition/forages/forage-quality-physical/separator. Accessed November 7, 2013.

60. Baker S, Herrman T. Evaluating particle size. KSU Ag Expt. Station and Coop. Extension Service. MF-2051. 2002. Available at: http://www.ksre.ksu.edu/bookstore/pubs/mf2051.pdf. Accessed March 18, 2014.

61. Nuzback LJ, Seglar WJ, Laubach M, et al. Geometric mean diameter fails to reflect particle size diversity in processed maize. J Anim Sci 2013;91(E-Suppl 2)/J Dairy Sci 96(E-Suppl 1):T81, P 30.

62. Kung L, Shaver R. Interpretation and use of silage fermentation analysis reports. 2000. Available at: http://www.uwex.edu/ces/crops/uwforage/fermentaion.html. Accessed August 22, 2013.

63. Bennett OL, Doss BO. Effects of Soil Moisture Requirements on Yield and Evapotranspiration For Cool-Season Perennial Forage Species. Agronomy Journal 1963;55(3):275–8.

64. Martin JH, Leonard WH, Stamp DL. Principles of field crop production. New York: Macmillan Publishing Co., Inc; 1976.

Feeding, Evaluating, and Controlling Rumen Function

Ian J. Lean, BVSc, DVSc, PhD, MANZCVS[a,b,*],
Helen M. Golder, BAgSci (Hons.)[a,b], Mary Beth Hall, PhD[c]

KEYWORDS

- Rumen function • Carbohydrates • Proteins • Acidosis • Evaluating nutrition

KEY POINTS

- The interactions of feeds within the rumen ensure that feed and nutritional assessment systems must be relatively complex and integrated to effectively capture and understand the effects on cattle.
- To understand the dynamics of digestion of protein and carbohydrates, it is necessary to understand the interactions between the rates of passage of feeds through the rumen and the rates of digestion of feeds in the rumen.
- Optimal production of microbial protein is the key goal for efficient dairy production.
- Ruminal acidosis can be a major risk in dairy production systems.
- Control of rumen function derives from good ration design and management, and can be supported by use of production modifiers.

A Video of the methodology to collect a sample of rumen contents for analysis accompanies this article at http://www.vetfood.theclinics.com/

INTRODUCTION

This article takes the approach of providing an overview of feeding, evaluating, and controlling the rumen in a clinical context. Pivotal references are included in each section for further reading to allow readers to improve their knowledge of each area, should an area interest them. The authors have also drawn attention to new work on the rumen that is changing our understanding of how to improve production and health of cattle through better management of the rumen.

Disclosures: None.
[a] SBScibus, PO Box 660, Camden, New South Wales 2570, Australia; [b] Dairy Science Group, Faculty of Veterinary Science, The University of Sydney, Brownlow Loop Road, Camden, New South Wales 2570, Australia; [c] USDA-ARS, U.S. Dairy Forage Research Center, 1925 Linden Drive West, Madison, WI 53706, USA
* Corresponding author. PO Box 660, Camden, New South Wales 2570, Australia.
E-mail address: ianl@sbscibus.com.au

The rumen is a large fermentation chamber containing a complex microbial ecosystem that works in a dynamic, symbiotic relationship with the host to convert feed into energy and protein. This microbial ecosystem consists of bacteria, protozoa, archaea, fungi, and bacteriophages (**Table 1**). The system is highly responsive to dietary changes.[1,2] Individual cows seem to have a unique rumen ecosystem comprising a core rumen microbiome[3] that adapts to different feed substrates.[4,5] The composition of the rumen microbiome reflects the diet, feed additives, health, age, condition, season, and geographic conditions.[6,7] The dominant bacteria belong to the Bacteroidetes and Firmicutes phyla, which account for approximately 80% to 95% of bacterial sequences.[3,8,9] The ratio of these varies with diet, other bacteria being less dominant but still of significance. The uniqueness of the interaction between cattle and their ruminal microbiome was strikingly highlighted by Weimer and colleagues,[10] who evacuated and swapped greater than 95% of the rumen fluid between two cattle. Within 24 hours the rumen pH and volatile fatty acids (VFA) concentration had returned to their original state, and bacterial community composition returned near to its original profile within 14 days for one cow and 61 days for the second.[10] The diverse synergies and antagonism of ruminal microbes allow ruminants to efficiently use a range of feeds (see **Table 1**).[2,11,12]

There are 3 levels at which one can assess the efficacy of the diet.

1. Feeds as tested (quality of base ingredients)
2. Feeds as evaluated in the bunk, parlor, or pasture (consistency of formulation with delivery)
3. In the cow: production outcomes (milk, milk constituents, weight, body condition score)
   - Output measures including fecal composition and urine
   - Blood measures

Feeding the rumen is related to the evaluation and control of rumen function for optimal production and health outcomes.

FEED INTAKE

Feed intake is both an input and output of rumen function. It is an input from the perspective that the amount of feed on offer and the way it is offered (eg, feeding frequency) determines intake and influences rumen outflow.

Feed Intake is influenced by:

- Feed availability and palatability
- Stage of lactation and nutritional demand (eg, when growing)

Table 1		
Concentration and function of microorganisms in the rumen		
Microorganism	**Number**	**Function in the Rumen**
Bacteria	10^{10} cells/mL	Ferment/degrade a range of substrates and reproduce
Protozoa	10^5–10^6 cells/mL	Ferment/degrade substrates, engulf starch, bacteria, and particles, and reproduce
Archaea	10^7–10^9 cells/mL	Metabolize hydrogen
Fungi	10^3–10^5 zoospores/mL	Source of cellulolytic enzymes Fiber degradation and digestion
Bacteriophages	10^8–10^9 cells/mL	Infect bacteria

Data from Refs.[2,11–17]

- Weight of the animal
- Milk production
- Weight gain
- Feed characteristics, particularly fiber estimates influencing rumen fill and digestibility
- Environment (temperature, humidity)
- Feeding systems and feed access

In general, nutritional models predict dry matter intake (DMI) as a function of body weight to the power of 0.66 to 0.75. The National Research Council[18] used a computer model to generate tables predicting DMI for cattle of different weights, production levels, and stages of lactation. The Institut National de la Recherche Agronomique[19] described feed intake in terms of forage fill values and fill units per kilogram of dry matter (DM). The Feed Into Milk Consortium[20] produced empirical equations to predict DMI across a range of diets. These equations included the variables concentrate feed level, milk energy output, silage intake potential, week of lactation, forage intake potential, and forage starch content.

Feed intake is depressed when:

- Highly fibrous, bulky food is fed
- When abdominal organs are competing for space (eg, uterus)
- Diets are deficient in essential components such as protein, nitrogen, minerals, vitamins, and amino acids, which are precursors for microbial growth, muscle, milk, or bone synthesis
- Feed access is restricted by time, bunk space, or competition
- Environmental temperatures and humidity increase and create heat stress

Keys to Achieving High Intake on Total Mixed Rations

- Increase feeding frequency in early lactation for diets of moderate to high energy density, especially when feeding management is not optimal.[21] The better the other aspects of feeding management, the less the benefit of increased frequency of feeding. Pushing up feeds between feedings is important to ensure that cattle get access to the feed and to stimulate feeding behavior.
- Ensure adequate access time to feed (feed bunks should not be empty of feed nor time off pasture excessive).
- Group by parity and production level. Primiparous and multiparous cows differ in feed intake and feeding behavior.
- Provide palatable feeds, which should include cleaning the bunks at least once a day to ensure clean feed.
- Avoid spoiled feeds. The importance of the impact on individual cattle and the herd in general can be substantial. Bolsen and colleagues[22] demonstrated significant decreases in DMI in addition to apparent digestibility of DM, organic matter, and neutral detergent fiber (NDF) in cattle fed silage that consisted of 25% aerobically surface-spoiled silage. In addition, the investigators noted that rumen fiber mats in treated cattle were either partially or totally destroyed.
- Provide adequate feed bunk space.
- Ensure that cows are comfortable (ie, relaxed, not heat stressed, socially adapted). Rapid changes in cow groupings are not advisable.
- Feed should not be hot in the bunk, silage stacks, or commodity bunks (indicates the deleterious action of yeasts and molds).
- Monitor moisture in the feed. Excessively wet feeds can sour and reduce DMI.

- Cows need adequate time to rest.
- Water access and quality need to be high.

Indicators of spoiled silage:

- Spoilage (mold or blackening, foul smell) in the stack or on the face with slow feeding
- Dropped, black cud in bunks or near silage
- Spoiled orts
- Changes to feces: often scant, slow passage, undigested, or "slimy," sometimes liquid diarrhea
- Low rumen scores: variable across the group. Rumen scores are a useful tool, but need to be assessed with some caution[23]

Keys for Achieving High Intake for Grazing Cattle

With grazing cows, availability of feed is influenced by varying the stocking rate, stocking intensity (grazing pressure, which is a function of appetite of cattle and supplementary feeding rates), herbage height, or time available for grazing. Changes in digestibility and composition that occur at different stages of the growing cycle must be understood if optimum use of grass is to be made.[24]

Of crucial importance is that more DMI can be achieved by offering more pasture; feed intake increases in a curvilinear manner, but pasture residuals then also increase. The residuals that are left influence the rate of grass production in the future, and the quality of grass. Put simply, leaving too much residual (typically >1600 kg/DM per hectare for temperate pastures, eg, ryegrass, fescues) can reduce pasture quality for the next grazing; leaving less than 1300 kg/DM per hectare for temperate grasses will reduce pasture growth rates. Consequently, ideal residuals are between 1300 and 1500 kg/DM/ha.

To achieve high production from pasture supplementary feed is provided, which should be of high digestibility, highly palatable, and free of antinutritional factors (eg, toxic endophyte alkaloids, high levels of nitrates), with the ration balanced by use of supplements (complementary feeds). Intake of forage is determined by selection, physical form, and substitution rates when forage is fed ad libitum.

Keeping Production Up and Rumen Function Stable on Pasture

- If pasture residuals are too short, some cattle are not achieving optimal DMI (and grass growth is depressed).
- Grazing short pasture or pasture high in legume may not provide sufficient physically effective fiber for rumen stability.
- If pasture residuals are too long, pasture quality will decline in the future.
- Provide simultaneous access of the herd to the pasture (releasing cattle to pasture as they are milked disadvantages less dominant cattle and heifers).
- Provide ample water access at pasture.
- Meet mineral requirements.

Increase DMI at pasture by:

- Increasing pasture available (stocking rate change, rotation change, fertilizer use)
- Increasing time of access to pasture
- Improved pasture quality (cultivar selection, fertilizer use)
- Moving hot wires (electric fences) to provide fresh pasture
- When weather is hot and humid, providing access to pasture in the cooler parts of the day

Summary

Management to achieve high DMI is critical, and additional details can be found in the key reviews listed.

Key Reviews

Forbes JM. Voluntary food intake and diet selection in farm animals. Oxfordshire (United Kingdom): CABI; 2007.

Grant RJ, Albright J. Feeding behavior and management factors during the transition period in dairy cattle. J Anim Sci 1995;73:2791–803.

FEEDING THE RUMEN

The strength of ruminant production is the capacity of ruminants to use resources that are not well used by monogastric animals, particularly the extensive and intensive grasslands of the world, highly productive silage crops such as maize, and by-products of human food manufacture that are not suitable for human consumption. Understanding and optimizing rumen function is pivotal to cattle production.

The outcomes of optimizing rumen function can be summarized as:

- Harvesting the optimal energy output from fermentable feeds (optimal meaning sufficient to meet requirements without causing acidosis or providing excess available rumen fat)
- Optimizing metabolizable protein (MP) supply to the small intestine
- Ensuring the cofactor production is sufficient for optimal metabolic processes (ie, producing enough B vitamins and other cofactors for enzyme function)

Cofactors for microbial growth in the rumen include sulfur, phosphorus, cobalt, biotin, para-aminobenzoic acid, thiamin, folic acid, and riboflavin. These agents are essential for bacteria to grow at optimal rates.

Concepts inherent to optimal nutrition of the herd include:

- An understanding that although the rumen is vital, maximizing output for any of the aforementioned (energy, protein, or cofactor), may be detrimental to the overall optimal function
- The rumen needs to be stable for optimal function, and rapid changes in diet are detrimental to good rumen function
- Small intestinal digestive efficiencies are important especially in regard of starch, fats, and nitrogen sources providing specific amino acids

Therefore, optimal ruminal function needs to be considered in the context of total tract digestion, including intestinal digestion.

Nutritional science has moved from concepts whereby cattle are fed "energy" and "crude protein" to one whereby there is a much greater focus on the specific substrates provided. Net or metabolizable energy are outputs of diets rather than inputs. Similarly, MP represents the output of ruminal microbes, produced from rumen degradable protein (RDP) and rumen undegraded protein (RUP) (more specifically RUP available in the small intestine). This article uses the nomenclature for feed fractions based on the Cornell Net Carbohydrate and Protein System.[25] The categories of this system are outlined in **Tables 2** and **4**. **Fig. 1** shows the different dietary chemical measures in relation to the plant cell.

Table 2
Carbohydrate fractions in feed

Dietary Component (CNCPS Fraction)	Detail and Structure	Speed of Fermentation (~rate per hour)	Feed Analysis	Fermentation Outcomes	Impact on Microbial Protein Production
Organic acids (not CHO) (A1)	Malate, citrate, oxalates, acetate, butyrate, propionate, valerate	Mostly prefermented ~1%–2%	Water soluble HPLC	Interconversion among acids, mainly results in acetate formation	Nil
Lactic acid (A1)		~5%	Water soluble HPLC	Propionate, valerate, acetate	Nil unless in excess
Simple sugars (A2)	Fructose, glucose, sucrose, lactose	Very rapid ~20% in fermented feeds and 40% in others[a]	Water soluble CHO/NSC/NFC	Propionate, butyrate, valerate, acetate, lactic acid	Generally positive, negative if in excess; responds to true protein or peptides
Starches (fructans) (B1)[a]	Glucose chains in starch, fructose chains in fructans	Moderate ~10%–40%	Starch/NSC/NFC HPLC	Propionate, butyrate, valerate, acetate, lactic acid	Generally positive, negative if in excess or overprocessed
Soluble fiber including pectins, B-glucans (B2)	Polysaccharides of galacturonic acid with neutral sugar side chain, and mixed linkage chains of glucose	Rapid ~40%–60% (except in soy hulls <10%)	NFC	Acetate, propionate, butyrate	Positive

Insoluble fiber hemicellulose, cellulose (B3)	Hemicellulose includes polymers of D-xylose and of glucose and mannose, known respectively as xylans and glucomannans; Arabinose, uronic acids, and galactose; Cellulose includes β-1,4 glucans but is combined with lignin, hemicellulose, cutin, minerals	Moderate to slow ~2%–15%	NDF	Acetate, propionate, butyrate	Positive; requires ammonia and branched-chain VFA
Unavailable fiber (lignin and fiber associated with lignin) (C)	Lignin	Nil	ADF (CNCPS lignin × 2.4)	Nil	Nil

Abbreviations: ADF, acid detergent fiber; CHO, carbohydrate; CNCPS, Cornell Net Carbohydrate and Protein System; HPLC, high-performance liquid chromatography; NDF, neutral detergent fiber; NFC, nonfiber carbohydrate; NSC, nonstructural carbohydrate; VFA, volatile fatty acid.

[a] As per CNCPS 6.5, but estimated at 100% to 200% per hour in CNCPS 6.1.

Data from Sniffen CJ, O'Connor JD, Van Soest PJ, et al. A net carbohydrate and protein system for evaluating cattle diets: II. Carbohydrate and protein availability. J Anim. Sci 1992;70:3562–77.

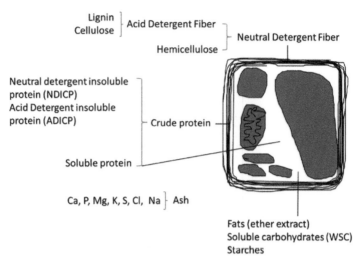

Fig. 1. Origins of dietary chemical measures in the plant cell. (*Courtesy of* Westwood CT, BVSc, PhD with permission).

To understand the dynamics of digestion of protein and carbohydrates, it is necessary to understand the interactions between the rate of passage of feeds through the rumen and the rate of digestion of feeds in the rumen.

The competing rates of fermentation (kd) and passage from the rumen (kp) dictate how much of a fermentable fraction is fermented in the rumen and how much passes undigested to the abomasum. The equation to calculate how much of any fraction is fermented in the rumen is kd/(kd + kp).[26] For example, if starch in a feed ferments at 10% per hour (10%/h) and the passage rate is 4%/h, then the amount of the starch in that feed predicted to ferment in the rumen equals 10/(10 + 4) = 71%. If the kd was only 4%/h, the amount would be 4/(4 + 4) = 50%. If kp is increased to 7%/h at kd = 4%/h, the amount fermented in the rumen is 4/(4 + 7) = 36%. The amounts of carbohydrate and protein fermented in the rumen form the basis for the amounts of microbial protein, fermentation acids, and greenhouse gases produced. In vitro fermentation methods, preferably with multiple time points, have been used to approximate fermentation rates. At present there is no method outside of research protocols to directly measure rates of liquid and solid passage.

The impact of digestion rates needs to be looked at from the perspective that kd are applied to fractions within feeds, such as water-soluble carbohydrates, starch, or NDF crude protein, and the feeds are themselves fractions of diets. The impact of a single rate on a single fraction will only be large if that fraction provides a sizable portion of the rumen degradable carbohydrate or protein. The sum of all fermented fractions determines the amount of carbohydrate and feed protein used to support fermentation. Ultimately, a balance among amounts of rapidly, intermediately, and slowly fermented materials is desired to provide enough fermentable materials to meet the cow's energy and protein needs but to avoid producing too much acid too quickly in the rumen, which could depress pH and fiber fermentation and lead to digestive upset.

Rates of carbohydrate fermentation are not necessarily single values even for a given feedstuff. Fermentation rates of NDF decrease at acidic relative to almost neutral pH.[27] The kd of starch has been reported to increase as the amount of starch in the diet is increased from 21% to 32%, with a greater increase seen with high moisture corn (17%–28%/h) than with dry ground corn (12%–15%/h).[28] The rate of fermentation of water-soluble carbohydrates and starch is also affected by the amount of RDP available.[29] Increases in the amount of RDP relative to readily available carbohydrates result in reduced amounts of carbohydrate stored as glycogen by the microbes, which means that the carbohydrate from the diet is fermented more immediately rather than stored. The increased rate of carbohydrate fermentation can result in greater production of lactic acid.[30] Another effect of increasing RDP relative to available carbohydrate is an increase in yield of microbial protein per unit of carbohydrate.[31] Despite the potentially positive effect of RDP on carbohydrate fermentation and microbial yield, gross increases in protein feeding are not recommended. In this regard, reductions in protein levels in dairy cattle diets have not always had a negative impact on production, but have improved efficiency of nitrogen use and have reduced the impact of dairies on the environment. It would seem that to make effective use of this information, we need to learn more about how protein and carbohydrate feeding integrate into maintaining a healthy rumen environment, and how to assure passage of microbes from the rumen without unduly increasing the passage of feed from the rumen and reducing its digestibility.

SUBSTRATES AND THEIR FATES IN THE RUMEN
Carbohydrates

Dietary carbohydrate is composed of fiber (ie, NDF) and nonfiber carbohydrate (NFC) fractions. Within these categories fractions are further divided, reflecting the chemical structure of the components and feed analytical methods (see **Table 2**). **Fig. 2** shows the main pathways for carbohydrate digestion in the rumen.

However, not only pure substrates are fed, and the complex structure of plants ensures that while an understanding of substrate is essential, understanding feeds is just as important. For example, different concentrate feeds have different effects on fermentation; despite very similar starch content among grains, these have very different effects on fermentation rates[32] and on the risk of ruminal acidosis (**Fig. 3**).[33] These grains do not operate in an independent context, and outcomes of fermentation of concentrates are influenced by the fiber and protein content of the diet. Furthermore, processing of grains has a profound effect on rumen function (see the articles on feed analysis by Hall, and ensiled feeds by Seglar and Shaver, elsewhere in this issue for further details).

Most rumen microbes depend on carbohydrates as a source of energy. Optimal fermentation requires a continuous supply of fermentable carbohydrates and cofactors to maintain microbial growth. Thus, a blend of carbohydrates of varying fermentation rates and compositions can serve well to provide such a supply while avoiding issues

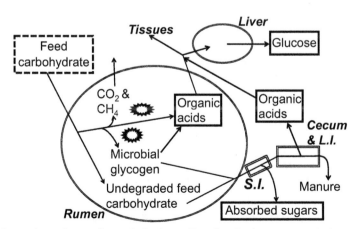

Fig. 2. The main pathways for carbohydrate digestion in the rumen. L.I., large intestine; S.I., small intestine.

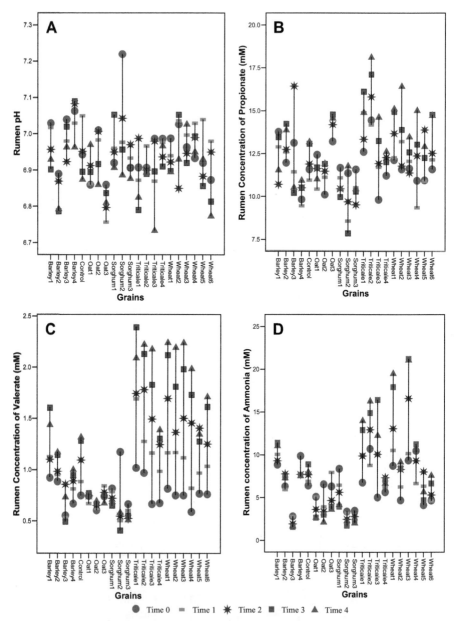

Fig. 3. Mean ruminal pH (*A*), mean ruminal concentration of propionate (*B*), mean ruminal concentration of valerate (*C*), and mean rumen concentration of ammonia (*D*) for 20 grain cultivars and control at 5 time points over a 3.6-hour period after consumption of grain. (*From* Lean IJ, Golder HM, Black JL, et al. In vivo indices for predicting acidosis risk of grains in cattle: comparison within vitro methods. J Anim Sci 2013;91:2823–35; with permission.)

of too rapid a fermentation with excessive acid production, or too slow a fermentation that does not meet animal nutrient requirements. Plant polysaccharides (starch, cellulose, hemicellulose, and pectins) are fermented by the extracellular enzymes of rumen bacteria, fungi, and some protozoa into monosaccharides and to 3 to 10 sugars (oligosaccharides). These sugars are converted by intracellular bacterial enzymes to pyruvate. Pyruvate is reduced to VFA, mainly acetate, propionate, and butyrate, plus CO_2, H_2, and CH_4. Although fermentation of starch produces 20% less energy than its conversion to glucose by endogenous enzymes,[34] microbial fermentation of structural carbohydrates is an advantage to animals on high-fiber diets. However, it is possible to process concentrates (eg, fine ground corn) to increase starch bypass to the small intestine and thus take advantage of the greater efficiency of use.

The rate of VFA production depends on the substrate: soluble carbohydrate (starches and sugars) > pectin > cellulose. This order also determines the VFA end product.

- Acetate and butyrate production is favored by the degradation of NDF, pectins, and sugars
- High levels of butyrate are found in some silages and are ingested
- Propionate production is favored by the degradation of sugars, starch, and soluble carbohydrate
- Lactic acid production is favored by the degradation of sugars and starches

Target intakes for feed components are outlined in **Table 3**. Targets are only one indication of appropriateness of a diet. Consistency of delivery, form of delivery, capacity of cattle to be selective, and antinutritional aspects of the diet all influence whether a diet is effective or not. Furthermore, diet formulation is influenced by the need for cost-effective solutions.

The key monitors for appropriate concentrations of fermentable carbohydrates in the diet are provided in **Table 3**.

Fiber

Fiber is needed to provide:

- A site for bacterial attachment
- Stimulation of chewing and salivation, which buffers the rumen and reduces risk of ruminal acidosis
- Stimulation for mixing of rumen content and controlling digesta flow rates for less coarse feeds
- Maintenance of health and function of rumen papillae
- Maintenance of milk fat production and content. It is important to be aware that fiber content of the diet is only one of many factors that influences milk fat production and content[35,36]
- Substrates (acetate and butyrate) for fat production

Ideal fiber intake is outlined for fresh, lactating cows in **Table 3**; ideally, 80% of the fiber is derived from long forage.[37] The function of fiber is influenced by:

- The chemistry of the fiber: older, more fibrous forages stimulate more chewing.
- The physical form of the fiber: chop length or grazing height.
- The other feeds in the diet (eg, fats and rapidly fermentable carbohydrate). Fats increase the energy density of the diet and allow a lower physically effective NDF (peNDF) to be used, whereas highly fermentable carbohydrate (eg, sugars and highly processed starches) increase the need for peNDF.
- The mixing and processing of the diet (in total mixed rations [TMR] diets). Poor mixing and selective eating can reduce the peNDF markedly. Ideally forages chopped no more than 5 cm (2 inches) long incorporated into a moist diet ($\sim$50% DM) will reduce sorting and enhance consumption of the diet as formulated. Molasses or other liquid feeds can be mixed in with diets to prevent sorting.

Table 3
Diet composition targets for early-lactation cows: effects of deficiency and excess on production and indicators in the field

Diet Composition (% Dry Matter)	Fresh Cow Targets	Effect of Deficiency	Deficiency Key Indicators	Effect of Excess	Excess Key Indicators
Dry matter intake	3.5%–4% body weight+	Weight and BCS loss	Weight loss >75 kg and BCS loss >0.75 (calving to nadir), high blood NEFA and high ketones (urine, blood, milk)	Reduced feed efficiency; suggests diet is imbalanced; targets for FCE (energy corrected milk/DMI) for day 150 of lactation Lot fed >1.3, ideally >1.4 Pasture and TMR >1.2, ideally >1.4 Pasture and concentrate >1.2, ideally >1.3	High residuals in bunk >2% or pasture >1600 kg (ryegrass). Marked increase in body weight or body condition in herds with adequate weight and BCS. Target BCS 3–3.25 peak and 3.25–3.5 at calving
Neutral detergent fiber (NDF) (%)	28–32	Increased risk of acidosis; reduced feed efficiency	Low NDF in diet. Loose, low fiber content of feces, fiber >1 cm long, undigested feed observed in feces, low fat test <3.5), low rumen fill <3.5, decreased rumination <50% chewing cud at rest, lameness prevalence may be high >25% of cows 2+	Body weight loss, lower milk, production, higher butterfat percentage, lower protein production	High NDF in diet. Low or declining BCS or weight. High fat, low protein test, high rumen fill, large firm feces, high fecal fiber, high blood NEFA and high ketones (urine, blood, milk)
Physically effective NDF (%)	19–21	Increased risk of acidosis; reduced feed efficiency	Usually low fiber content of feces, low fat test, low rumen fill, decreased rumination <50% chewing cud at rest, lameness prevalence may be high (depends on the environment)	Lower production, higher butterfat percentage, lower protein production	Firm feces, high fiber content of feces, high rumen fill, unlikely to be excessively high without high NDF%, decreased rumination <50% chewing cud at rest

Crude protein (CP) (%)	15.5–19	Lower milk production, body protein mobilization, increased acidosis risk	Pale green feces, slow passage rates, can have high rumen fill, lower fiber digestion, low MUN, low milk protein production, low milk protein content	Lower pregnancy rates with high soluble protein intake	Dark green loose feces although color can be variable, variable passage rates, high MUN, low production, possible weight loss
Degradability of CP (%)	65%–70% of CP; ie, 13% RDP of diet dry matter	Lower production depending on the amino acid composition of the RUP fraction of CP	Lower fiber digestion, can have high rumen fill, low BUN or MUN, low milk protein production, low milk protein %	Lower production, lower pregnancy rates with high soluble protein intake, can increase BCS mobilization	High BUN or MUN
Estimated metabolizable protein (MP) (g/d)	Positive MP balance	Lower production depending on the amino acid composition	Poor production with increase in weight gain and BCS over lactation, poor feed efficiency	Loss of income, inefficient use of protein	
Estimated metabolizable energy (MJ/ME)	11.5–12	Weight and BCS loss	Weight and BCS loss, high blood NEFA and high ketones (urine, blood, milk)	Weight and BCS gain if imbalanced	Low MUN (if high NFC)
Estimated net energy lactation (Mcal/lb)	0.76–0.79	Weight and BCS loss	High blood NEFA and high ketones (urine, blood, milk)	Weight and BCS gain if imbalanced	
Starch (%)	20–26, depending on NDF and forage NDF content of diet	Low production (not an absolute, but often the case)	Low milk protein, can test fecal starch	Increased risk of acidosis and lameness	Loose, bittersweet-smelling feces (may be low MUN depending on protein in diet), often contain bubbles of trapped gas, high prevalence of cattle with pH <6.5 on stomach tube or 6.0 on ruminocentesis indicates presence of acidosis

(continued on next page)

Table 3
(continued)

Diet Composition (% Dry Matter)	Fresh Cow Targets	Effect of Deficiency	Deficiency Key Indicators	Effect of Excess	Excess Key Indicators
Sugar (%)	6–8	Low production	Low milk protein	Increased risk of acidosis and lameness	Loose, bittersweet-smelling feces, high prevalence of cattle with pH <6.5 on stomach tube or 6.0 on ruminocentesis indicates presence of acidosis
Ether extract (%)	4–5	Lower efficiency of production		Decreased fiber digestion, lower fat percentage especially rumen degradable	Feces less well digested and turn white after drying
Dietary cation-anion difference (mEq/100 g)	25–40	Lower production	Urinary pH in lactation low <7	Decreased milk production	Urinary pH in lactation high >8.5, high K & Na and low Cl & S in feed

Abbreviations: BCS, body condition score; BUN, blood urea nitrogen; DMI, dry matter intake; FCE, feed conversion efficiency; MUN, milk urea nitrogen; NEFA, nonesterified fatty acids; RDP, rumen degradable protein; RUP, rumen undegraded protein.

- The way that the diet is fed: cattle at pasture can be highly selective. Allowing differential access to feed ensures that both available feed and fiber differ among cows. In cows fed component-based diets, feeding order can make a difference; for example, feeding forage for several hours after a large allocation of grain may not provide an optimal feeding order. It is preferable to feed forage before grain to maintain rumination and provide salivary buffering.
- Frequency of feeding: infrequent feeding and hungry cows engorge, increasing the risk of ruminal acidosis.

Means of assessing fiber in the cow are presented in **Table 3**.

Mertens[38] proposed the following definition for peNDF: The peNDF of a feed reflects the physical properties of the fiber (primarily particle size) that stimulates chewing activity and establishes biphasic stratification of ruminal contents (floating mat of large particles on a pool of liquid and small particles).

A challenge with peNDF is that, except in laboratory settings, there have not been readily available ways to assess feeds that take into account the physical form and digestibility that influence peNDF. Forage NDF has been used as a proxy for peNDF, but this still does not tell the complete story. The gold standard for evaluating whether peNDF in a diet is adequate is to observe the cows. For non–heat-stressed cows, approximately 5 out of 10 cows not eating, drinking, sleeping, or in heat should be ruminating. If fewer cows are ruminating, evaluate residual feed in the feed bunk for evidence of sorting against forage (see the articles on TMR audit and diagnostic investigation elsewhere in this issue for further discussion of evaluating dietary particle separation). If cows are fed forage and concentrate separately, verify that consumption of forage is adequate. Evaluate the diet weighing, mixing, and formulation, and verify that the feeds being included in the diets match the feed analyses being used.

Chemical analysis of pasture is not necessarily a good indicator of fiber function. Estimates of peNDF fiber in pasture range from as low as 40% to 75% of NDF, but are simply estimates because testing has not been done, in contrast to estimates derived from conserved forages that have been tested against chewing indices and milk fat percentage[38,39] and have a long history of development. As with cows fed TMR, 50% of cows fed on pasture and supplemented with other feeds should be ruminating when resting. **Table 3** provides indicators for inadequate peNDF intake.

Rules of thumb for pasture peNDF:

- Lush winter grass (**Fig. 4**A), approximately 40% of NDF
- Lush spring grass (see **Fig. 4**B), approximately 60% of NDF
- Summer grass (see **Fig. 4**C), approximately 75% of NDF
- Testing the strength of grass by testing its shear strength gives an indication of pasture-effective fiber (see **Fig. 4**D)

Key Reviews

Allen MS. Relationship between fermentation acid production in the rumen and the requirement for physically effective fiber. J Dairy Sci 1997;80:1447–62.

Mertens DR. Creating a system for meeting the fiber requirements of dairy cows. J Dairy Sci 1997;80:1463–81.

Mertens DR. Measuring fiber and its effectiveness in ruminant diets. In Proc. Plains Nutr. Cncl. Spring Conf. San Antonio (TX), 2002; p. 40–66.

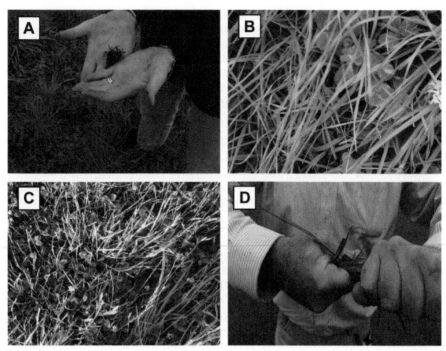

Fig. 4. (*A*) Lush winter grass. (*B*) Lush spring grass. (*C*) Summer grass. (*D*) Testing the strength of grass.

Van Soest PJ. Nutritional ecology of the ruminant. 2nd edition. Ithaca (NY): Cornell University Press; 1994.

Protein and Nitrogen

In many respects, the key task in feeding the rumen is to produce microbial protein (see the article on protein feeding by Paton et al. elsewhere in this issue for further discussion). Systems that assess protein requirements in dairy cattle need to reflect:

- Ruminal degradation of dietary protein (ie, RDP)
- The capacity of the rumen to use nonprotein nitrogen (NPN) sources for the synthesis of microbial protein
- The degree to and efficiency with which RDP can be synthesized into microbial protein
- The variation in value to the animal of different proteins that escape ruminal degradation (RUP or "bypass protein")
- Endogenous protein losses

Fig. 5 shows the main pathways for protein breakdown and metabolism in the rumen.

The ultimate purpose of supplementing feeds high in protein is to meet the MP requirements of the cattle.[18] RDP from the diet is broken down into peptides and amino acids by proteolytic bacteria in the rumen, and is later further digested to ruminal VFA and ammonia, while NPN provides ruminal ammonia.[40,41] The RUP portion of the diet escapes the rumen and the digestible portion is absorbed as amino acids in the small intestine. Critically, microbial protein has a very high biological value.

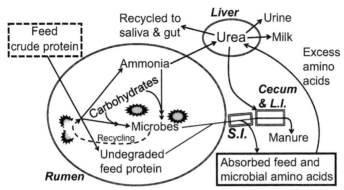

Fig. 5. Fates of protein breakdown and metabolism in the rumen. Feed protein may escape fermentation in the rumen, be incorporated into microbial protein, or be degraded to ammonia. Ruminal ammonia and nonprotein nitrogen from the feed can be converted to amino acids by the microbes if enough energy from carbohydrates is available. Digestible amino acids from microbes and escape (bypass) feed protein is absorbed in the small intestine. Nitrogen from excess ruminal ammonia and excess absorbed protein is converted to urea to be excreted or recycled. L.I., large intestine; S.I., small intestine.

Protein is required by the cow:

- To support the maintenance and growth requirements of rumen microbes. Feed proteins are hydrolyzed to peptides, amino acids, and ammonia using energy released from the degradation of fermentable organic matter.
- For the maintenance and synthesis of body tissue proteins (and conceptus) as an alternative source of energy, and the synthesis of milk proteins. The absorbed amino acids used for these purposes are termed MP or total digestible true protein, providing amino acids to the animal after digestion and absorption of the feed in the small intestine.

Table 4 provides details of the nitrogen fractions fed to cattle. The practical importance of these understandings is that the site of digestion of the B2 fraction in particular is subject to other influences in the diet, such as rate of fermentation and rate of passage. The A and B1 fractions are almost all RDP, and the B3 and C fractions are RUP. However, the influence of rate of degradation in the rumen and rate of passage can ensure that the B3 fraction can also contribute substantially to RDP. The C fraction is not digestible and escapes digestion in the total tract. There is marked variability in the production of microbial protein,[42] and systems to predict MP requirements and production provide very similar results,[43] but are likely subject to relatively large errors of prediction. Again, however, practical management of protein nutrition should not be unduly influenced by this, as careful monitoring of consistently fed herds should indicate whether the protein nutrition is appropriate.

Energy for the proteolytic bacteria to ferment RDP is required from readily fermentable carbohydrates (especially sugars and starches); therefore, increased synchrony of ruminally available protein and carbohydrate has the potential to increase the efficiency of microbial nitrogen production and animal productivity.[44] Increases in RDP have increased organic acid concentrations regardless of ruminally available carbohydrate.[45] In part this may be due to RDP increasing the fermentation rate of carbohydrate by reducing the amount of feed carbohydrate that is stored as microbial glycogen.[29] Reduction in glycogen storage reduces the energy cost of converting

Table 4
Nitrogen and protein fractions in feed

Dietary Component as per CNCPS Fraction	Digestion (% per hour) (Intestinal Digestibility of That Escaping the Rumen)	Feed Analysis	Digestion Outcomes	Impact on Metabolizable Protein Production
A Fraction Amino acids, peptides, nitrates, ammonia and urea	Very rapid, 200% (100%)	TCA-soluble nitrogen	NPN, very rapidly available nitrogen	Provides ammonia and BCVFA for structural carbohydrate fermenting bacteria, and peptides and amino acids for bacteria that ferment NSC. Nitrates are used for protein production and reduce methane production (but can be toxic)
B1 Fraction Globulins and some albumins	Very rapid, 50%–100% (100%)	TCA-precipitable protein from the buffer-soluble protein minus the A fraction	Rapidly degraded true protein	Provides ammonia and BCVFA for structural carbohydrate fermenting bacteria, and peptides and amino acids for bacteria that ferment NSC
B2 Fraction Most albumins, glutelins	Slow, 5%–15% (100%)	The B2 fraction is the remaining protein once the A, B1, B3, and C fractions are accounted for	Intermediate degradation rates true protein	Provides some ammonia for structural carbohydrate fermenting bacteria, and peptides and amino acids for bacteria that ferment NSC. Provides amino acids to the small intestine
B3 Fraction Prolamins, extensin proteins, denatured proteins	Low, 0.1%–1.5% (80%)	Neutral detergent–insoluble nitrogen minus the C fraction	Slowly degraded true protein	Provides amino acids to the small intestine
C Fraction Maillard proteins, protein bound to lignin	Nil (0%)	Acid detergent-insoluble nitrogen	True protein, unavailable to the tract	No contribution (based on CNCPS)

Abbreviations: BCVFA, branched-chain volatile fatty acids; NPN, nonprotein nitrogen; TCA, trichloroacetic acid.
Data from Sniffen CJ, O'Connor JD, Van Soest PJ, et al. A net carbohydrate and protein system for evaluating cattle diets: II. Carbohydrate and protein availability. J Anim Sci 1992;70:3562–77.

glucose to glycogen, and thus increases the energy available to grow more microbes. However, the increase in microbial production or yield only benefits the cow if the microbes pass to and from the rumen.

> Maximizing production of microbial protein is an essential strategy in most dairy production systems.

Indicators of good protein nutrition are given in **Table 3**. The output of microbial protein is maximized under the following conditions.

- Ruminal ammonia concentrations exceed 5 mg/dL,[46] which equates to approximately 13% RDP. Higher concentrations may be of benefit with high intakes of rapidly fermentable carbohydrates. Many herds have successfully fed diets that contain a concentration of RDP lower than 13% as part of an approach to lower protein concentrations in diets of lactating cows; this suggests that the optimal concentration of RDP can be lower than 13% and achieve high yields of microbial protein.
- For bacteria that use peptides, these pools are available at amounts that exceed nonstructural carbohydrate (NSC) in the diet by 14%.[47]
- There is sufficient energy available derived from fermentable carbohydrate for optimal bacterial maintenance and growth (many of the equations expressing flow of microbial nitrogen to the small intestine have related this back to organic matter digested in the rumen).
- Cofactors are not limiting for production of bacteria, especially those dependent on phosphorus and sulfur.
- There are branched-chain (isobutyric, 2-methylbutyric, isovaleric) VFA available.[48,49] These VFA are usually obtained from deamination of proteins and amino acids (these should be available if 13% RDP is available).[46] Book values for RDP and RUP of feeds are provided in several documents and are useful as a guide,[18] remembering that the RDP and RUP for a feed are specific to a particular diet and animal.
- There is no excess of rapidly fermentable carbohydrate leading to energy spilling and loss of efficiency.[50]

Feeds supplemented to dairy cattle to increase dietary crude protein intake include: legume grains and legume forages, canola and soybean meals, and brewers' and distillers' by-products including gluten feeds, meals, and grains. In some countries, including the United States, nonruminant-derived animal and blood meals and marine proteins can be fed. These feedstuffs vary widely in their relative proportions of RDP and NPN, extent of rumen degradation, and intestinal digestibility of RUP,[18] and also vary markedly in their amino acid composition.

The strategies of feeding of RUP or bypass protein to supply additional protein (more specifically, rate-limiting amino acids) to the small intestine have been long developed, and the strengths and weaknesses of these strategies are now well understood.

- Reducing the amount of RDP and increasing the amount of RUP can decrease microbial protein production and not have a net positive effect on MP supply.
- Supplying proteins with poor-quality amino acid profiles that reach the small intestine may not increase MP availability, as the amino acids may not be limiting

production. Of note, the overall amino acid profile of protein in a feed may not be the same as in the B2 and B3 fractions that reach the small intestine.

- Not recognizing the lack of availability of the C fraction can overestimate the value of a bypass protein.
- Therefore, the strategy pivotal to successful protein nutrition is to maximize microbial protein harvest and to supply rate limiting amino acids to the small intestine.

However, the precise effects of the bypass protein remain somewhat controversial. Part of the reason for this controversy relates to limitations in study designs used to evaluate production responses.

There are 3 pools that absorbed amino acids are partitioned to:

1. Gluconeogenesis and ketogenesis (oxidized for energy)
2. Milk protein
3. Body (and conceptus) proteins

The relative partitioning among these pools will depend on:

- The mix of nutrients entering the body (ie, the abundance and concentrations of other sources of energy and cofactors)
- The availability or need to replenish body tissue stores (ie, whether the cow can draw on body tissue pools or needs to contribute to body tissue pool)
- Other physiologic influences on the cow (stage of lactation, phenotypic and genetic capacity for milk production, environmental conditions, age, growth stage, previous nutrition)

Consequently, given the complexity of factors that need to be considered, estimating milk or growth responses to changes in protein nutrition will be best managed through modeling approaches.[18,20,25] Systems for assessing nutritional requirements of cattle used throughout the world are highly convergent in their estimates of protein needs for cattle[43]; however, there is considerable variance regarding estimates of microbial nitrogen outflow from the rumen.[42] The latter and the effects of other physiologic influences ensures that nutritional management, while based on the sound application of the principles outlined in this article, must be matched with keen observation of the cattle and their responses to nutritional change. The indicators for failure to achieve good microbial nitrogen production and effective production of MP overall are provided in **Table 3**. Monitoring these indicators, especially milk production, milk protein, milk urea nitrogen, and body condition indicators, is an essential part of effectively feeding the rumen.

In practical terms, the optimal output of microbial protein from the rumen will often be near the maximum, because NSC, ruminally available nitrogen, and peptides are (almost always) less expensive than RUP. Targets for protein nutrition are given in **Table 3**.

Key References

Lean IJ. Systems of describing nutritional requirements of dairy cattle. In: Rojinski H, editor. Encyclopedia of dairy science. 2nd edition. Atlanta (GA): Elsevier Science Ltd; 2011.

Nocek J, Russell J. Protein and energy as an integrated system. Relationship of ruminal protein and carbohydrate availability to microbial synthesis and milk production. J Dairy Sci 1988;71: 2070–107.

Water

Cows will drink 40 to 70 L of water per day but may require up to 200 L of water per day. Cows will go to water from 6 up to even 40 times a day, and water sources should be made readily available. Providing adequate amounts of water and adequate drinking space to cattle at pasture is critical, as is providing adequate access for housed cattle.

Water intake will decrease if:

Chemical Quality is Poor:
- Intake of water that is too acidic (pH <5.1–5.5; optimal is 7.0) has been associated with poor milk production, low milk fat test, poor weight gains and growth, low DMI and increased rates of disease
- Too alkaline pH (>8.5–9.0)
- Contains hydrogen sulfide (rotten egg odor); this may also interact with copper or selenium/vitamin E, and may cause anemia
- High sulfate content (>1450 ppm) may reduce water intake and could increase the need for selenium, vitamin E, and copper in the diet
- Too much salinity[18] can be a problem in some areas where dry land or irrigation salinity are problems, and needs to be assessed in regard of water intake, and the potential for changing dietary cation/anion balance and increasing the risk of udder edema and milk fever

Water is Polluted With:
- Bacteria. Effluent problems in particular can decrease water intake, increase the risk for ketosis and enteric diseases. Effluent contamination has been associated with epidemics of calf death
- Algae, especially blue-green (eg, *Microcystis aeruginosa*)
- Chemical or industrial pollution such as contamination with copper or mine effluent (eg, sulfates, molybdenum, manganese, iron)
- Fecal soiling from birds or other stock, or human effluent

Stray Voltage Greater Than 4 V
- To the trough may reduce water intake
- To the surface that the animal is standing on may reduce water intake

Excessive Water Intake Will Occur With:
- High dietary salt levels (feed and water)

Increased Urine Production and Water Intake Occurs With:
- Mercury pollution
- Excessive protein, NPN, or nitrates

Signs of Inadequate Water Intake:
- Firm, constipated feces (horse-like droppings)
- Low urinary output
- Infrequent drinking
- Increased packed cell volume greater than 37%
- Decreased milk production
- Drinking urine, puddles

Signs of Excessive Water Intake:
- Excessive urine production
- Cattle appear bloated

Key Review
  Beede DK. What can we do about water quality? In: Cornell nutrition conference for
  feed manufacturers, East Syracuse (NY), 2012. p. 77–84.

COFACTORS (B VITAMINS)

The B vitamins are essential cofactors for rumen function and include thiamin, biotin, riboflavin, niacin, pantothenic acid, folic acid, vitamin B_{12}, and pyridoxine. Choline is also required. Girard[51] astutely noted that many of the pivotal studies on B vitamins had been conducted in the 1940s to 1950s with a view to determining the potential for deficiency states to arise. Since that review there has been a considerable reevaluation in the context of improving production and influencing subclinical disease. The vitamins reviewed here are those with broadest clinical application and with most implications for rumen function.

Schwab and colleagues[52] examined diets containing 30% and 40% NFC and 60% or 35% forage to evaluate the effects of diet on the apparent synthesis (AS) of B vitamins. Increasing dietary forage content decreased ruminal AS of pyridoxine, folic acid, and B_{12}. Increasing dietary NFC content increased ruminal AS of nicotinic acid, nicotinamide, niacin, pyridoxine, B_6, and folic acid but decreased the AS of B_{12}, suggesting that the AS of B_{12} was optimal with 35% forage and 30% NFC. Amounts of B vitamins synthesized were, in order of highest to lowest: niacin, riboflavin, B_{12}, thiamin, B_6, and folic acid. Biotin AS values were negative for all diets, suggesting either no ruminal synthesis or that destruction by ruminal microflora was greater than synthesis.

> There is considerable loss of many of the B vitamins (thiamin, nicotinamide, folic acid, riboflavin, and choline) before the small intestine,[53] suggesting the need to consider use of protected forms of these if supplementing.

Thiamin

Cattle synthesize thiamin in the rumen, and normally microbial synthesis is sufficient to supply needs. However, under certain circumstances thiaminases that will lead to thiamin deficiency are produced or ingested. Thiaminase I acts to substitute a nitrogen-containing ring for the thiazole ring, and thiaminase II cleaves the methylene bridge to create free pyrimidine and thiazole.

Causes or sources of thiaminases include:

- Thiaminase-producing bacteria. *Clostridium sporogenes* and *Bacillus thiaminolyticus* produce thiaminase I. Acidification of the rumen increase thiaminase I reactivity, and diets high in starches also increase *Bacillus aneurinilyticus* growth with thiaminase II activity
- Plant thiaminases (eg, bracken fern)
- Amprolium, a coccidiostat: thiaminase I
- Thiabendozale: thiaminase I
- Molasses feeding
- Intensive grain feeding
- Possibly excessive sulfur intake, as sulfite can cleave thiamin

The result of such diets is the development of the condition of polioencephalomalacia (PEM) or cerebrocortical necrosis. There is little capacity to store thiamin in the body, and signs of thiamin deficiency include weight loss, poor growth rates, and scouring.

Studies in feedlot steers fed on a 100% concentrate diet showed marked responses in production when supplemented by thiamin. However, such responses were not consistent. Shaver and Bal[54] supplemented dairy cows with thiamin 150 mg per cow per day, and found a significant increase of 2.7 L per cow per day in milk production in one trial, a tendency toward higher milk 0.7 L per cow per day in a second trial, and significantly lower milk fat yield in a third study based on a different forage base. The variable responses suggest a need for further studies on responses of milking cows to thiamin. Thiamin supplementation has been recommended as a treatment to address endophyte toxicosis in the United States; however, data are equivocal and more information is required.

Niacin

Niacin plays a vital role in energy metabolism through the coenzymes nicotinamide adenine dinucleotide and nicotinamide adenine dinucleotide phosphate. These compounds are hydrogen-carrying agents or electron donors in the oxidative phosphorylation chain. The coenzymes are also involved in the Krebs cycle, glycolysis, fatty acid synthesis and oxidation, and the synthesis and breakdown of glycerol and amino acids. The results obtained from supplementation of niacin have been variable. Kung and colleagues[55] found that lactation persistency improved in cows fed on niacin. Dufva and colleagues[56] found increased milk production in niacin-supplemented cows, but Jaster and colleagues[57,58] found no significant production response to niacin. Milk production responses to niacin supplementation trials were reviewed by Hutjens[59] and Girard[51] with similar outcomes. There was a −2.2% to +8.8% increase in milk yield (mean +2.0%) and a range of milk fat increase of −0.0 to +0.5% (mean +0.17%).

Biotin

Biotin is involved in the use of adenosine triphosphate bond energy to activate carboxyl groups, and plays important roles in glucose and fatty acid metabolism. It is present in acetyl-coenzyme A (CoA) carboxylase, pyruvate carboxylase, propionyl-CoA carboxylase, and methylcrotonyl-CoA carboxylase, and is crucial for gluconeogenesis. Milk production responses to biotin for dairy cattle were evaluated using meta-analysis and 2 studies produced very similar results.[60,61] Biotin increased milk production by 1.29 kg per head per day (95% confidence interval [CI] 0.47–2.11 kg), but no significant effect was found on milk fat and protein percentages or yields.[60] Milk production and composition results were not influenced by duration of treatment before calving or supplementation before or after calving, or by parity.[60] The authors also evaluated articles that examined the effects of biotin on hoof health, and reported that biotin supplementation can lower the incidence and prevalence of hoof disorders in cattle.[60]

THE RUMEN OUT OF CONTROL: ACIDOSIS

Ruminal acidosis is not simply one disorder, but rather a continuum of conditions that reflect the degree of generation and safe sequestration of hydrogen in the rumen. The degree of severity reflects the substrates available to cattle, for example, sugar and starch that predispose cattle to acidosis, and the balance of the diet including fiber that reduces risk and protein that may have a bidirectional risk. The risk of acidosis is present in all milk production systems, but especially when concentrates are fed.

A large Australian study found that 10% of dairy cows less than 100 days in milk had acidosis, as defined by assessment of ruminal VFA, ammonia, lactic acid, and pH when sampled.[62] Studies in Wisconsin found that 20.1% and 23% of cows had subacute acidosis as defined by rumen pH.[63,64] Therefore, it is likely that many cows will experience some level of acidosis during lactation and, indeed, some may be affected many times. It can be estimated that if the prevalence of subacute acidosis is 10% and the duration of a case is 2 days, there would be an incidence of approximately 1500 cases over a 300-day lactation in a herd of 100 cows.

It is important to recognize that lactic acid is usually only present in situations where sugars are present, whereas acidosis with high concentrations of VFA, especially propionate and valerate, is associated with excess starch ingestion.[65]

Acidosis is a continuum of conditions of varying severity that reflect the challenge of safely sequestering hydrogen that accumulates from carbohydrate fermentation. Safe pools to "hide hydrogen" include starch engulfment by protozoa, bacterial glycogen formation, growth of bacteria, methane, and weak organic acids (VFA). Less safe pools include lactic acid. Alternatively, decreasing the hydrogen supply by increasing the more slowly fermenting fiber content of the diet and enhancing rumination can also reduce risk.

Clinical Signs

The clinical signs of ruminal acidosis usually reflect the severity of the case, and are frequently not recognized or are subtle for milder cases of ruminal acidosis, as their onset can occur after a time lag from a predisposing event.[66] The occurrence of milder ruminal acidosis is often a herd problem[67] and is difficult to diagnose in individuals. Many of the clinical signs associated with ruminal acidosis have many differential diagnoses[68]; therefore, collective interpretation of all clinical signs observed is important.

Individual cattle

In individual cattle suspected of ruminal acidosis, a physical examination should be performed that includes measurements of heart rate, respiration rate, rate of rumen contractions, and body temperature. Locomotion, body condition, perineal staining, fecal consistency, and rumen fill should also be scored.[69–71] Demeanor, dehydration, and sites of pain should be assessed. Samples of rumen fluid can be taken to support clinical indicators of acidosis in the herd; the authors prefer to use stomach-tube methods, as these are quick and less invasive than ruminocentesis.

Cattle with rumen perturbations consistent with subacute acidosis may present with a range of clinical and subclinical signs that include diarrhea, poor body condition, a dull and lethargic demeanor, dehydration, lack of rumen fill, lameness, weak rumen contractions, depression in milk fat, and inappetence.

In acute acidosis ruminal distension, diarrhea (often with grain in the feces and a sickly, sweet smell), abdominal pain, tachycardia, tachypnea, staggering, recumbency, coma, a marked decline in milk yield, and death may occur.[72,73]

The key considerations in the diagnosis of acute cases of acidosis are the history of the following.

Access to sugars Sources of sugars include forage beets, turnips, cereals that are frosted (eg, oats, wheats), sugar, fruit, and molasses.

Access to rapidly fermentable starch Grains have the following order of risk of acidosis: wheat, triticale, barley, oats, maize, and sorghum, roughly based on rate of starch fermentation.[32] Finely ground grains have a greater rate of starch fermentation than more coarsely ground grains.[74] Ensiled high-moisture grains ferment more rapidly than do equivalent dry grains, and increasing amounts of dietary starch may also increase the rate of starch fermentation.[28]

Adaptation The less that cows are adapted to the substrate, the greater is the risk to the cows. Most acute cases result from unlimited access to rapidly fermentable substrate and are usually obvious (eg, beef cattle breaking into a grain silo).

Diet structure The lower the fiber in the diet, the greater the risk of acidosis (ie, over-hot TMR rations or lush pastures with grain feeding). The risk is higher for dairy cows fed twice daily in the parlor than for cows on partial mixed ration (PMR) or TMR. Excellent access to water may also be important in reducing the risk of acidosis.

Confirmation of diagnosis should occur through the observation of the clinical signs as per the aforementioned criteria and a sample of rumen fluids consistent with acute acidosis: low pH less than 5 and changes in the rumen fluid, including a milky-white appearance containing grain (if grain overload is the cause) and sickly-sweet smell, can be present.

Herd diagnosis: subacute acidosis
Although access to fermentable feeds is important to the diagnosis of subacute cases, the focus must be on the herd examination, as clinical signs of acidosis can be relatively subtle in the individual animal.

Check the latest herd test results. Milk fat-to-protein ratios of less than 1.02 to 1 for cows in the first 100 days in milk provide a weak, but useful, indication of acidosis. It is not true that all cows with a low test are likely to have acidosis, but cows with acidosis are very likely to have low fat test. Unsaturated fatty acids have also been implicated in milk fat depression without any relationship to ruminal acidosis.[75] The sensitivity and specificity for using a fat/protein ratio as a predictor of acidosis is 0.54 and 0.81, respectively.[76]

The herd should be examined for the following.

Dung check If a high percentage of cattle are scouring, especially if the dung bubbles and contains grain, the risk of acidosis is high. The dung can contain undigested fiber particles larger than 1.5 cm. Differential diagnoses include very lush grass and parasites.

Lameness check Only swelling of the coronary band occurs at the same time as ruminal acidosis, but herds that have had acidosis causing other typical foot problems that arise with acidosis often have active acidosis, especially if there has been no effort to control it. Changes observed in hooves such as "poverty or hardship lines" and paint-brush hemorrhage indicate acidosis, but the acidosis has occurred sometime before examination.

Check on bulk vat A low fat/protein test on a herd basis is similar to that in an individual cow. Again it is only a rough guide, but a low herd fat/protein test is a cause to consider the possibility of acidosis or concerns with excessive intake of dietary unsaturated fatty acids.

History Have cattle bled from the mouth (or nose) or have liver abscesses been reported for the farm? Both of these indicate that the cows very likely have had acidosis in the past. Some acidotic herds have a history of increased respiratory disease, but there are many other causes of respiratory disease apart from acidosis.

Ration An essential step is to check the ration and feeding systems to see whether the following problems are present. Highly fermentable diets (eg, NSC >36% and NDF <32%) need not be enough alone to provide a problem, and acidosis can be present with less NSC and more NDF. Chemical analysis should be performed on individual feed components and residual TMR after feeding to obtain the percentage of DM, NDF, acid detergent fiber, crude protein, starch, sugar, and NSC content.[77] This analysis will allow estimation of the overall chemical composition of diet for comparison with recommended requirements. This information, combined with the evaluation of the physical characteristics of the feed, will indicate possible suboptimal rumen function and ruminal acidosis.[77] Often the way that the diet is fed, for example, short chop or sorting in PMR or TMR herds, access by cows to extra grain in the milking parlor, and very lush pastures or young grass, plays an important role. Feeding behavior will be the best indicator of adequacy of dietary fiber and physical form.

Feeding behavior Feeding behavior of the herd, including the following, should be observed: the percentage of cows chewing cud at rest (should be >50%), sorting behavior of a TMR and DMI; and whether cows are allowed to go straight to pasture after milking or are held to provide even access. Cows that have a low rumination time, are sorting their feed, have a cyclic feeding pattern, or low DMI may be at risk for ruminal acidosis.[78,79] Cows that are low in the social order, which are frequently first-lactation cows, often eat last and therefore can be exposed to feed with a different effective fiber content or chemical composition resulting from sorting from the previous cows, and may increase their risk for ruminal acidosis.[80] The animal's increased risk for ruminal acidosis will be dictated by what they sort for: concentrate (increased risk) or forage (typically decreased risk). All feed sources should be assessed for forage, chop length, or particle size if applicable, and for quality, using relevant characteristics (ie, stage of maturity of pasture, type of pasture or forage).

Physical examination Cattle should be checked for acidosis between 2 and 4 hours after feeding in the milk parlor or after receiving a PMR or TMR. These animals can be checked for ruminal pH: stomach-tubing of cattle is a quick and easy method for checking rumen contents (Video 1). If more than 4 out of 10 cows have a pH of less than 6.5 on stomach tube or less than 6.0 on rumenocentesis then, because these findings are present with other signs of acidosis, it is worth undertaking preventive steps to control acidosis. Within a herd, groups of cattle may be diagnosed with different ruminal conditions.[70] The sensitivity and specificity of using rumen pH values as a predictor of acidosis from rumen fluid collected using a stomach tube is 0.68 and 0.84, respectively, and from rumenocentesis is 0.74 and 0.79, respectively.[76]

Effects of Concentrates and Grains on Fermentation and Ruminal Acidosis Risk

Concentrates differ in rates of fermentation owing to the following.

- Chemical composition (higher rates for sugars and starches; see earlier discussion)
- Level of processing (finer flake, smaller particle size; more rapid)
- The physical structure of starch is also important; for example, maize starch is less available than wheat starch
- Nonstarch polysaccharides influence the availability of starches; grain sorghum or milo is less rapidly available

The extent of ruminal fermentation is also influenced by rumen outflow rates: the higher the rate of outflow, the less that is fermented.

Differences in ruminal responses to different grain species and cultivars are shown in **Fig. 3**. The grains differ markedly in pH response over time, in propionate, valerate, and ammonia concentrations in the rumen, and in risk for acidosis.[33]

Effects of Protein on Ruminal Acidosis

The potential for dietary protein content to influence rumen function and be involved in the pathogenesis of nutritional disorders such as ruminal acidosis has been largely unexplored. The supply of RDP has influenced organic acid and lactate pool sizes.[29] However, 8% of the dry weight of bacteria is hydrogen,[81] therefore providing a considerable sink for hydrogen generated in ruminal catabolism of carbohydrates. Consequently it may be possible that protein can be either beneficial for or detrimental to the risk of ruminal acidosis, depending on substrate availability, concentration, and dietary management.

THE RUMEN OUT OF CONTROL: BLOAT

Risk of ruminal bloat or tympany is predominantly confined to cattle grazing legume dominant or very lush grass pastures, but individual cattle can bloat on almost any diet. Bloat is particularly associated with the legumes, alfalfa, ladino, and white and red clovers. Factors that promote bloating lead to the formation of stable foam in the rumen. Failure to regurgitate the foam and entrapped gases in the foam leads to greatly increased intraruminal pressure. Initial rumen hypermotility ceases as the condition progresses, and is replaced by hypomotility. If relief is not provided, ruminal tympany becomes marked. Severe respiratory distress is noted, feces are often expelled, and even vomiting of foam has been noted. Cattle are extremely distressed and may kick at their sides, their eyes bulge and their tongue is protruded, and death can be very rapid (within 15 minutes of exposure).

Concerns regarding bloat management have been greatly reduced since the introduction of the ionophore, monensin, to dairy diets.[82] However, the efficacy of the detergent poloxalene in legume bloat may be higher.[83] The single most important plant factor predisposing cattle to bloat is the presence of highly soluble plant protein, especially ribulose-1,5-bisphosphate carboxylase/oxygenase (RuBisCO). These proteins are particularly associated with the leaves of the plants (particularly lucerne *Medicago sativa*, white clover *Trifolium repens*, and red clover *Trifolium pratense*). Factors in plants that suppress bloat include condensed tannins, larger stem to leaf ratios, and plant lipids.

Rainfall and water management of crops appears to have a significant impact on the bloating capacity of pastures. In part this may be explained by increased pasture growth and increased solubility of protein in the pastures. The use of nitrogenous fertilizers tends to increase the incidence of bloat, probably in association with increased plant-soluble protein concentrations.

Agronomic strategies that limit the legume content of dairy pastures are a particularly effective form of control. Feeding strategies are very important in effective control: excessive restriction of pastures, especially strip-grazed pasture, can lead to cattle breaking through fences into potentially bloating pastures. Ensuring that cattle have adequate access to effective fiber, excellent access to pasture, and the use of bloat-controlling agents such as ionophores, detergents, and bloat oils, will reduce the risk.

FATS

The metabolic and energetic importance of fats to the diet of cattle and humans is being increasingly recognized. The metabolism of fats in the rumen is well covered in the article by Jenkins and Harvatine elsewhere in this issue. Although there is little apparent need to supply fats to the rumen for optimal rumen function, consideration needs to be given to the negative effects of ruminally unsaturated fatty acid load (RUFAL). The RUFAL reflects the total unsaturated fatty acid supply entering the rumen each day from feed. Sources of these include lush pastures, distillers' by-products, oil seeds, and fat and oil sources, and it is recommended that intake of these should not generally exceed 3.5% of dietary DM. However, there are important theoretic metabolic benefits in the supply of fats that should encourage their use and protection of fats through the use of calcium soaps, formation of prills, and particle size to minimize RUFAL while supplying fats.

The negative effects of RUFAL include a marked reduction in ruminal digestion of fiber when concentrations of RUFAL are high. The lipids are toxic to some rumen bacteria. The RUFAL is effective in reducing methane production. However, caution should be exercised in interpreting the effects of fats and oils on metabolism, because in general, DMI is lower and efficiency of milk production is higher with fat feeding.[75] Feeding of RUFAL can disrupt microbial protein production; however, feeding of oil seeds significantly decreased milk protein percentage and tended to increase milk protein yields.[75]

In the field, indicators of an excess of RUFAL include a low milk fat percentage (although this is definitely not a specific or sensitive indicator), evidence of oil or fat in the feces (an oily sheen especially when wet, water pools on top of the manure), and feces turning "white" in the sun.

Key Reviews

Jenkins T. Lipid metabolism in the rumen. J Dairy Sci 1993;76:3851–63.

Jenkins TC, Harvatine KJ. Lipid feeding and milk fat depression. This issue of Vet Clin North Am Food Anim Pract.

Rabiee AR, Breinhild K, Scott W, et al. Effect of fat additions to diets of dairy cattle on milk production and components: a meta-analysis and meta-regression. J Dairy Sci 2012;95:3225–47.

CONTROLLING THE RUMEN

Individual cattle seem to have unique ruminal responses to changes in diet for several reasons that are largely based on the type of substrate fed and feeding strategy. This aspect poses challenges for developing effective control strategies to maintain optimal rumen function and prevent disorders such as ruminal acidosis. Control strategies are likely to vary between herds. It is clear from recent research[84] that substrate challenge dominates the capacity of antimicrobial agents to control either lactic acidosis or acidosis associated with substantial intake of wheat. Therefore, the following sections should be perused in the context of the other control strategies of ensuring careful adaptation to diets, well-processed and well-integrated TMR diets, adequate peNDF, and limiting and optimizing preformed lactic acid (from silages or high moisture grains and earlage), sugar and starch, and protein.

Rumen Modifiers

The base approach for maintaining good rumen function is to provide and properly manage a balanced diet containing adequate forage and fiber. However, rumen function can also be manipulated by the inclusion of rumen modifiers such as antibiotics, buffers and neutralizing agents, yeasts, direct-fed microbials, and enzymes. These agents potentially control rumen function and prevent ruminal acidosis; however, they need to overcome individual animal variation in rumen microbiomes and responses to changes in diet. These vehicles seem to influence the rumen by different mechanisms, but our understanding of these mechanisms is largely based on in vitro ruminal responses, which may not reflect in vivo responses. Further work is required to elucidate these mechanisms, particularly during different feeding situations.

Prudent use of strategies using approved feed additives are important for countries where antimicrobial agents are available; however, animal variation suggests that no single feed additive will be capable of controlling disorders such as ruminal acidosis in all cattle.[84] Different feed additives may need to be used depending on feed substrates; however, a degree of ruminal acidosis may be inevitable in some cattle.[67] Feeding combinations of feed additives such as monensin and direct-fed microbials may have synergistic effects, but the literature is limited and further research is required.

Several antibiotics such as monensin are used in the ruminant industries. However, the use of antibiotics as feed additives in animal nutrition has been banned in the European Union.[85]

Buffers and neutralizing agents

A buffer, by definition, reduces the decrease in pH without causing an increase in pH.[86] Sodium bicarbonate, derived from natural deposits of trona,[86] is a weak base that buffers hydrogen ions of organic acids[87] and is the most common buffer used in the dairy industry.[88] Other buffers include potassium carbonate, potassium bicarbonate, and sodium sesquicarbonate,[89] and the skeletal remains of the seaweed *Lithothamnium calcareum*.

Sodium bicarbonate's primary mode of action may not be as a buffer, but through indirect increases in DM and water intakes caused by sodium, facilitated though a higher ruminal fluid dilution rate and lower starch digestion rate.[90,91] Moreover, production responses to sodium bicarbonate, potassium carbonate, potassium bicarbonate, and sodium sesquicarbonate may reflect corrections in the dietary cation-anion difference (DCAD) to a positive optimum of +250 to 400 mEq/kg.[92] Quantitative reviews demonstrate that the effects of buffers and neutralizing agents on ruminal fermentation and milk production in dairy cattle varies among substrates, with benefits being primarily observed in maize silage-fed cattle.[86,88,89] Furthermore, under heat-stress conditions the need for potassium and sodium in the diet increases, and alkalinizing diets provide benefits for milk production.[93]

Sodium bicarbonate has additive effects with magnesium oxide,[94,95] hence this combination is often incorporated in dairy rations. Magnesium oxide is an alkalizing agent; however, it is not established as to whether the mode of action is through alkalizing ability,[96] alleviation of magnesium deficiency,[86] or improved digestibility.[95]

Responses of dairy cattle to the addition of buffers to the diet may not simply reflect responses to controlling rumen function. Inclusion rates of these products will reflect considerations of acidosis risk, DCAD, exposure to maize silage, and level of heat stress.

Key References also for Feeding in Hot Weather:

West J. Nutritional strategies for managing the heat-stressed dairy cow. J Anim Sci 1997;77:21–35.

Erdman RA, Botts RL, Hemken RW, et al. Effect of dietary sodium bicarbonate and magnesium oxide on production and physiology in early lactation. J Dairy Sci 1980;63:923–30.

Wu W, Murphy MR. Dietary cation-anion difference effects on performance and acid-base status of lactating dairy cows: a meta-analysis. J Dairy Sci 2004;87:2222–9.

Monensin

Monensin is a carboxylic polyether ionophore produced by a naturally occurring strain of *Streptomyces cinnamonensis*.[97] It is approved for use in lactating cattle in several countries including Australia, Argentina, Brazil, New Zealand, South Africa, and the United States.[98] The effects of sodium monensin are primarily to increase ruminal propionate production, reflecting an increase in propionate-producing bacteria in comparison with those producing formate, acetate, lactate, and butyrate. There is a concomitant decrease in methane production from the rumen and a sparing effect on ruminal protein digestion.[99,100] Monensin is also proposed to selectively inhibit grampositive bacteria, in particular inhibition of lactate-producing bacteria, in the rumen without affecting most lactate-utilizing bacteria[101,102]; however, lactate concentrations have been rarely reported in in vivo cattle studies with monensin, and monensin does not always suppress gram-positive bacteria.[102] There is a large disparity in ruminal fermentation responses between monensin studies that may result from differences in monensin dose rates, cattle management, physiologic state of the cattle, and diet.[65]

The effects of monensin on blood metabolites, production, reproduction, and health were examined in a series of meta-analyses.[103–105] Monensin use in lactating dairy cattle significantly reduced blood concentrations of β-hydroxybutyrate by 13%, acetoacetate by 14%, and free fatty acid by 7%, and increased blood glucose by 3% and urea by 6%, but had no significant effect on cholesterol, calcium, milk urea, or insulin.

Monensin use in lactating dairy cattle significantly decreased DMI by 0.3 kg, but increased milk yield by 0.7 kg and improved milk production efficiency by 2.5%. Monensin decreased milk fat percentage by 0.13%, but had no effect on milk fat yield; however, there was significant heterogeneity between studies for both of these responses. Milk protein percentage was decreased 0.03%, but protein yield increased 0.016 kg/d with treatment. Monensin increased body condition score by 0.03 and similarly improved body weight change (0.06 kg/d). These findings indicate a benefit of monensin for improving milk production efficiency while maintaining body condition. The effect of monensin on milk fat percentage and yield was influenced by diet.

Over all the trials analyzed by Duffield and colleagues,[105] monensin decreased the risk of ketosis (relative risk [RR] = 0.75), displaced abomasum (RR = 0.75), and mastitis (RR = 0.91). No significant effects of monensin were found for milk fever, lameness, dystocia, retained placenta, or metritis. Monensin had no effect on firstservice conception risk or days to pregnancy.

In summary, monensin use increases the production of milk and milk protein, and the efficiency of production, and reduces the risk of ketosis.

Direct-fed microbials

Several different terms have been used for supplementing microbes in the rumen.[106] The term probiotic was first used by Parker,[107] and was more clearly defined by Fuller[108] as "a live microbial feed supplement, which beneficially affects the host animal by improving its intestinal microbial balance." In The United States probiotics are considered to include viable microbial cultures, culture extracts, enzyme preparations, or their combinations.[106] To avoid confusion regarding several terminologies for probiotics, in 1989 the US Food and Drug Administration redefined probiotics as directfed microbials (DFM), with the definition "a source of live (viable) naturally occurring microorganisms."[106]

Several products of single or mixed bacterial cultures are used in the ruminant industries, largely strains from the following bacterial genera: *Bifidobacterium*, *Enterococcus*, *Streptococcus*, *Prevotella*, *Bacillus*, *Lactobacillus*, *Megasphaera*, and

Propionibacterium.[109] *Lactobacillus acidophilus* and *Propionibacterium freudenreichii* are the primary bacterial DFM used in the dairy industry.[110] The primary yeast and fungal products used contain *Saccharomyces cerevisiae* and *Aspergillus oryzae* strains, respectively.[106,109] Most exogenous enzyme products incorporated in ruminant feeds are fiber-degrading enzymes that are products of microbial fermentation from bacterial (mostly *Bacillus* spp) or fungal (mostly *Trichoderma longibrachiatum*, *Aspergillus niger*, *A oryzae*) origin,[111] and many do not contain live microorganisms,[112] so may not be classified as DFM. There is a need to optimize dosage, timing, strains of DFM, and animal conditions under which these are optimized.[109] The DFM that target the rumen must be active in the rumen and must remain viable during delivery.[109]

Animal responses to DFM have been inconsistent, reflecting supplementation with many different organisms, strains of organisms, and combinations of organisms, and differences in microorganism inclusion level, diet, feeding management, and animal factors.[110] Hence the evaluation of DFM performances is a challenge. Ruminal fermentation and production responses to individual DFM have been recently reviewed.[106,109,112–114] Some reviews of DFM have found increased milk production in dairy cattle and improved health and performance in calves, and ruminal responses indicated that they could reduce the risk of ruminal acidosis.[113] However, results are inconsistent. Responses to DFM in the rumen include a decrease in the area below ruminal pH defined for subacute ruminal acidosis, an increase in propionate concentrations, increased protozoa counts, and altered counts of bacteria such as those of lactate-producing and lactate-utilizing bacteria.[113] More work on DFM is warranted, but support for any particular product is very limited at present.

Yeasts

Yeasts are a large, but not homogeneous, group of additives. In contrast to DFM, there is a large body of literature published on yeast products. Assumptions of equivalency of action in the rumen or responses to supplementation within the group should not be made. There are 2 major types of yeast marketed: live yeast containing greater than 15 billion live yeast cells per gram, and yeast fermentation by-products (cultures). The action of the live yeast depends on the function of live yeast cells in the rumen, whereas the fermentation by-products act through the supply of products of fermentation using yeasts. Actions that have been identified with yeasts include small increases in rumen pH, reductions in lactic acid, enhanced fiber digestion, and small increases in VFA production.

The effects of yeast fermentation products, specifically Diamond V products, were assessed using meta-analysis. The raw mean differences between treated and untreated cattle reported in peer-reviewed publications were 1.18 kg/d (95% CI 0.55–1.81) and 1.61 kg/d (95% CI 0.92–2.29) for milk yield and 3.5% fat-corrected milk (FCM), respectively.[115] Milk fat yield and milk protein yield for peer-reviewed studies showed an increase in the raw mean difference of 0.06 kg/d (95% CI 0.01–0.10) and 0.03 kg/d (95% CI 0.00–0.05), respectively.[115] DMI increased in early lactation studies and was lower in later lactation studies for treated cows.[115]

In a multistudy evaluation of the effects of a live yeast (Levucell SC; Lallemand Animal Nutrition, Milwaukee, WI, USA; *Saccharomyces cerevisiae* CNCMI-1077; 10×10^9 cfu/d) it significantly improved 3.5% FCM yield by 0.96 kg/d, with the effect being greater for cows less than 100 days in milk.[116] Feed efficiency (3.5% FCM/kg DMI) was improved, but there was no overall effect of this live yeast on DMI.[116] Both milk fat yield (0.03 kg/d) and milk true protein yield (0.02 kg/d) increased with live yeast supplementation.[116]

Enzymes

Fiber digestion in ruminants is not maximal because between 20% and 70% of cellulose alone remains undigested.[117] The application of exogenous fibrolytic enzymes to forages has been investigated as a method of enhancing fiber digestion and production.

The milk production responses to the use of fibrolytic enzymes have been assessed, and averaged 2.3 L per cow per day, but had substantial variation (standard deviation 6.5 L) (Brad Granzin, Wollongbar, NSW, Australia, personal communication, 2004). Adesogan and colleagues[118] also found an increase. The variable responses in in vitro and in vivo studies to exogenous feed enzymes might suggest that enzyme additives are not effective at enhancing fiber digestion. However, it is more likely that the exogenous fibrolytic enzymes are effective, and the high level of variability can be accounted for by differences in enzyme type, enzyme-substrate specificity, level of supplementation, method of application, and the energy balance of the animal.[112]

SUPPLEMENTARY DATA

Supplementary data related to this article can be found online at http://dx.doi.org/10.1016/j.cvfa.2014.07.003.

REFERENCES

1. Tajima K. Diet-dependent shifts in the bacterial population of the rumen revealed with real-time PCR. Appl Environ Microbiol 2001;67:2766–74.
2. Kamra DN. Rumen microbial ecosystem. Curr Sci 2005;89:124–35.
3. Jami E, Mizrahi I. Composition and similarity of bovine rumen microbiota across individual animals. PLoS One 2012;7:e33306.
4. Dougherty RW, Riley JL, Baetz AL, et al. Physiologic studies of experimentally grain-engorged cattle and sheep. Am J Vet Res 1975;36:833–5.
5. Brown MS, Krehbiel CR, Galyean ML, et al. Evaluation of models of acute and subacute acidosis on dry matter intake, ruminal fermentation, blood chemistry, and endocrine profiles of beef steers. J Anim Sci 2000;78:3155–68.
6. Stewart CS, Flint JF, Bryant MP. The rumen bacteria. In: Hobson PN, Stewart CS, editors. The rumen microbial ecosystem. 2nd edition. London (United Kingdom): Blackie Academic and Professional; 1997. p. 10–72.
7. Pers-Kamczyc E, Zmora P, Cieślak A, et al. Development of nucleic acid based techniques and possibilities of their application to rumen microbial ecology research. J Anim Feed Sci 2011;20:315–37.
8. Khafipour E, Li S, Plaizier JC, et al. Rumen microbiome composition determined using two nutritional models of subacute ruminal acidosis. Appl Environ Microbiol 2009;75:7115–24.
9. de Menezes AB, Lewis E, O'Donovan M, et al. Microbiome analysis of dairy cows fed pasture or total mixed ration diets. FEMS Microbiol Ecol 2011;78:256–65.
10. Weimer PJ, Stevenson DM, Mantovani HC, et al. Host specificity of the ruminal bacterial community in the dairy cow following near-total exchange of ruminal contents. J Dairy Sci 2010;93:5902–12.
11. Bergen WG. Quantitative determination of rumen ciliate protozoal biomass with real-time PCR. J Nutr 2004;134:3223–4.
12. Ferrer M, Golyshina OV, Chernikova TN, et al. Novel hydrolase diversity retrieved from a metagenome library of bovine rumen microflora. Environ Microbiol 2005;7:1996–2010.

13. Slyter LL. Influence of acidosis on rumen function. J Anim Sci 1976;43:910–29.
14. Janssen PH, Kirs M. Structure of the archaeal community of the rumen. Appl Environ Microbiol 2008;74:3619–25.
15. Lynd LR, Weimer PJ, van Zyl WH, et al. Microbial cellulose utilization: fundamentals and biotechnology. Microbiol Mol Biol Rev 2002;66:506–77.
16. Krause DO, Denman SE, Mackie RI, et al. Opportunities to improve fiber degradation in the rumen: microbiology, ecology, and genomics. FEMS Microbiol Rev 2003;27:663–93.
17. Guttman B, Raya R, Kutter E. Basic phage biology. In: Kutter E, Sulakvelidze A, editors. Bacteriophages: biology and applications. New York: CRC Press; 2004. p. 29–66.
18. National Research Council (NRC). Nutrient requirements of dairy cattle. 7th edition. Washington, DC: National Academic Press; 2001.
19. Institut National de la Recherche Agronomique I. Ruminant nutrition. Recommended allowances and feed tables. London; Paris: John Libbey Eurotext; 1989.
20. Thomas C. Feed into milk: a new applied feeding system for dairy cows. Nottingham (United Kingdom: Nottingham University Press; 2004.
21. Grant R, Albright J. Feeding behavior and management factors during the transition period in dairy cattle. J Anim Sci 1995;73:2791–803.
22. Bolsen KK, Huck GL, Siefers MK, et al. Silage management: five key factors. Manhattan (KS): Kansas State University; 1999.
23. Burfeind O, Sepúlveda P, von Keyserlingk MA, et al. Technical note: evaluation of a scoring system for rumen fill in dairy cows. J Dairy Sci 2010;93:3635–40.
24. Forbes JM. Voluntary food intake and diet selection in farm animals. Oxfordshire (United Kingdom): CABI; 2007.
25. Sniffen CJ, O'Connor JD, Van Soest PJ, et al. A net carbohydrate and protein system for evaluating cattle diets: II. Carbohydrate and protein availability. J Anim Sci 1992;70:3562–77.
26. Waldo DR, Smith LW, Cox EL. Model of cellulose disappearance from the rumen. J Dairy Sci 1972;55:125–9.
27. Bossen D, Mertens D, Weisbjerg MR. Influence of fermentation methods on neutral detergent fiber degradation parameters. J Dairy Sci 2008;91:1464–76.
28. Oba M, Allen MS. Effects of corn grain conservation method on feeding behavior and productivity of lactating dairy cows at two dietary starch concentrations. J Dairy Sci 2003;86:174–83.
29. Hall MB. Dietary starch source and protein degradability in diets containing sucrose: effects on ruminal measures and proposed mechanism for degradable protein effects. J Dairy Sci 2013;96:7093–109.
30. Malestein A, Vantklooster AT, Prins RA, et al. Concentrate feeding and ruminal fermentation.3. Influence of concentrate ingredients on pH, on dl-lactic acid concentration in rumen fluid of dairy-cows and on dry-matter intake. Neth J Agr Sci 1984;32:9–21.
31. Argyle J, Baldwin R. Effects of amino acids and peptides on rumen microbial growth yields. J Dairy Sci 1989;72:2017–27.
32. Opatpanakit Y, Kellaway R, Lean I, et al. Microbial fermentation of cereal grains in vitro. Aust J Agric Res 1994;45:1247–63.
33. Lean IJ, Golder HM, Black JL, et al. In vivo indices for predicting acidosis risk of grains in cattle: comparison with in vitro methods. J Anim Sci 2013;91:2823–35.
34. Baldwin RL. Modeling ruminant digestion and metabolism. London: Chapman and Hall; 1995.

35. Bauman DE, Griinari JM. Nutritional regulation of milk fat synthesis. Annu Rev Nutr 2003;23:203–27.
36. Moate P, Chalupa W, Boston R, et al. Milk fatty acids II: Prediction of the production of individual fatty acids in bovine milk. J Dairy Sci 2008;91:1175–88.
37. Mertens D. Effect of fiber on feed quality for dairy cows. In: 46th Minnesota Nutrition Conference. St Paul (MN): University of Minnesota; 1985. p. 209.
38. Mertens DR. Creating a system for meeting the fiber requirements of dairy cows. J Dairy Sci 1997;80:1463–81.
39. Armentano L, Pereira M. Measuring the effectiveness of fiber by animal response trials. J Dairy Sci 1997;80:1416–25.
40. France J, Dijkstra J. Volatile fatty acid production. In: Dijkstra J, Forbes JM, France J, editors. Quantitative aspects of ruminant digestion and metabolism. Wallingford (United Kingdom): CABI Publishing; 2005. p. 157–76.
41. Chalupa W, Rickabaugh B, Kronfeld D, et al. Rumen fermentation in vitro as influenced by long chain fatty acids. J Dairy Sci 1984;67:1439–44.
42. Firkins J, Allen M, Oldick B, et al. Modeling ruminal digestibllity of carbohydrates and microbial protein flow to the duodenum. J Dairy Sci 1998;81:3350–69.
43. Lean IJ. Systems of describing nutritional requirements of dairy cattle. In: Rojinski H, editor. Encyclopedia of dairy science. 2nd edition. Atlanta (GA): Elsevier Science Ltd; 2011. p. 418–28.
44. Johnson RR. Influence of carbohydrate solubility on non-protein nitrogen utilization in the ruminant. J Anim Sci 1976;43:184–91.
45. Herrera-Saldana R, Huber JT. Influence of varying protein and starch degradabilities on performance of lactating cows. J Dairy Sci 1989;72:1477–83.
46. Satter LD, Roffler RE. Nitrogen requirement and utilization in dairy cattle. J Dairy Sci 1975;58:1219–37.
47. Russell JB, O'Connor JD, Fox DG, et al. A net carbohydrate and protein system for evaluating cattle diets: I. Ruminal fermentation. J Anim Sci 1992;70:3551–61.
48. Griswold K, Hoover W, Miller T, et al. Effect of form of nitrogen on growth of ruminal microbes in continuous culture. J Anim Sci 1996;74:483–91.
49. Russell J, Sniffen C. Effect of carbon-4 and carbon-5 volatile fatty acids on growth of mixed rumen bacteria in vitro. J Dairy Sci 1984;67:987–94.
50. Nocek J, Russell J. Protein and energy as an integrated system. Relationship of ruminal protein and carbohydrate availability to microbial synthesis and milk production. J Dairy Sci 1988;71:2070–107.
51. Girard C. B-complex vitamins for dairy cows: a new approach. Can J Anim Sci 1998;78(suppl):71–90.
52. Schwab EC, Schwab CG, Shaver RD, et al. Dietary forage and nonfiber carbohydrate contents influence B-vitamin intake, duodenal flow, and apparent ruminal synthesis in lactating dairy cows. J Dairy Sci 2006;89:174–87.
53. Santschi D, Berthiaume R, Matte J, et al. Fate of supplementary B-vitamins in the gastrointestinal tract of dairy cows. J Dairy Sci 2005;88:2043–54.
54. Shaver R, Bal M. Effect of dietary thiamin supplementation on milk production by dairy cows. J Dairy Sci 2000;83:2335–40.
55. Kung L, Gubert K, Huber JT. Supplemental niacin for lactating cows fed diets of natural protein or nonprotein nitrogen. J Dairy Sci 1980;63:2020–5.
56. Dufva GS, Bartley EE, Dayton AD, et al. Effect of niacin supplementation on milk production and ketosis of dairy cattle. J Dairy Sci 1983;66:2329–36.
57. Jaster EH, Bell DF, McPherron TA. Nicotinic acid and serum metabolite concentrations of lactating dairy cows fed supplemental niacin. J Dairy Sci 1983;66:1039–45.

58. Jaster EH, Hartnell GF, Hutjens MF. Feeding supplemental niacin for milk production in six dairy herds. J Dairy Sci 1983;66:1046–51.
59. Hutjens M. Role of niacin in minimizing nutritional stress. Anim Hlth Nutr 1987;42: 23–9.
60. Lean I, Rabiee A. Effect of feeding biotin on milk production and hoof health in lactating dairy cows: a quantitative assessment. J Dairy Sci 2011;94:1465–76.
61. Chen B, Wang C, Wang YM, et al. Effect of biotin on milk performance of dairy cattle: a meta-analysis. J Dairy Sci 2011;94:3537–46.
62. Bramley E, Lean IJ, Fulkerson WJ, et al. The definition of acidosis in dairy herds predominantly fed on pasture and concentrates. J Dairy Sci 2008;91:308–21.
63. Oetzel GR, Nordlund KV, Garrett EF. The effect of ruminal pH and stage of lactation on ruminal concentrations in dairy cows. J Dairy Sci 1999;82(Suppl 1): 38–9.
64. Oetzel GR. Monitoring and testing dairy herds for metabolic disease. Vet Clin North Am Food Anim Pract 2004;20:651–74.
65. Golder HM. Increased understandings of ruminal acidosis in dairy cattle. Camden (New South Wales): University of Sydney; 2013.
66. Nordlund KV, Garrett EF. Rumenocentesis: a technique for collecting rumen fluid for the diagnosis of subacute rumen acidosis in dairy herds. Bovine Pract 1994; 28:109–12.
67. Enemark JM. The monitoring, prevention and treatment of sub-acute ruminal acidosis (SARA): a review. Vet J 2008;176:32–43.
68. Britton RA, Stock RA. Acidosis, rate of starch digestion and intake. In: Proceedings of the Symposium of Feed Intake by Beef Cattle, MP 121, Agicultural Experiment Station, Oklahoma; 1986. p. 125–136.
69. Sprecher DJ, Hostetler DE, Kaneene JB. A lameness scoring system that uses posture and gait to predict dairy cattle reproductive performance. Theriogenology 1997;47:1179–87.
70. Bramley E, Lean IJ, Fulkerson WJ, et al. Feeding management and feeds on dairy farms in New South Wales and Victoria. Anim Prod Sci 2012;52:20–9.
71. Atkinson O. Guide to the rumen health visit. Practice 2009;31:314–25.
72. Krause KM, Oetzel GR. Understanding and preventing subacute ruminal acidosis in dairy herds: a review. Anim Feed Sci Technol 2006;126:215–36.
73. Oetzel GR. Clinical aspects of ruminal acidosis in dairy cattle. Proceedings of the Thirty-Third Annual Conference, American Association of Bovine Practitioners. Rapid City (SD), September 21–23, 2000. p. 46–53.
74. Galyean M, Wagner D, Owens F. Dry matter and starch disappearance of corn and sorghum as influenced by particle size and processing. J Dairy Sci 1981; 64:1804–12.
75. Rabiee AR, Breinhild K, Scott W, et al. Effect of fat additions to diets of dairy cattle on milk production and components: a meta-analysis and meta-regression. J Dairy Sci 2012;95:3225–47.
76. Rabiee AR, Lean IJ. Evaluation of diagnostic tests used for ruminal subacute acidosis using receiver-operating characteristic (ROC) analysis. 2012.
77. Reference Advisory Group on Fermentative Acidosis of Ruminants (RAGFAR). Ruminal acidosis - aetiopathogenesis, prevention and treatment. A review for veterinarians and nutritional professionals. Australian Veterinary Association, editor. Carlton (Victoria): Blackwell Publishing Asia Pty. Ltd; 2007. p. 45–47.
78. Britton R, Stock R, Cornell U. Acidosis - a continual problem in cattle fed high grain diets. Proceedings: 1989 Cornell Nutrition Conference for Feed Manufacturers Syracuse Marriott, Oct 24-26, 1989. p. 8–15.

79. Maekawa M, Beauchemin KA, Christensen DA. Effect of concentrate level and feeding management on chewing activities, saliva production, and ruminal pH of lactating dairy cows. J Dairy Sci 2002;85:1165–75.
80. Kleen JL, Hooijer GA, Rehage J, et al. Subacute ruminal acidosis (SARA): a review. J Vet Med A Physiol Pathol Clin Med 2003;50:406–14.
81. Todar K. Nutrition and growth of bacteria in Todar's online textbook on bacteriology. In. 2012. http://textbookofbacteriology.net/nutgro.html.
82. Lowe L, Ball G, Carruthers V, et al. Monensin controlled-release intraruminal capsule for control of bloat in pastured dairy cows. Aust Vet J 1991;68:17–20.
83. Majak W, Hall J, McCaughey W. Pasture management strategies for reducing the risk of legume bloat in cattle. J Anim Sci 1995;73:1493–8.
84. Golder HM, Celi P, Rabiee AR, et al. Effects of feed additives on rumen and blood profiles during a starch and fructose challenge. J Dairy Sci 2014;97: 985–1004.
85. Anadón A. WS14 the EU ban of antibiotics as feed additives (2006): alternatives and consumer safety. J Vet Pharmacol Ther 2006;29:41–4.
86. Staples CR, Lough DS. Efficacy of supplemental dietary neutralizing agents for lactating dairy cows. A review. Anim Feed Sci Technol 1989;23:277–303.
87. Ha J, Emerick R, Embry L. In vitro effect of pH variations on rumen fermentation, and in vivo effects of buffers in lambs before and after adaptation to high concentrate diets. J Anim Sci 1983;56:698.
88. Hu W, Murphy MR. Statistical evaluation of early- and mid-lactation dairy cow responses to dietary sodium bicarbonate addition. Anim Feed Sci Technol 2005;119:43–54.
89. Erdman RA. Dietary buffering requirements of the lactating dairy cow: a review. J Dairy Sci 1988;71:3246–66.
90. Russell JB, Chow JM. Another theory for the action of ruminal buffer salts: decreased starch fermentation and propionate production. J Dairy Sci 1993; 76:826–30.
91. Valentine SC, Clayton EH, Judson GJ, et al. Effect of virginiamycin and sodium bicarbonate on milk production, milk composition and metabolism of dairy cows fed high levels of concentrates. Aust J Exp Agr 2000;40:773–81.
92. Hu W, Murphy M. Dietary cation-anion difference effects on performance and acid-base status of lactating dairy cows: a meta-analysis. J Dairy Sci 2004; 87:2222–9.
93. West J. Effects of heat-stress on production in dairy cattle. J Dairy Sci 2003;86: 2131–44.
94. Thomas JW, Emery RS. Additive nature of sodium bicarbonate and magnesium oxide on milk fat concentrations of milking cows fed restricted-roughage rations. J Dairy Sci 1969;52:1762–9.
95. Erdman RA, Botts RL, Hemken RW, et al. Effect of dietary sodium bicarbonate and magnesium oxide on production and physiology in early lactation. J Dairy Sci 1980;63:923–30.
96. Herod EL, Bechtle RM, Bartley EE, et al. Buffering ability of several compounds in vitro and the effect of a selected buffer combination on ruminal acid production in vivo. J Dairy Sci 1978;61:1114–22.
97. Haney ME Jr, Hoehn MM. Monensin, a new biologically active compound. I. Discovery and isolation. Antimicrob Agents Chemother (Bethesda) 1967;7:349–52.
98. Gallardo MR, Castillo AR, Bargo F, et al. Monensin for lactating dairy cows grazing mixed-alfalfa pasture and supplemented with partial mixed ration. J Dairy Sci 2005;88:644–52.

99. Richardson LF, Raun AP, Potter EL, et al. Effect of monensin on rumen fermentation in vitro and in vivo. J Anim Sci 1976;43:657–64.
100. Russell JB, Houlihan AJ. Ionophore resistance of ruminal bacteria and its potential impact on human health. FEMS Microbiol Rev 2003;27:65–74.
101. Dennis SM, Nagaraja TG, Bartley EE. Effect of lasalocid or monensin on lactate-producing or using rumen bacteria. J Anim Sci 1981;52:418–26.
102. Weimer P, Stevenson D, Mertens D, et al. Effect of monensin feeding and withdrawal on populations of individual bacterial species in the rumen of lactating dairy cows fed high-starch rations. Appl Microbiol Biotechnol 2008;80:135–45.
103. Duffield TF, Rabiee AR, Lean IJ. A meta-analysis of the impact of monensin in lactating dairy cattle. Part 2. Production effects. J Dairy Sci 2008;91:1347–60.
104. Duffield TF, Rabiee AR, Lean IJ. A meta-analysis of the impact of monensin in lactating dairy cattle. Part 1. Metabolic effects. J Dairy Sci 2008;91:1334–46.
105. Duffield TF, Rabiee AR, Lean IJ. A meta-analysis of the impact of monensin in lactating dairy cattle. Part 3. Health and reproduction. J Dairy Sci 2008;91: 2328–41.
106. Yoon IK, Stern MD. Influence of direct-fed microbials on ruminal microbial fermentation and performance of ruminants: a review. Asian Australas J Anim Sci 1995;8:533–55.
107. Parker R. Probiotics, the other half of the antibiotic story. Anim Nutr Health 1974; 29:4–8.
108. Fuller R. Probiotics in man and animals. J Appl Bacteriol 1989;66:365–78.
109. Seo JK, Kim SW, Kim MH, et al. Direct-fed microbials for ruminant animals. Asian Australas J Anim Sci 2010;12:1657–67.
110. Raeth-Knight ML, Linn JG, Jung HG. Effect of direct-fed microbials on performance, diet digestibility, and rumen characteristics of Holstein dairy cows. J Dairy Sci 2007;90:1802–9.
111. Pendleton B. The regulatory environment. In: Muirhea S, editor. Direct-fed microbial, enzyme and forage additive compendium. Minnetonka (MN): The Miller Publishing Co.; 2000. p. 49.
112. Beauchemin KA, Colombatto D, Morgavi DP, et al. Use of exogenous fibrolytic enzymes to improve feed utilization by ruminants. J Anim Sci 2003;81:E37–47.
113. Krehbiel CR, Rust SR, Zhang G, et al. Bacterial direct-fed microbials in ruminant diets: performance response and mode of action. J Anim Sci 2003;81:E120–32.
114. Beauchemin KA, Krehbiel CR, Newbold CJ. Enzymes, bacterial direct-fed microbials and yeast: principles for use in ruminant nutrition. In: Mosenthin R, Zentek J, Żebrowska T, editors. Biology of nutrition in growing animals. Elsevier Science Health Science Division; 2006. p. 251–84.
115. Poppy GD, Rabiee AR, Lean IJ, et al. A meta-analysis of the effects of feeding yeast culture produced by anaerobic fermentation of Saccharomyces cerevisiae on milk production of lactating dairy cows. J Dairy Sci 2012;95:6027–41.
116. de Ondarza MB, Sniffen CJ, Dussert L, et al. Case study: multiple-study analysis of the effect of live yeast on milk yield, milk component content and yield, and feed efficiency. Prof Anim Sci 2010;26:661–6.
117. Varga GA, Kolver ES. Microbial and animal limitations to fiber digestion and utilization. J Nutr 1997;127:819S–23S.
118. Adesogan AT, Romero JJ, Ma ZX. Improving cell wall digestion and animal performance with fibrolytic enzymes. J. Anim. Sci. Vol. 91, E-Suppl. 2/J. Dairy Sci. Vol. 96, E-Suppl. 1 2013:165.

Carbohydrate Nutrition

Managing Energy Intake and Partitioning Through Lactation

Michael S. Allen, PhD[a],*, Paola Piantoni, Veterinaria, MS[b]

KEYWORDS

- Energy intake • Energy partitioning • Energy balance • Feeding behavior
- Grouping cows • Maintenance group • Ruminal starch fermentability
- Fiber digestibility

KEY POINTS

- Energy intake and partitioning are affected by the interaction between diet and the physiological state.
- Control of feed intake is complex and involves the integration of multiple signals by brain feeding centers; dominant control mechanisms vary within a day and across diets and physiological states.
- Energy partitioning is affected by insulin concentration, insulin sensitivity, and the type and temporal supply of fuels provided by the diet.
- Concentration and digestion characteristics of forage fiber affect the filling effect of diets and feed intake, especially when ruminal distention dominates control of feed intake around peak lactation.
- Concentration and ruminal fermentability of starch are primary factors related to metabolic control of feed intake, which likely dominates in the transition period and midlactation to late lactation.
- The optimal diet will vary with the physiological state; therefore, different rations must be offered through the lactation cycle to maximize milk yield, efficiency of production, and cow health.

INTRODUCTION

Carbohydrates normally compose more than 60% of the diets of lactating cows and can have large effects on energy intake and partitioning. These effects depend on the type and digestion characteristics of carbohydrates, which interact with the

Disclosures: None.
[a] Department of Animal Science, Michigan State University, 474 South Shaw Lane, Room 2265A, East Lansing, MI 48824, USA; [b] Department of Animal Science, Michigan State University, 474 South Shaw Lane, Room 2200, East Lansing, MI 48824, USA
* Corresponding author.
E-mail address: allenm@msu.edu

Vet Clin Food Anim 30 (2014) 577–597
http://dx.doi.org/10.1016/j.cvfa.2014.07.004
0749-0720/14/$ – see front matter © 2014 Elsevier Inc. All rights reserved.

physiological state of cows. Forage fiber is more filling than other diet fractions because of its initial bulk and because it is digested more slowly over time. Therefore, concentration of forage fiber in diets can limit feed intake during periods when control of feed intake is dominated by ruminal distention. Feed intake can also be limited by ruminal fermentability of starch, through fuels that stimulate hepatic oxidation and increase hepatic energy status, especially during the transition and midlactation to late-lactation periods. Starch supplies glucose and glucose precursors for synthesis of milk lactose, the production of which is the primary determinant of milk yield. However, some starch sources are rapidly fermented; excessive ruminal fermentability can decrease ruminal pH and alter ruminal biohydrogenation pathways, reducing milk fat concentration and yield. Milk fat depression (MFD) spares glucose, potentially increasing plasma insulin concentration and energy partitioned to body reserves. The objective of this article is to discuss carbohydrate type and digestion characteristics and how they interact with the physiological state of cows to affect energy intake and partitioning and ultimately milk yield and cow health.

CONTROL OF FEED INTAKE

Energy-intake control mechanisms are complex and involve multiple signals, redundancies, and levels of integration. Signals related to hunger and satiety are integrated in brain feeding centers to control feeding behavior and, consequently, energy intake.[1] It is important to understand that there is rarely, if ever, a single signal controlling feeding behavior but rather multiple signals that are integrated to determine feeding. At times, certain signals dominate control of feeding; these signals vary temporally, within days, as well as across physiological states and diets. Feeding behavior is determined by meal size and frequency and is not only affected by physical, metabolic, and endocrine signals but also by management and environment (**Fig. 1**).

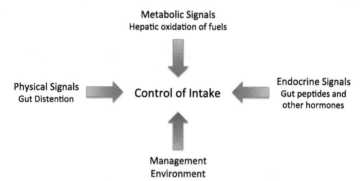

Fig. 1. Intake is controlled by signals from physical, metabolic, and endocrine origin as well as by the environment and management. Metabolic signals likely predominate during the transition period and midlactation to late lactation: increased hepatic oxidation of fuels can increase energy status of the liver, inducing satiety and the end of a meal. Signals from gut distension start to predominate as lactation progresses after the fresh period and during peak lactation, when milk production is greatest, and are affected by concentration and digestion characteristics of forage neutral detergent fiber (NDF). Endocrine signals contribute to the control of feed intake throughout lactation and are affected by nutrients in the chyme (eg, cholecystokinin, glucagon-like peptide 1) and energy balance of the cow (eg, leptin). Management (eg, competition, access to feed, availability of feed) and the environment (eg, heat index) can also affect feed intake, especially during periods of stress (ie, transition period). All signals can occur simultaneously and are integrated in brain feeding centers to affect control of feed intake within a meal, within a day, and in the long-term.

Physical Control

Physical constraints to feed intake in ruminants have been previously reviewed.[2] Ruminal distension stimulates tension receptors located in the reticulum and cranial sac of the rumen,[3] and the resulting signal is conveyed to brain feeding centers via vagal afferents. Rumen distension is affected by both the volume and weight of digesta,[4] which is primarily determined by forage neutral detergent fiber (NDF) concentration and NDF digestion characteristics[5] (eg, fragility, rates of digestion and passage). Signals from ruminal distention likely dominate control of feeding when milk yield is greatest (peak lactation, high-producing cows) and when high forage rations are fed and have relatively less effect during the fresh and late-lactation periods (**Fig. 2**A, B).

Metabolic Control

Research in laboratory animals suggests that meals can be terminated by signals carried to the brain via hepatic vagal afferents.[6] A decrease in the firing rate of the vagus nerve, associated with increased oxidation of various metabolites, induces satiety, whereas an increase in the firing rate causes hunger. The signal likely originates in the liver because vagotomy of the hepatic branch of the vagus nerve decreased hypophagic effects of propionate in sheep.[7] Moreover, the signal is likely related to hepatic energy charge (phosphorylation potential), which is determined by the balance between the rate of production of high-energy phosphate bonds from oxidation of fuels and the rate of utilization by energy-consuming reactions, and not only by oxidation of fuels.[8] We call this the Hepatic Oxidation Theory (HOT) of the control of feed intake.[9] Briefly, meal size and frequency, which determine feeding behavior, are altered by temporal patterns of fuel absorption, mobilization of body reserves, and hepatic oxidation.[9] Fuels that can be oxidized in the ruminant liver include those mobilized from body reserves and provided by the diet, such as nonesterified fatty acids (NEFA), glycerol, amino acids, and lactate as well as fuels exclusively derived from the diet, such as propionate and butyrate. Fatty acids (FA) are the primary fuel oxidized in the liver, and their supply varies both within the day (negatively related with plasma insulin concentration) as well as throughout lactation, as the physiological state of cows changes. Of fuels derived from the diet, propionate is most likely the one to stimulate satiety because it can be rapidly produced in the rumen, absorbed, extracted by the liver, and oxidized.[5] Readers interested in a more detailed discussion of HOT are referred to reviews for ruminants,[9] a comparison across species,[10] and its relationship with metabolic disease in the postpartum period in dairy cows.[11]

Endocrine Control

Besides insulin, other hormones can potentially contribute to both short- and long-term control of feed intake. Gut peptides, such as cholecystokinin (CCK) and glucagon-like peptide 1, have been implicated in the short-term control of feed intake,[12,13] whereas leptin has been implicated in the long-term control of feed intake.[14] Gut peptides are usually secreted in the small intestine in response to different nutrients in the chyme and have been related to decreased gastric emptying (potentially increasing gut distention) and increased digestive enzyme release, which might improve nutrient digestibility. Leptin is secreted by adipocytes, and its secretion is correlated to the size of the body fat depots.[14] Leptin induces satiety and might help maintain body weight over the long-term. Signals related

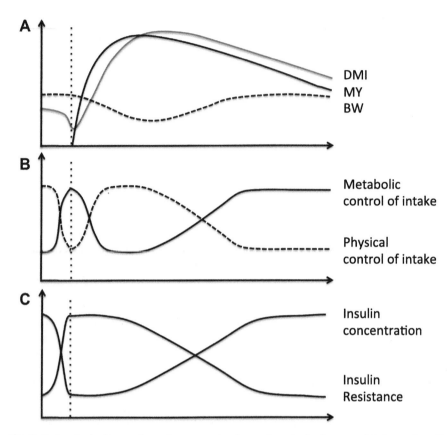

Fig. 2. Suggested schemes for primary mechanisms of control of energy intake and partitioning through lactation. The vertical doted line in each panel indicates parturition. (*A*) Dry matter intake (DMI) is generally depressed in the peripartum period and increases postpartum, driven by milk production. Milk yield (MY) increases postpartum until it reaches peak and then declines. The difference between milk energy output and feed energy input determines energy balance and body weight (BW) loss, which increases as lactation progresses and decreases after peak production. (*B*) Metabolic control of intake is likely dominant during the dry, early postpartum, and midlactation to late-lactation periods; physical control of intake is likely dominant during peak lactation. Note that as one control mechanism increases in dominance, the other one decreases; but both may occur at all times. (*C*) As insulin concentration decreases during the dry period, insulin resistance increases. During early postpartum, the cow goes through a phase of insulin resistance and low insulin concentration, mobilizing body energy reserves. As lactation progresses, insulin concentration increases and insulin resistance decreases, which allow the cow to replenish body energy reserves while producing milk.

to gut peptides are integrated in brain feeding centers with other signals originated in the gastrointestinal tract and the environment to determine feeding behavior.

Other Factors

Other factors that affect feed intake include the environment (eg, heat index) and management (eg, competition, access to feed).

CONTROL OF ENERGY PARTITIONING
Insulin Concentration and Insulin Sensitivity

The effects of insulin on the metabolism of carbohydrates, proteins, and lipids play an essential role in energy partitioning in the dairy cow.[15] Energy partitioning between milk and body condition is affected by both insulin concentration and the sensitivity of tissues to insulin (**Fig. 3**). Low plasma insulin concentration results in greater lipolysis in adipose tissue, increasing plasma NEFA concentration, and potentially energy in milk. Muscle, adipose tissue, and liver are insulin-sensitive tissues, whereas the mammary gland is not. Insulin resistance of insulin-sensitive tissues varies through the lactation cycle and has been associated with increased plasma concentrations of adipokines and NEFA and overconditioning.[16] Somatotropin also decreases insulin sensitivity of adipose tissue.[17] Insulin resistance might be associated with excessive accumulation of visceral fat, which is related to increased secretion of adipokines, such as resistin, interleukin 6 (IL-6), and tumor necrosis factor (TNF)-alpha.[18,19] These molecules are thought to increase insulin resistance by altering insulin signaling in the cell, but their mechanisms have not been fully elucidated. Overconditioning induces a state of systemic chronic inflammation, evidenced by increased plasma concentrations of TNF-alpha, IL-6, and NEFA, and increased oxidative stress,[20] all of which have been related to the alteration of the insulin signaling pathway.[19] Around parturition, the excessive lipid mobilization usually observed in overconditioned cows

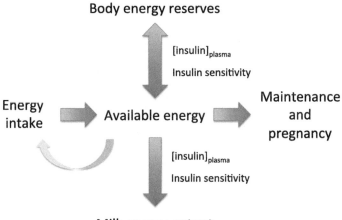

Fig. 3. Available energy in excess of that required for maintenance and pregnancy will be partitioned to milk and body reserves depending on plasma insulin concentration and adipose tissue sensitivity to insulin. During the postpartum and early lactation periods, low plasma insulin concentration and low sensitivity of adipose tissue to insulin result in a lipolytic state. Body energy reserves are mobilized, and this increases energy available for milk production but can also decrease energy intake by metabolic signals (eg, hepatic oxidation). As lactation progresses, the lipolytic state ceases and energy intake gradually increases; at peak lactation, energy partitioning to milk is greatest. As lactation proceeds past peak lactation and milk yield declines, available energy increases and body energy reserves begin to be restored as plasma insulin concentration and insulin sensitivity of adipose tissue increase. The increase in plasma glucose and insulin concentrations and downregulation of gluconeogenesis increase the availability of fuels for oxidation in the liver, decreasing energy intake. A reduction in milk energy output (eg, milk fat depression) can increase energy partitioning to body reserves and reduce energy intake by metabolic mechanisms (eg, hepatic oxidation) by increasing available energy and insulin concentration.

increases the risk of metabolic disorders; accumulation of NEFA in plasma can contribute to oxidative stress and increased expression of TNF-alpha and, therefore, elicit inflammatory responses[20] and insulin resistance.[21]

Recombinant Bovine Somatotropin

Recombinant bovine somatotropin (rbST) favors partitioning of energy to milk by increasing nutrient uptake for milk synthesis, decreasing the loss of secretory cells in the mammary gland, increasing gluconeogenesis in the liver, decreasing uptake of glucose in muscle, and decreasing lipogenesis in positive-energy balance and increasing lipolysis in negative energy balance in adipose tissue.[17] With proper management, supplementation of rbST increases milk production, persistency of lactation, dry matter intake (DMI), and production efficiency, with no effect on milk composition.[22] Besides diluting maintenance requirements by increasing milk yield and efficiency of production, rbST is useful for managing energy reserves through lactation in individual cows.

Milk Fat Depression

MFD is characterized by a decrease in milk fat concentration and yield, with no change in other components, milk yield, or DMI (see Chapter 6 on Lipids and Milk Fat Depression).[23] Fuels spared by the reduction in milk fat synthesis are partitioned to body reserves[24] or might increase energy balance and reduce feed intake[25] by hepatic oxidation of fuels. MFD is caused by altered microbial biohydrogenation of unsaturated long-chain fatty acids (LCFA) to specific conjugated linoleic acid (CLA) isomers in the rumen. Several LCFA isomers that cause MFD have been identified, including trans-10, cis-12 C18:2.[23] This CLA isomer inhibits milk fat synthesis in the mammary gland by downregulating the expression of several genes involved in lipogenesis, decreasing de novo FA synthesis in milk.[26] Furthermore, this CLA isomer has the opposite effect in adipose tissue, increasing the expression of genes involved in lipogenesis, likely because MFD increases energy balance by sparing energy for lipid synthesis, suggesting a role of trans-10, cis-12 CLA in energy partitioning. Feeding highly fermentable starch sources can cause MFD, likely by reducing ruminal pH. Concentration of fat in milk is positively related to ruminal pH,[27] and a reduction in ruminal pH could favor ruminal microorganisms with alternative biohydrogenation pathways, increasing the synthesis of trans-10 intermediates and, therefore, MFD.[28] However, low ruminal pH is not a prerequisite for the shift in biohydrogenation.[29] Factors that can potentially increase the amount of trans-10, cis-12 CLA reaching the duodenum for absorption and, therefore, MFD are related to diet formulation (eg, concentration of unsaturated LCFA,[30] low fiber/high concentrate, the use of ionophores) and management (eg, slug feeding, mixing errors).

CHANGES IN PHYSIOLOGICAL STATE THROUGH LACTATION

Several weeks prepartum, insulin concentration decreases[31] and insulin resistance of adipose tissue increases (see **Fig. 2C**)[32] resulting in lipolysis and increased plasma NEFA concentration. The decrease in plasma insulin concentration and the increase in insulin resistance are associated with a decrease in glucose uptake by maternal muscle and adipose tissue and an increase in NEFA supply to the liver and extrahepatic tissues. Using NEFA as a fuel spares glucose for the fetus when conceptus growth and metabolic activity are maximal. Export of acetyl coenzyme A (CoA) (derived from β-oxidation of NEFA) from the liver as ketone bodies spares glucose for the fetus in late gestation and for production of milk lactose in early lactation.

Insulin resistance and low concentration of plasma insulin persist during early lactation causing sustained elevation of plasma NEFA concentration. High plasma NEFA concentration will increase milk fat concentration to allow for the survival of the neonate. The plasma concentration of bovine somatotropin increases around parturition and decreases as lactation progresses, and insulin sensitivity of tissues gradually increases. As milk production begins to decline and energy intake increases, euglycemia is restored and plasma insulin concentration increases. As energy balance improves, the lipolytic state ceases and restoration of body energy reserves begins. Great variation exists among cows for the duration of the lipolytic state depending on the extent to which energy intake is limited by metabolic mechanisms.

EFFECTS OF DIET ON FEED INTAKE

Dietary characteristics that determine the filling effect and type and temporal absorption of fuels vary greatly across dietary ingredients and can affect voluntary feed intake. The filling effect of diets is largely affected by the concentration and digestion characteristics of forage NDF, and absorbed fuels vary mainly with concentration and ruminal fermentability of starch as well as with concentration and type of supplemental fat.[5]

Filling Effects of Diets

The filling effect of a diet is determined primarily by the initial bulk density of feeds as well as their filling effect over time in the rumen. The overall filling effect is determined by forage NDF concentration, forage particle size, fragility of forage NDF (determined by forage type: legumes, perennial grasses, annual grasses), and NDF digestibility within a forage family.[5] Forage NDF is less dense initially, digests more slowly, and is retained in the rumen longer than other diet components. Increasing the diet forage NDF concentration can dramatically reduce feed intake of high-producing cows that are limited by fill to the greatest extent. Several studies in the literature reported a decrease in DMI of up to 4 kg/d when the diet NDF concentration was increased from 25% to 35% by substituting forages for concentrates.[5] Although most studies reported a significant decrease in DMI as forage NDF increased, the DMI response was variable, depending on the degree to which intake was limited by ruminal fill.

Experiments that have evaluated the effects of forage particle size have generally shown small effects on DMI.[5] In one experiment, alfalfa silage particle size showed little effect on DMI when fed in high-grain diets; but when fed in a high-forage diet, alfalfa silage with a longer chop length reduced DMI.[33] Feed intake might have only been limited by ruminal fill in the high-forage diet, which could explain the interaction observed. Increasing the diet NDF concentration by substituting nonforage fiber sources (NFFS) for concentrated feeds has shown little effect on DMI in studies reported in the literature.[5] NFFS include byproduct feeds with high NDF concentrations, such as soyhulls, beet pulp, cottonseeds, corn gluten feed, almond hulls, and distillers grains. Fiber in NFFS is likely less filling than forage fiber both initially (smaller particle size) and over time in the rumen (faster fermentation and passage rates).

Forage NDF has a much longer ruminal retention time than other major dietary components. The retention time in the rumen is longer because of the longer initial particle size and a slow rate of comminution, which differs greatly across forages. As forages mature, the NDF fraction generally becomes more lignified. Lignin is a component of plant cell walls that helps stiffen the plant and prevents breakage of the stalk. It is also essentially indigestible by ruminal microbes and limits fermentation of cellulose and hemicellulose. Within a forage type, the degree to which NDF is lignified is related to the filling effects of the NDF. Fiber that is less lignified clears from the rumen faster, allowing more space for the next meal. However, the ruminal retention time of NDF from perennial grasses is generally longer than for legume NDF despite being less lignified.[34–37] Because of this, perennial grasses are more filling and should be limited in diets when feed intake is controlled by distension, unless it is of exceptionally high quality. Corn is an annual grass, and corn silage NDF digests and passes from the rumen quickly compared with perennial grasses and can be an excellent source of forage NDF for high-producing cows.

Importance of maintaining rumen fill

Although ruminal distention becomes a primary limitation to feed intake as milk yield increases, it normally has little effect on feed intake during the transition period, when feed intake is likely controlled by hepatic oxidation.[9] Glucose demand of fresh cows is high when glucose utilization for milk production outpaces gluconeogenesis. Although cows require diets with adequate glucose precursors (ie, starch from grains), it is important to also maintain rumen fill. Formulating diets to maintain rumen fill with ingredients that are retained in the rumen longer, and have moderate rates of fermentation and high ruminal digestibility, will likely benefit cows through the transition period. Increased ruminal digesta mass can provide more energy over time when feed intake decreases at parturition or from metabolic disorders and infectious diseases. This increase will help maintain euglycemia and prevent even more rapid mobilization of body reserves. In addition, ruminal digesta is very important to buffer fermentation acids, and the buffering capacity is directly related to the amount of digesta in the rumen.[2] Therefore, diets formulated with ingredients that increase the amount of digesta in the rumen will have greater buffering capacity and will maintain buffer capacity longer if feed intake decreases. Inadequate buffering can result in low ruminal pH, decreasing fiber digestibility and acetate production, and increasing propionate production, possibly stimulating propionate oxidation in the liver and decreasing feed intake. Low ruminal pH can increase the risk of health problems, such as ruminal ulcers, liver abscesses, and laminitis, likely increasing stress and mobilization of body reserves even further during the postpartum period. Moreover, diets formulated with ingredients that maintain digesta in the rumen longer when feed intake decreases will likely decrease the risk of abomasal displacement.

Physically effective fiber

Diets must contain adequate effective fiber for proper rumen function at all stages of lactation, and this can be achieved with the inclusion of low-energy roughages in diets. However, when the drive to eat is high, signals from ruminal distension dominate control of feed intake over metabolic mechanisms (eg, cows at peak lactation); therefore, high concentrations of low-energy forages can limit feed intake. Optimum particle length of individual forages depends on several factors, including forage type, silo type (if ensiled), other forages in the diet, diet fermentability, the physiological state of the cow consuming the forage, and stocking density/competition for feed. An adequate concentration of long particles is required to form a rumen mat to retain small particles that would otherwise escape the rumen, increasing diet digestibility, efficiency of feed utilization, rumen fill, and buffering capacity. Some forages that are particularly fragile (eg, brown midrib corn silage) benefit from a longer chop length; but forages that are resilient to packing might have to be chopped shorter, particularly when packing is difficult (eg, upright silos). Forages lacking physically effective fiber must be limited in diets and combined with forages with adequate particle length. When overcrowding causes competition at the feed bunk and slug feeding, diets with more physically effective fiber can limit the rate of feeding, decreasing the risk of low ruminal pH, especially for highly fermentable diets.

Starch Concentration and Ruminal Fermentability

Starch is a highly digestible and energy dense feed component that typically ranges from less than 20% to more than 28% of dietary DM in rations fed to lactating dairy cows. Starch is composed of polymers of glucose (amylose and amylopectin) with bonds that are readily cleaved by mammalian enzymes. However, starch is packaged in the seed endosperm in granules that are embedded in a protein matrix, which varies in solubility and resistance to digestion.[38] The endosperm type affects the ruminal fermentability of starch, which ranges from less than 30% to more than 90% across starch sources.[39,40] Altering the concentration and ruminal fermentability of starch in rations affects the digestibility of starch,[41] ruminal pH and fiber digestibility, and the type, amount, and temporal absorption of fuels (eg, acetate, propionate, lactate, glucose) available to the cow,[5] and therefore, has great effects on the lactational performance by affecting energy intake and partitioning as well as absorbed protein.[9] Diets with greater ruminal starch fermentability can depress feed and energy intakes. Increasing ruminal starch fermentation by substituting a more fermentable starch source for a less fermentable starch source decreased feed intake of cows by more than 3 kg/d in several studies reported in the literature.[5] Oba and Allen[42] showed that a more rapidly fermentable starch source (high-moisture corn) reduced feed intake of cows in midlactation 8% compared with a less fermentable starch source (dry ground corn) by decreasing meal size. The more fermentable starch source nearly doubled the rate of starch digestion in the rumen, increasing propionate production, compared with the less fermentable starch source. The reduction in meal size and DMI by the more fermentable starch source is likely because of a more rapid flux of propionate to the liver stimulating oxidation and satiety.[9]

Factors affecting ruminal starch fermentability

Ruminal fermentability of starch is affected by grain type (eg, corn, wheat, barley, sorghum), processing (eg, rolling, grinding, steam flaking), conservation method (eg, dry, ensiled), ration composition, and animal characteristics (eg, rumen microbial population, rate of passage). Starch in wheat, barley, and oats is generally more readily fermented than starch in corn; starch in sorghum is most resistant to fermentation in the rumen and digestion by the animal.[43] These differences are primarily because of differences in the endosperm type rather than differences in starch composition (amylose vs amylopectin) per se. Floury endosperm contains proteins that are readily solubilized, allowing greater access of enzymes to starch granules, whereas vitreous endosperm contains prolamin proteins that are insoluble and resistant to digestion, decreasing access of the enzymes to starch granules.[44] Starch sources vary in amount and proportion of the two types of endosperm, and there is large variation in vitreousness of the endosperm (percent of the total endosperm that is vitreous) among varieties within certain grain types. Endosperm vitreousness in corn harvested at physiological maturity ranges from 0% to more than 75%, and corn with a more vitreous endosperm is more resistant to both particle size reduction (by grinding) and digestion[45] than corn with a more floury endosperm. Vitreousness increases with increasing maturity at harvest,[46] so differences among corn hybrids are greatest when field dried. Because corn silage is harvested earlier than high-moisture corn, the grain will have less vitreous endosperm and more moisture if harvested as a whole plant for silage than as high-moisture corn from the same field. However, there can be large differences in vitreousness within corn silage harvested between 30% and 40%

DM and within high-moisture corn harvested between 60% and 75% DM (40% and 25% moisture) from the same field.

When grains are ensiled, ruminal fermentability of starch can be greatly affected by both the grain moisture concentration and storage time because ensiling solubilizes endosperm proteins over time, increasing starch fermentability. The increase in protein solubility and starch fermentability over time is greatest for grains with higher moisture concentration.[47] Therefore, the change is greatest for wetter corn silage and least for drier, high-moisture corn. The greatest change occurs over the first few months of ensiling and must be anticipated and accounted for when formulating rations. Because of this, it is recommended to wait several months after ensiling before feeding corn silage. However, proteolysis continues for months at a slower rate, and corn silage and high-moisture corn stored for long periods (1 or 2 years or even more) can be difficult to feed in high concentrations because they are so readily fermented.

Processing increases the rate of starch digestion; the effects are greater for grains with more vitreous endosperm, such as sorghum and corn.[43] Steam flaking causes swelling and disruption of the kernel structure, increasing access of the enzymes to starch granules. Rolling or grinding whole grains, or processing silage to crush kernels, reduces the particle size, increasing the surface area. Dry grains can be finely ground, greatly reducing the effects of endosperm vitreousness on ruminal fermentability. Processing (rolling) corn silage is not as effective at increasing the surface area as fine grinding; however, it can reduce differences in digestibility of sources varying in vitreousness.

Measurement of starch concentration and fermentability

Starch concentration is relatively consistent within cereal grain types but varies greatly within forages containing starch, such as corn silage and small grain silages. Therefore, book values for starch concentration may be acceptable for cereal grains; but starch concentration must be measured for forages from grain crops. For instance, the starch concentration of corn silage varies from less than 20% to more than 50% of DM depending on grain concentration, which, in turn is dependent on genetics, environment, and maturity at harvest.[48] The starch concentration of corn silage is inversely related to NDF concentration; the fibrous stover fraction of the plant is enriched if kernels are not filled.

The nonfiber carbohydrate (NFC) concentration of diets is not an accurate measure of starch concentration. The NFC fraction is calculated by subtracting measured components (NDF, crude protein (CP), ether extract, ash) from total DM. It contains other carbohydrates, such as sugars and pectin, and can be underestimated to the extent that nonprotein nitrogen is present. Although starch, sugars, and pectin are generally highly digestible, their effects on rumen microbial populations and fuels available to the animal differ greatly. Starch that is ruminally fermented increases propionate production in the rumen,[49] and starch that escapes ruminal fermentation provides glucose that is absorbed or metabolized to lactate in the small intestine.[50] Sugars are nearly completely fermented in the rumen and generally increase butyrate production.[51] Most strains of pectin-degrading rumen bacteria produce acetic and formic acids and relatively little propionic acid.[52] Propionic and lactic acids are glucose precursors, whereas formic, acetic, and butyric acids are not. In addition, propionate can decrease feed intake under some conditions[5]; starch, sugars, and pectin can affect fiber digestion and ruminal biohydrogenation of FA through different effects on ruminal microbial populations. Therefore, NFC is not a useful proxy for starch when formulating rations for lactating cows.

Relative differences in rate of starch digestion can be determined by in vitro starch digestion (IVSD) with ruminal microbes. This process can be done by incubating samples over time in rumen fluid with buffered media and evaluating the rate of starch disappearance or, less costly and equally informative, by evaluating starch disappearance over a period of time (eg, 7 hours). A 7-hour incubation time seems to be a reasonable mean residence time of starch in rumens of lactating cows; therefore, it is used to predict in vivo ruminal digestibility of starch. However, it is naïve to think this technique (or any other) can provide an absolute number for starch digestibility because ruminal digestibility of starch in vivo is highly affected by the enzyme activity of the rumen fluid and particle size of the starch source and because residence time of starch in the rumen is extremely variable, not only across cows but also across sources of starch.[53] Nevertheless, 7-hour retention time IVSD provides useful information about the relative rates of fermentation among starch sources. Samples must be ground before analysis, which removes important variation for many comparisons (eg, processed vs unprocessed corn silage). Because IVSD of the same sources are highly variable across runs, comparisons must be done in the same in vitro run (at the same time). This requirement is because enzyme activities (amylases and proteases) of rumen fluid are highly variable from cow to cow, time relative to feeding, and diet consumed. For example, in our laboratory, the coefficient of variation for 7-hour IVSD across runs can be as high as 25% even after attempting to minimize variation by taking rumen fluid from several cows fed a specific diet at the same time of day relative to feeding. This is much higher than our coefficient of variation for 30-hour in vitro NDF digestibility of less than 3%.

Insoluble endosperm proteins inhibit starch digestion, and the solubility of protein has been measured as an indicator of relative differences in starch digestibility. Like IVSD, the determination of protein solubility requires grinding samples, which remove variation among sources. Because it is a chemical rather than a biological measure, it is less variable across runs than IVSD. The accuracy of ruminal starch digestibility prediction from protein solubility is limited by the relationship between protein solubility and rate of starch digestion as well as our limited knowledge of the passage rate of starch from the rumen. Therefore, like IVSD, measures of protein solubility provide some information related to ruminal starch digestion but cannot be used to measure in vivo ruminal starch digestibility accurately.

Fat Type and Concentration

Fat sources are often added to dairy cattle diets with the goal of increasing energy intake to increase milk energy output or energy balance. However, fat supplements have had inconsistent effects on energy intake in dairy cows, partly because of the differences in type and amount of fat included in the diet. Feed intake is often decreased and rarely increased with the addition of fat to diets.[5] In several experiments, the depression in feed intake by dietary fat more than offset the increased energy density of the diet resulting in decreased energy intake. The extent of intake depression by dietary fat is related to unsaturated FA reaching the duodenum.[5,24] The mechanism by which dietary fat affects feed intake is complex and likely involves the effects of FA on gut peptides and pancreatic hormones and direct and indirect effects on the hepatic oxidation of fuels. Unsaturated FA are more likely to be oxidized, whereas saturated FA are more likely to be stored,[54] consistent with greater hypophagic effects of unsaturated compared with saturated fats. Gut peptide responses likely affect hepatic oxidation through their effects on pancreatic hormones, and CCK may directly affect the firing rate of the vagal afferents causing satiety.[55]

EFFECTS OF DIET ON ENERGY INTAKE AND PARTITIONING THROUGH LACTATION

Diet composition interacts with the physiological state of cows to affect energy intake and partitioning because differences in the supply and fate of fuels depend on the lipolytic state and glucogenic capacity. In the periparturient period, feed intake is limited primarily by metabolic mechanisms; but as lactation progresses, feed intake increases and distention increasingly dominates control of feed intake. As lactation proceeds and the milk yield decreases, signals from distention diminish and feed intake is increasingly dominated by signals derived from the metabolism of fuels.

Effect of Diet and Physiologic State on Energy Intake

The extent to which ruminal distention limits feed intake is positively related to milk yield. This relationship was shown in two studies in which groups of cows with a wide range of milk yield were offered diets differing in their filling effects. The first study compared brown midrib corn silage to a control corn silage.[56] Both silages had similar DM and NDF concentrations, but in vitro NDF digestibility (30 hours) was nearly 10% higher for the low-lignin brown midrib corn silage than for the control silage. When both forages were offered to a group of cows with a wide range of milk yield, DMI and fat-corrected milk (FCM) responses to the brown midrib corn silage compared with the control corn silage increased linearly with initial milk yield of cows. Silage hybrid did not affect DMI or FCM for the lower-producing cows (~32 kg/d), but brown midrib corn silage increased FCM by approximately 8 kg/d for the highest-producing cows (~55 kg/d) compared with the control corn silage. The second study compared diets differing in forage to concentrate ratio.[57] Diets contained either 44% forage (24.3% NDF and 33.8% starch) or 67% forage (30.7% NDF and 23.1% starch). The low-forage diet increased DMI linearly with milk yield of cows (up to ~4.5 kg/d for the highest producing cows) compared with the high-forage diet, and FCM yield increased approximately 2.2 kg for each kg increase in DMI for cows producing more than approximately 40 kg FCM/d. Although the low-forage diet increased DMI across production level of cows, the forage level of the diets did not affect FCM in cows producing less than approximately 40 kg/d.

The effects of starch fermentability on DMI[58] and production[59] responses are affected by the physiological state of cows. Increased ruminal starch fermentability of rations had opposite effects on milk production depending on the initial milk yield of cows: high-moisture corn increased concentration of milk fat and FCM yield of cows producing more than approximately 40 kg of milk per day but decreased both for cows with lower milk yield.[59] Propionate flux to the liver increases when more fermentable starch is fed, which likely stimulates oxidation more quickly within the time frame of meals, increasing hepatic energy status and satiety, and decreasing meal size and DMI. However, the rate of increase in hepatic energy status depends on glucogenic flux, which varies among cows and for individual cows across lactation. Propionate carbon will increasingly oxidize acetyl CoA as propionate uptake by the liver exceeds glucogenic capacity, increasing energy charge and ultimately stimulating satiety.[9] A more rapidly fermentable starch source (high-moisture corn) depressed feed intake compared with a less-fermentable starch source (dry ground corn) for cows with greater plasma insulin concentration[58] likely because glucogenic flux is downregulated by chronically elevated plasma insulin concentration and propionate stimulates oxidation of acetyl CoA sooner during meals, stimulating satiety.

Effect of Diet and Physiological State on Energy Partitioning

Early postpartum cows are in a lipolytic state and differ greatly from cows in positive energy balance. Propionate is more hypophagic for fresh cows than cows in midlactation despite the greater glucose demand and the lower plasma insulin concentration,[60] likely because of a consistent supply of acetyl CoA derived from β-oxidation of NEFA.[9] Although high glucose demand and low plasma insulin concentration result in greater glucogenic flux, making it unlikely for propionate to be oxidized per se, uptake of propionate by the liver and entry into the tricarboxylic acid cycle increases oxidation of the pool of acetyl CoA within meals, increasing energy charge and causing satiety.[61,62] Feed intake of high-producing cows is less likely affected by propionate from highly fermentable diets because plasma glucose and insulin concentrations are low, hepatic gluconeogenesis is upregulated, and hepatic acetyl CoA concentration is low. Therefore, stimulation of oxidation within meals by propionate is likely delayed compared with fresh cows and cows in late lactation. Consequently, feed intake increases until signals from ruminal distention trigger the end of the meal. As lactation proceeds past peak and milk yield declines, feed intake is increasingly dominated by metabolic signals once again. In midlactation to late-lactation cows, highly fermentable diets often decrease feed intake and FCM yield, whereas reducing ruminal starch fermentability often increases energy intake and partitioning to milk.

Fuels derived from starch digestion include glucose precursors that are needed in greater supply as milk yield increases, whereas fermentation of fibrous feeds yields fuels that can spare glucose (eg, acetate) but provide little glucose precursors. Glucose precursors are more limiting as milk yield increases, and rations that provide more glucose precursors result in a more positive response in milk yield for higher-producing cows. Milk yield response to dry ground corn substituted for soyhulls at 30% of the diet DM increased linearly with initial milk yield of cows ranging from 28 to 62 kg/d.[63] However, there was no benefit for additional starch from corn for cows at the lower end of the range in milk yield. In an experiment mentioned previously in which the starch concentration of the ration offered to lactating cows was increased from approximately 23% to approximately 34% by decreasing the forage NDF concentration of the diet (from 24% to 16% forage NDF, respectively), DMI response to the high-starch, low-forage NDF ration increased linearly with increasing milk yield of cows, but FCM response increased only for cows producing more than approximately 40 kg/d of FCM.[57]

Energy partitioning between milk production and body condition varies depending on the fuels available and as the physiological state changes throughout lactation (see **Fig. 3**). Substitution of fiber for starch greatly alters the fuels available for intermediary processes and often results in greater partitioning of energy to milk rather than body reserves in midlactation to late-lactation cows with a low to moderate milk yield. Ipharraguerre and colleagues[64] showed that substitution of up to 40% of diet DM of soyhulls for dry ground corn increased milk fat percent (linearly from 3.60% to 3.91%) and decreased body weight gain (linearly from 1.02 to −0.14 kg/d) with no effect on milk yield (~29 kg/d) and a slight decrease in DMI (tendency, linearly from 23.8 to 22.7 kg/d). In addition, Voelker and Allen[65] demonstrated that beet pulp decreased body condition score (BCS) without decreasing yields of milk or milk fat when substituted for high-moisture corn up to 12% of the diet DM. Furthermore, a 69% forage diet (0% corn grain) containing brown midrib corn silage increased energy partitioned to milk, decreasing body weight gain while numerically increasing FCM yield compared with a 40% forage diet (29% corn grain) containing a control corn silage.[66]

In contrast, DMI and milk yield were reduced when the control corn silage, which had approximately 20% lower in vitro NDF digestibility than the brown midrib corn silage (46.5% vs 55.9%), was fed in the higher-forage diet.

As lactation proceeds, insulin concentration and sensitivity of tissues increase and energy is increasingly partitioned to body reserves. Increasing the supply of glucose precursors beyond that required for milk production increases energy partitioning to body reserves. Intravenous glucose infusion of up to 30% of the net energy requirement linearly increased plasma insulin concentration, energy balance, body weight, and back fat thickness, without affecting DMI or milk yield of midlactation cows.[67] An experiment conducted with cows in the last 2 months of lactation showed that the substitution of beet pulp for barley grain linearly decreased BCS and back fat thickness, maintained milk yield, and linearly increased milk fat yield and milk energy output.[68] The decrease in BCS and the increase in milk fat yield were associated with a linear decrease in plasma insulin concentration as well as with a linear increase in plasma NEFA concentration. High-starch diets might result in greater insulin concentration, increasing the partitioning of energy to adipose at the expense of milk; but they can also result in lower ruminal pH, decreasing fiber digestibility, and inducing MFD and, therefore, reducing milk energy output. The energy spared from the reduction in milk fat synthesis during MFD will likely be partitioned to body energy reserves, possibly by altering gene expression in adipose tissue.[25] Decreasing fermentability of diets by increasing fiber from forages or NFFS can maintain the milk yield while decreasing gain in body condition.

RECOMMENDATIONS

All forages should be tested for concentrations of DM, NDF, CP, as well as lignin or in vitro NDF digestibility. Most laboratories report lignin as a percentage of DM, which is not directly useful because lignin only limits digestion of fiber. Therefore, lignin (percentage of DM) should be divided by NDF (percentage of DM) to determine the extent to which the NDF is lignified. There are several measures of lignin used although the predominant measure is acid detergent sulfuric acid lignin (ADL). Acid detergent lignin as a percent of NDF ranges from approximately 3% to 9% for corn silage and from approximately 11% to 20% for alfalfa (hay and silage). Within a forage type, forage NDF with the lowest ADL/NDF is the least filling. Additionally, mixed grass-legume forages should be tested for acid detergent fiber (ADF) to help determine the fraction of grass and legume in the forage; ADF/NDF is approximately 0.8 for legumes and approximately 0.6 for grasses. Mixed forages with more grass should be limited for high-producing cows with intake limited by rumen fill. The following recommendations focus on meeting the energy needs through lactation by considering the concentration and digestibility of fiber and starch and their interaction with stage of lactation.

Far-off Dry Cows (8 Weeks–3 Weeks Prepartum)

The goal is to meet, but not exceed, energy requirements and maintain BCS.

Allocation of forages

Use forages with high NDF and low crude protein concentrations, such as mature grass hay or silage and straw, to limit the energy intake to requirements. Forages with low NDF digestibility and long ruminal retention times can be used. Limit corn silage with high grain concentrations.

Supplementation

Add grain only to meet the energy requirements, limiting body condition gain.

Close-up Dry Cows (3 Weeks Prepartum to Parturition)

The goal is to meet, but not exceed, energy requirements and maintain rumen fill through the transition period. The pool of ruminal digesta will provide energy, buffering capacity, and distention to reduce the risk of ketosis, acidosis, and displaced abomasum, respectively, following parturition.

Allocation of forages
Wheat straw digests and likely passes from the rumen slowly and it can be used to dilute energy density of corn silage in total mixed rations (TMRs) for dry cows. Grass silage or hay might be more beneficial because the fiber is more digestible and it provides energy for a longer time when feed intake decreases around calving. However, the use of grasses with high potassium concentrations should be limited to reduce milk fever in the postpartum period. Avoid finely chopped silages (to ensure adequate rumen retention time) and forages with high protein concentrations (to decrease nitrogen excretion).

Supplementation
Include a limited amount of moderately fermentable starch to stimulate insulin secretion and limit fat mobilization while maintaining rumen fill. NFFS do not provide glucose precursors or rumen fill and should be limited. Measure and record BCS at dry-off and at parturition to adjust the energy concentration of dry cow diets.

Fresh Cows (Parturition to ~2 Weeks Postpartum)

These cows require glucose precursors, and rations should contain higher starch concentrations to the extent possible. However, they also have lower rumen digesta mass, which increases the risk of low ruminal pH as well as displaced abomasum. Therefore, the goal with this diet is to maintain rumen fill and to provide glucose precursors in a form that will maximize energy intake. Cows should be switched to the high-group ration when they are cleared of health problems, have increasing milk production, and are aggressive at the feed bunk following feeding. Most cows will be in this group for less than 2 weeks, but cows with excessive body condition at parturition might be in this group for longer.

Allocation of forages
Use forages with a moderate to high NDF concentration and high NDF digestibility but long ruminal retention times, such as grass hay or silage. The use of forages with high NDF concentrations will allow adequate dietary space for grain while maintaining rumen fill. Avoid finely chopped silages. Consider that long fiber particles are necessary to form a mat and increase digesta retention in the rumen; but excessive length of cut can increase sorting, particularly in dry diets. Corn silage can be used; but limit highly fermentable corn silage (eg, aged corn silage ensiled for more than 1 year, corn silage less than 30% DM, overprocessed corn silage) because it might be too fermentable and, therefore, limit feed intake during this period.

Supplementation
Avoid feeding very highly fermentable starch sources (eg, wheat, barley, low-density steam-flaked corn, and aged [>1 year old] high-moisture corn and corn silage) to fresh cows because rapid production and absorption of propionate can stimulate hepatic oxidation and suppress feed intake, particularly for cows in a lipolytic state.[9,61] Starch sources with moderate ruminal fermentability and high digestibility in the small intestine, such as dry ground corn, can be fed at higher concentrations in the diet to provide more glucose precursors without suppressing feed intake or decreasing ruminal pH. Reduction in ruminal pH can reduce fiber digestibility and energy intake. Dry ground

corn (finely ground) is the preferred starch source because of its moderate rumen fermentability (~60%) but high whole-tract digestibility (>90%). Supplementing corn silage–based diets with dry ground corn works well for this ration, with a total starch concentration of 22%–25% (DM basis). Starch concentration must be decreased when feeding highly fermentable starch sources. Because feed intake is less limited by ruminal distention and greater rumen digesta mass is desirable during this period, the forage NDF concentration should be relatively high (~22% of diet DM) and NFFS should be limited to diluting starch concentration when necessary. NFFS can be used to dilute starch when high NDF forages are used but should otherwise be limited because they provide few glucose precursors and little rumen fill.

High-Producing Cows (~2 Weeks Postpartum to ~3 Body Condition Score)

Cows in early to midlactation have a high glucose requirement for milk production and partition relatively little energy to body reserves. They respond well to rations with low forage NDF concentration (low fill) and highly fermentable starch. Therefore, the goal is to feed a low-fill, highly fermentable diet as gut fill begins to dominate control of feed intake. Gut-fill might begin to dominate control of feed intake beginning 2 weeks after calving for some cows in the herd or after 3 weeks for others, and is likely indicated by low plasma NEFA and ketone concentrations, increasing milk production, and aggressive intake. Cows should be switched to the maintenance ration when BCS exceeds 3.0 on a 1-to-5 scale.

Allocation of forages
Use forages with high fiber fragility, such as brown-midrib corn silage and legume hay or silage; these forage sources will clear from the rumen at a faster rate and will allow greater feed and energy intakes compared with forages that have longer retention times in the rumen (eg, mature grasses). Adequate long particles are needed to retain potentially fermentable particles, increasing the overall diet digestibility. Forages with low NDF concentrations (except for corn silage) might limit the diet space for starch, which is needed to provide glucose precursors; therefore, it should be used sparingly. For instance, it is difficult to meet the requirements for physically effective fiber and include an adequate starch concentration in the ration using alfalfa silage with 35% NDF.

Supplementation
High-producing cows respond favorably to highly fermentable diets. Starch sources, such as low-density steam-flaked corn, high-moisture corn, or rolled barley, work well in these diets. However, starch sources that are very rapidly fermented, such as ground wheat, should be limited. Starch concentration of rations should be in the range of 25% to 30% (DM basis), although the optimum concentration depends on competition for bunk space, forage/effective NDF concentration, and starch fermentability. Higher-starch, lower-fill rations generally increase peak milk yield and decrease the loss of body condition in early lactation. Once the body condition that was lost in early lactation is replenished, cows should be switched to a maintenance diet with a lower starch concentration and ruminal fermentability. NFFS can be used to dilute starch, if needed, but should otherwise be limited because they provide few glucose precursors. Restoration of body condition will occur sooner in lactation for diets with lower forage NDF and greater starch concentrations because the extent and duration of the negative energy balance will be lessened. Therefore, the number of cows receiving both this and the maintenance diet is affected by the composition of this ration; this diet must be adjusted according to the number of stalls and bunk space available for cows in each diet group.

Maintenance Group (>150 Days Postpartum and ~3 Body Condition Score)

The maintenance ration is the key component of a ration formulation/grouping system to increase the health and production of cows. The goal is to maintain the BCS (preventing further body weight gain) while also maintaining or increasing milk yield. Cows should be offered the maintenance ration when they have replenished body reserves, reaching a BCS of 3. Cows gain body condition when offered rations with greater starch concentrations than required for milk production, which increases plasma glucose and insulin concentrations and partitions energy to body reserves. If they continue receiving a high-starch diet, BCS will continue to increase and they will be at increased risk of metabolic disease following parturition. Moreover, as lactation progresses past midlactation, the highly fermentable diet that is optimal for high-producing cows can depress feed intake as milk yield and glucose demand decreases, increasing the risk of abomasal displacement and MFD. It is, therefore, suggested to feed a more filling, less fermentable diet as milk yield declines. This practice will increase feed intake and provide a more consistent supply of fuels, partitioning more energy to milk rather than body reserves.

Allocation of forages
Forages with a wide range of NDF concentration can be used in these diets, but the NDF should be potentially digestible. More grass can be included in these diets; although grass fiber may have longer retention time in the rumen and be more filling, it is generally more digestible than fiber from legumes. High-protein forages should be limited to avoid feeding excess protein.

Supplementation
Lowering ration starch concentration should limit the body condition gain while maintaining and possibly improving feed intake and yields of milk and milk fat. The optimal concentration of starch depends on the milk yield of the herd and possible physical groups but will likely be in the range of 18% to 22% (DM basis). The BCS should be determined and recorded when cows are moved to the maintenance group and again at dry-off. Monitoring BCS is essential to adjust the starch concentration of the maintenance diet over time. Highly fermentable starch sources (eg, aged corn silage, high-moisture corn, bakery waste, ground barley, wheat) should be limited, if not avoided, by substituting less fermentable feeds, such as dry ground corn or NFFS. Nonforage fiber sources (beet pulp, corn gluten feed, soyhulls, and so forth) can be used to dilute starch to the target concentration. These flex-fuel cows have lower requirements for glucose precursors and can better use nonstarch feeds to provide energy in a form to spare glucose. Unsaturated fats likely decrease feed intake and increase the risk of MFD and subsequent partitioning of energy to body reserves and should, therefore, be limited.

SUMMARY

The management of energy balance through lactation is necessary to maximize milk yield, efficiency of milk production, and animal health. Carbohydrates compose the largest fraction of diet DM of lactating cows and vary greatly in physical form and products of digestion.

The type and temporal supply of fuels interact with the physiological state of cows to affect the energy intake and partitioning. Consideration of the physical and digestion characteristics of diets beyond their nutrient composition and how they interact with physiological stages as they change through lactation to affect energy intake and partitioning is of crucial importance to optimize forage allocation and supplementation for lactating cows as well as to formulate and adjust diets to maximize milk production and promote animal health.

REFERENCES

1. Forbes JM. A personal view of how ruminant animals control their intake and choice of food: minimal total discomfort. Nutr Res Rev 2007;20(2):132–46.
2. Allen MS. Physical constraints on voluntary intake of forages by ruminants. J Anim Sci 1996;74(12):3063–75.
3. Leek BF. Sensory receptors in the ruminant alimentary tract. In: Milligan LP, Grovum WL, Dobson A, editors. Control of digestion and metabolism in ruminants. 1986. p. 1–17. Prentice-Hall Englewood Cliffs, NJ.
4. Schettini MA, Prigge EC, Nestor EL. Influence of mass and volume of ruminal contents on voluntary intake and digesta passage of a forage diet in steers. J Anim Sci 1999;77(7):1896–904.
5. Allen MS. Effects of diet on short-term regulation of feed intake by lactating dairy cattle. J Dairy Sci 2000;83(7):1598–624.
6. Langhans W, Damaske U, Scharrer E. Different metabolites might reduce food intake by the mitochondrial generation of reducing equivalents. Appetite 1985;6(2):143–52.
7. Anil MH, Forbes JM. The roles of hepatic nerves in the reduction of food intake as a consequence of intraportal sodium propionate administration in sheep. Q J Exp Physiol 1988;73(4):539–46.
8. Friedman MI, Harris RB, Ji H, et al. Fatty acid oxidation affects food intake by altering hepatic energy status. Am J Physiol 1999;276(4 Pt 2):R1046–53.
9. Allen MS, Bradford BJ, Oba M. Board invited review: the hepatic oxidation theory of the control of feed intake and its application to ruminants. J Anim Sci 2009;87(10):3317–34.
10. Allen MS, Bradford BJ. Control of food intake by metabolism of fuels: a comparison across species. Proc Nutr Soc 2012;71(3):401–9.
11. Allen MS, Piantoni P. Metabolic control of feed intake: implications for metabolic disease of fresh cows. Vet Clin North Am Food Anim Pract 2013;29(2):279–97.
12. Bradford BJ, Harvatine KJ, Allen MS. Dietary unsaturated fatty acids increase plasma glucagon-like peptide-1 and cholecystokinin and may decrease pre-meal ghrelin in lactating dairy cows. J Dairy Sci 2008;91(4):1443–50.
13. Relling AE, Reynolds CK. Abomasal infusion of casein, starch and soybean oil differentially affect plasma concentrations of gut peptides and feed intake in lactating dairy cows. Domest Anim Endocrinol 2008;35(1):35–45.
14. Houseknecht KL, Baile CA, Matteri RL, et al. The biology of leptin: a review. J Anim Sci 1998;76(5):1405–20.
15. Brockman RP, Laarveld B. Hormonal regulation of metabolism in ruminants; a review. Livest Prod Sci 1986;14(4):313–34.
16. De Koster JD, Opsomer G. Insulin resistance in dairy cows. Vet Clin North Am Food Anim Pract 2013;29(2):299–322.
17. Bauman DE. Bovine somatotropin: review of an emerging animal technology. J Dairy Sci 1992;75(12):3432–51.
18. Gustafson B, Hammarstedt A, Andersson CX, et al. Inflamed adipose tissue: a culprit underlying the metabolic syndrome and atherosclerosis. Arterioscler Thromb Vasc Biol 2007;27(11):2276–83.
19. Qatanani M, Lazar MA. Mechanisms of obesity-associated insulin resistance: many choices on the menu. Genes Dev 2007;21(12):1443–55.

20. Sordillo LM, Raphael W. Significance of metabolic stress, lipid mobilization, and inflammation on transition cow disorders. Vet Clin North Am Food Anim Pract 2013;29(2):267–78.
21. Pires JA, Souza AH, Grummer RR. Induction of hyperlipidemia by intravenous infusion of tallow emulsion causes insulin resistance in Holstein cows. J Dairy Sci 2007;90(6):2735–44.
22. Soderholm CG, Otterby DE, Linn JG, et al. Effects of recombinant bovine somatotropin on milk production, body composition, and physiological parameters. J Dairy Sci 1988;71(2):355–65.
23. Baumgard LH, Sangster JK, Bauman DE. Milk fat synthesis in dairy cows is progressively reduced by increasing supplemental amounts of trans-10, cis-12 conjugated linoleic acid (CLA). J Nutr 2001;131(6):1764–9.
24. Harvatine KJ, Allen MS. Effects of fatty acid supplements on milk yield and energy balance of lactating dairy cows. J Dairy Sci 2006;89(3):1081–91.
25. Harvatine KJ, Perfield JW, Bauman DE. Expression of enzymes and key regulators of lipid synthesis is upregulated in adipose tissue during CLA-induced milk fat depression in dairy cows. J Nutr 2009;139(5):849–54.
26. Baumgard LH, Corl BA, Dwyer DA, et al. Effects of conjugated linoleic acids (CLA) on tissue response to homeostatic signals and plasma variables associated with lipid metabolism in lactating dairy cows. J Anim Sci 2002;80(5):1285–93.
27. Allen MS. Relationship between fermentation acid production in the rumen and the requirement for physically effective fiber. J Dairy Sci 1997;80(7):1447–62.
28. Bauman DE, Harvatine KJ, Lock AL. Nutrigenomics, rumen-derived bioactive fatty acids, and the regulation of milk fat synthesis. Annu Rev Nutr 2011;31:299–319.
29. Harvatine KJ, Allen MS. Effects of fatty acid supplements on feed intake, and feeding and chewing behavior of lactating dairy cows. J Dairy Sci 2006;89(3):1104–12.
30. Harvatine KJ, Allen MS. Fat supplements affect fractional rates of ruminal fatty acid biohydrogenation and passage in dairy cows. J Nutr 2006;136(3):677–85.
31. Zachut M, Honig H, Striem S, et al. Periparturient dairy cows do not exhibit hepatic insulin resistance, yet adipose-specific insulin resistance occurs in cows prone to high weight loss. J Dairy Sci 2013;96(9):5656–69.
32. Bell AW, Bauman DE. Adaptations of glucose metabolism during pregnancy and lactation. J Mammary Gland Biol Neoplasia 1997;2(3):265–78.
33. Beauchemin KA, Farr BI, Rode LM, et al. Effects of alfalfa silage chop length and supplementary long hay on chewing and milk production of dairy cows. J Dairy Sci 1994;77(5):1326–39.
34. Oba M, Allen MS. Evaluation of the importance of the digestibility of neutral detergent fiber from forage: effects on dry matter intake and milk yield of dairy cows. J Dairy Sci 1999;82(3):589–96.
35. Linton JA, Allen MS. Nutrient demand interacts with forage family to affect intake and digestion responses in dairy cows. J Dairy Sci 2008;91(7):2694–701.
36. Kammes KL, Allen MS. Nutrient demand interacts with forage family to affect digestion responses in dairy cows. J Dairy Sci 2012;95(6):3269–87.
37. Kammes KL, Allen MS. Rates of particle size reduction and passage are faster for legume compared with cool-season grass, resulting in lower rumen fill and less effective fiber. J Dairy Sci 2012;95(6):3288–97.
38. Kotarski SF, Waniska RD, Thurn KK. Starch hydrolysis by the ruminal microflora. J Nutr 1992;122(1):178–90.

39. Nocek JE, Tamminga S. Site of digestion of starch in the gastrointestinal tract of dairy cows and its effect on milk yield and composition. J Dairy Sci 1991; 74(10):3598–629.
40. Firkins J, Eastridge M, St-Pierre N. Effects of grain variability and processing on starch utilization by lactating dairy cattle. J Anim Sci 2001;79(E-Suppl):E218–38.
41. Ngonyamo-Majee D, Shaver RD, Coors JG, et al. Relationships between kernel vitreousness and dry matter degradability for diverse corn germ plasm. Anim Feed Sci Technol 2008;142(3–4):259–74.
42. Oba M, Allen MS. Effects of corn grain conservation method on feeding behavior and productivity of lactating dairy cows at two dietary starch concentrations. J Dairy Sci 2003;86(1):174–83.
43. Huntington GB. Starch utilization by ruminants: from basics to the bunk. J Anim Sci 1997;75(3):852–67.
44. Hoffman PC, Shaver RD. The nutritional chemistry of dry and high moisture corn. Reno(NV): Proc 10th Western Dairy Management Conference. March 9–11, 2011. p. 179–94.
45. Hoffman PC, Ngonyamo-Majee D, Shaver RD. Technical note: determination of corn hardness in diverse corn germ plasm using near-infrared reflectance baseline shift as a measure of grinding resistance. J Dairy Sci 2010;93(4):1685–9.
46. Philippeau C, Michalet-Doreau B. Influence of genotype and ensiling of corn grain on in situ degradation of starch in the rumen. J Dairy Sci 1998;81(8): 2178–84.
47. Allen MS, Grant RJ, Weiss WP, et al. Effects of endosperm type of corn grain on starch degradability by ruminal microbes in vitro. J Dairy Sci 2003;(86S):61.
48. Allen MS, Coors JG, Roth GW. Corn silage. In: Silage science and technology, Agronomy monograph, vol. 42. American Society of Agronomy, Crop Science Society of America, Soil Science Society of America, Madison, WI; 2003. p. 547–608.
49. Sutton JD, Dhanoa MS, Morant SV, et al. Rates of production of acetate, propionate, and butyrate in the rumen of lactating dairy cows given normal and low-roughage diets. J Dairy Sci 2003;86(11):3620–33.
50. Reynolds CK, Aikman PC, Lupoli B, et al. Splanchnic metabolism of dairy cows during the transition from late gestation through early lactation. J Dairy Sci 2003; 86(4):1201–17.
51. Oba M. Review: effects of feeding sugars on productivity of lactating dairy cows. Can J Anim Sci 2011;91(1):37–46.
52. Dehority BA. Pectin-fermenting bacteria isolated from the bovine rumen. J Bacteriol 1969;99(1):189–96.
53. Allen MS. Adjusting concentration and ruminal digestibility of starch through lactation. In: Proceedings of the Four-State Dairy Nutrition and Management Conference. Dubuque(IA), June 13–14, 2012. p. 24–30.
54. Leyton J, Drury PJ, Crawford MA. Differential oxidation of saturated and unsaturated fatty acids in vivo in the rat. Br J Nutr 1987;57(3):383–93.
55. Richards W, Hillsley K, Eastwood C, et al. Sensitivity of vagal mucosal afferents to cholecystokinin and its role in afferent signal transduction in the rat. J Physiol 1996;497(Pt 2):473–81.
56. Oba M, Allen MS. Effects of brown midrib 3 mutation in corn silage on dry matter intake and productivity of high yielding dairy cows. J Dairy Sci 1999;82(1):135–42.
57. Voelker JA, Burato GM, Allen MS. Effects of pretrial milk yield on responses of feed intake, digestion, and production to dietary forage concentration. J Dairy Sci 2002;85(10):2650–61.

58. Bradford BJ, Allen MS. Depression in feed intake by a highly fermentable diet is related to plasma insulin concentration and insulin response to glucose infusion. J Dairy Sci 2007;90(8):3838–45.
59. Bradford BJ, Allen MS. Milk fat responses to a change in diet fermentability vary by production level in dairy cattle. J Dairy Sci 2004;87(11):3800–7.
60. Oba M, Allen MS. Dose-response effects of intrauminal infusion of propionate on feeding behavior of lactating cows in early or midlactation. J Dairy Sci 2003; 86(9):2922–31.
61. Stocks SE, Allen MS. Hypophagic effects of propionate increase with elevated hepatic acetyl coenzyme A concentration for cows in the early postpartum period. J Dairy Sci 2012;95(6):3259–68.
62. Stocks SE, Allen MS. Hypophagic effects of propionic acid are not attenuated during a 3-day infusion in the early postpartum period in Holstein cows. J Dairy Sci 2013;96(7):4615–23.
63. Ploetz CJ, Burczynski SE, VandeHaar MJ, et al. Milk production responses to a change in dietary starch concentration vary by production level in dairy cattle. J Dairy Sci 2013;96(Suppl 1):252–3.
64. Ipharraguerre IR, Ipharraguerre RR, Clark JH. Performance of lactating dairy cows fed varying amounts of soyhulls as a replacement for corn grain. J Dairy Sci 2002;85(11):2905–12.
65. Voelker JA, Allen MS. Pelleted beet pulp substituted for high-moisture corn: 1. Effects on feed intake, chewing behavior, and milk production of lactating dairy cows. J Dairy Sci 2003;86(11):3542–52.
66. Oba M, Allen MS. Effects of brown midrib 3 mutation in corn silage on productivity of dairy cows fed two concentrations of dietary neutral detergent fiber: 1. Feeding behavior and nutrient utilization. J Dairy Sci 2000;83(6):1333–41.
67. Al-Trad B, Reisberg K, Wittek T, et al. Increasing intravenous infusions of glucose improve body condition but not lactation performance in midlactation dairy cows. J Dairy Sci 2009;92(11):5645–58.
68. Mahjoubi E, Amanlou H, Zahmatkesh D. Use of beet pulp as a replacement for barley grain to manage body condition score in over-conditioned late lactation cows. Anim Feed Sci Technol 2009;153(1–2):60–7.

Protein Feeding and Balancing for Amino Acids in Lactating Dairy Cattle

Robert A. Patton, MS, PhD, PAS[a],*,
Alexander N. Hristov, MSc, PhD, PAS[b], Hélène Lapierre, agr, MSc, PhD[c]

KEYWORDS

- Amino acids • Lactation • Metabolizable protein • Microbial protein • Limiting AA

KEY POINTS

- Amino acid (AA) nutrition of the dairy cow is complicated because of feeding 2 systems at the same time: one microbial and one mammalian.
- The cow must detoxify ammonia to urea; excess urea is secreted in urine.
- Several nutrition models can predict duodenal flow of protein and essential AA (EAA) with reasonable accuracy as well as the digestible flow of individual EAA leading to a prediction of metabolizable protein (MP).
- Metabolism of absorbed AA still has not been well characterized.
- All EAA can become limiting depending on the diet, but lysine, methionine, histidine, and leucine have been the most studied.
- Requirements for MP and AA for the lactating dairy cow have also not been well defined.
- Balancing for MP and AA should allow feeding of lower protein rations resulting in greater milk nitrogen efficiency and less environmental impact.
- AA balance for dairy cattle is still an evolving science.

INTRODUCTION

Nature has made the protein nutrition of the lactating dairy cow complicated. When dairy cows are fed, two systems are being fed: a microbial system that can use amino acid (AA) but whose basic requirement is for ammonia and nonprotein nitrogen (NPN),

Funding Sources: None.
Conflict of Interest: None.
[a] Nittany Dairy Nutrition Incorporated, 9355 Buffalo Road, Mifflinburg, PA 17844, USA; [b] Department of Animal Science, Pennsylvania State University, 324 Henning Building, University Park, PA 16802, USA; [c] Dairy and Swine Research and Development Centre, Agriculture and Agri-Food Canada, 2000 College Street, Sherbrooke, Québec J1M 0C8, Canada
* Corresponding author.
E-mail address: nittnut@aol.com

and a mammalian system that requires AA and must detoxify ammonia as in other mammalian species.

Interdependency of these systems complicates defining AA requirements and supply. First, the amount of microbial protein (MCP) must be determined, and then this amount must be separated from dietary AAs that escape rumen degradation. The sum of MCP and dietary AAs that escape rumen degradation and that flows to the small intestine is, after digestion in the small intestine, termed metabolizable protein (MP). The term MP is used to define the total AA available to the cow in support of all physiologic functions.

Studies that are needed to close gaps in the knowledge of these interactions, in order that cow MP requirements may be better defined, require costly and invasive techniques. Furthermore, animal studies are often of short duration, because both of the expense and the intensive labor needed to conduct such studies. This limitation should be considered when evaluating AA effects because in the short term, the animal may be able to use body protein to fulfill deficiencies. The body condition loss in early lactation is a good example. Conversely, the animal may respond to AA treatment in the short term but may adjust and show no response in the longer term.[1]

On a practical basis, dietary crude protein (CP) is often overfed to ensure a sufficient supply of all AA to support all biological functions. Balancing milking cow rations for AA can increase profitability by lowering protein cost and increasing production of milk and milk protein.[2,3] However, this does not occur in all circumstances.[4,5] Lowering CP intake by adequate balancing for AA will reduce urea excretion and therefore environmental pollution. Unfortunately, lowering the MP supply without regard to the AA composition of the MP can significantly reduce milk production.[3,5]

For a variety of reasons, there are many questions regarding the application of AA balancing. There is a need for specific field recommendations regarding the use of MP and AA concepts to achieve greater economy and efficiency of protein utilization.

The purpose of this article is to describe the current knowledge of protein and AA metabolism in lactating cows with an emphasis on information generated since National Research Council (NRC) 2001, discuss areas where the knowledge is incomplete, and suggest some recommendations to make AA balancing practical.

Amino Acids for Dairy Cows

Of the 20 AAs required to build proteins, 9 are considered essential because the cow cannot produce them: histidine (His), isoleucine (Ile), leucine (Leu), lysine (Lys), methionine (Met), phenylalanine (Phe), threonine (Thr), tryptophan (Trp), and valine (Val). Although arginine (Arg) can be synthesized by the cow, it should be considered provisionally essential because it can become limiting under conditions of high production or disease.[6]

The nonessential AAs (NEAA) are also required for protein synthesis, but in addition to dietary sources, they are all synthesized by tissues from other AAs, both essential and nonessential.[7] In addition to dietary sources of protein that escape rumen degradation, rumen bacteria produce both NEAA and essential AA (EAA). The AAs of rumen microbes are well-digested and reasonably well-balanced relative to the AA needs of the cow, whereas both the digestibility and the balance of dietary AA can vary considerably.

AMINO ACID FLOW TO THE SMALL INTESTINE

The flow of AA arriving at the duodenum with the potential to be digested and absorbed originates from 3 sources:

- MCP leaving the rumen
- Undegraded portion of feed protein
- Endogenous protein secreted by gut tissue

Microbial Protein Synthesis in the Rumen

The MCP provides most of the MP (including both EAA and NEAA), is lowest in cost, and has an AA distribution much like milk (**Table 1**). However, MCP is deficient relative to milk protein in His and Met. Providing a rumen environment that produces the optimum amount of MCP should be a major goal when balancing dairy rations.

The factors known to impact the amount of MCP production have been reviewed,[7,8] and little additional knowledge has been added since these studies. Briefly, the factors exerting the greatest influence on MCP synthesis are as follows:

- Presence of an adequate rumen fiber mat to provide a good microbial environment as well as to provide rumination and buffering
- Providing adequate fermentable organic matter; the amount of organic matter (ie, neutral detergent fiber [NDF], non-fiber carbohydrate [NFC], and true protein) that is fermented will determine the amount of MCP produced
- Maintaining a level of degradable protein that provides sufficient free rumen AA and ammonia concentration.[9]

The MCP has 2 sources: bacteria and protozoa. Protozoa contribute varying percentages of the MCP ranging from 5% to 20%.[10,11] Previously it was thought little protozoal protein reached the abomasum because protozoa were preferentially held in the rumen.

There are 3 sources of the free ammonia for rumen bacteria:

- Degraded feed protein
- Urea from saliva and from arterial blood passing directly through the rumen wall
- Ammonia that becomes available from microbial cell lysis.

Combinations of these processes along with the mixing of rumen contents provide stable levels of rumen ammonia, free AA, and peptides.[12] Stable ammonia levels along with multiple meals and different rates of carbohydrate degradation account for the modest success of timing protein and carbohydrate degradation, although in vitro studies suggest that the effect should be significant.[13]

Both the percentage of MCP that is true protein and the AA composition of that true protein have been the subject of debate.[7,14] Estimates between 50% and 80% of MCP as true protein are common. A review by Clark and colleagues[15] summarized the variation in reported AA composition. Some of this difference may be due to the contamination of bacterial protein with feed protein. Estimates of bacterial and protozoal AA composition are summarized in **Table 1** along with feed proteins.

Rumen Undegradable Protein

The other major source ($\sim$30%–45% of total AA flow to the duodenum) is feed protein that is not degraded in the rumen.[7] This proportion may be overestimated because of the presence of endogenous protein.

Overall, rumen undegradable protein (RUP) content of a feed is determined by:

- AA content of the feed protein
- Physical structure (folding) of the protein
- Amount of heating the protein has undergone.

Proteins with more cross-binding are more resistant to microbial degradation and tend to have a more compact physical structure. Proteins with more Lys and Arg residues are more susceptible to degradation because these residues are more easily attacked by bacterial enzymes. Proteins that have more tertiary folding are more

Table 1
Mean essential AA composition (% of CP) of milk, rumen microbes, bovine tissue, and various feedstuff

Item	AA										% EAA[a]
	Arg	His	Ile	Leu	Lys	Met	Phe	Thr	Trp	Val	
Milk[b]	3.3	2.8	5.7	9.9	7.9	3.0	5.0	4.1	1.4	6.6	49.7
Rumen bacteria[c]	5.1	2.0	5.7	8.1	7.9	2.6	5.1	5.8	—	6.2	48.5
Rumen protozoa[d,92]	3.5	1.5	5.5	6.7	8.2	1.7	4.7	4.4	—	5.2	42.4
Alfalfa hay, 18.1% CP[e]	4.2	1.9	3.9	6.7	4.8	1.3	4.6	4.0	1.4	5.0	37.8
Alfalfa silage, 19.3% CP	1.8	1.9	4.1	6.7	4.7	1.3	4.4	3.8	1.2	5.1	35.1
Corn silage, 8.2% CP	2.3	1.7	3.4	8.5	2.8	1.6	3.9	3.4	0.7	4.5	32.9
Grass silage, 18.8% CP	3.0	1.5	4.1	7.1	4.3	1.5	4.5	3.9	—	5.3	35.3
Grass pasture, 13.4% CP	4.1	1.9	4.0	7.4	4.9	1.6	4.8	4.1	2.1	5.2	40.1
Barley grain, 12.3% CP	4.9	2.2	3.4	6.8	3.6	3.6	5.1	3.3	1.2	4.8	39.0
Corn grain, 9.1% CP	4.8	2.9	3.4	12.0	3.0	2.0	4.9	3.6	0.8	4.6	41.9
Wheat grain, 11.9% CP	4.8	2.3	3.3	6.6	2.8	1.5	4.5	2.9	1.3	4.2	34.0
Corn distillers (distillers dried grains), 29.9% CP	4.3	2.7	3.7	11.7	2.8	2.0	4.9	3.7	0.8	4.9	41.3
Canola meal, 42.5% CP	6.4	2.9	4.2	6.8	5.9	2.1	4.2	4.5	1.5	5.4	43.7
Soybean meal, 53.3% CP	7.3	2.6	4.5	7.6	6.1	1.3	5.1	3.9	1.3	4.7	44.5
Blood meal, 93.4% CP	4.3	5.9	1.1	12.3	8.7	1.2	6.8	4.6	1.4	8.2	54.3
Pork meal, 59.1% CP	6.7	2.0	2.8	5.8	5.1	1.4	3.3	3.1	0.7	4.0	34.7
Poultry meal, 62.1% CP	6.6	2.2	3.8	7.0	5.9	1.9	3.9	3.9	1.0	4.7	41.0

a % of essential AAs of total.
b Data from Lapierre H, Lobley GE, Doepel L, et al. Triennial lactation symposium: mammary metabolism of amino acids in dairy cows. J Anim Sci 2012;90:1708–21.
c Data from Clark JH, Klusmeyer TH, Cameron MR. Microbial protein synthesis and flows of nitrogen fractions to the duodenum of dairy cows. J Dairy Sci 1992;75:2304–23.
d Data from Ibrahim EA, Ingalls JR. Microbial protein biosynthesis in the rumen. J Dairy Sci 1972;55:971–8.
e CP, % DM; all feed data from: AminoDat V5, 2013.

resistant to microbial degradation as are those proteins that have undergone more heating.[7] These factors are accounted for in estimates of CP rumen degradability as used by various nutritional models.

When proteins are heated, 3 physical processes occur:

- Compaction of the protein, making it more difficult for the microbes to attach
- AA residues bind to fiber of the feed, increasing the amount of RUP and reducing the overall digestibility of the protein
- Formation of Maillard products, which are indigestible.

Another factor that determines degradation is the physical form of the protein.[16] Proteins with smaller particle size are more degradable than larger particles within the same protein source. If the particle is not readily fermentable, the particle has the potential to pass out of the rumen more rapidly, reducing overall degradability. Any factors increasing the rate of passage reduce protein degradability.

Different systems have been developed for modeling the amount of a feed protein that is undegraded.[17] Models use 1, 3 (A, B, C), or 5 (A1, A2, B1, B2, C) protein fractions to calculate the protein degradability, with each feed ingredient having its own protein fractions.

Studies suggest there is little difference in EAA content between intact protein and RUP.[7,18,19] However, some data indicate there are significant differences in AA composition between the intact protein and the portion of protein that escapes degradation.[8] Most of this difference appears to be in Arg, Lys, and NEAA. However, for the feeds that are highly resistant to degradation, such as animal protein meals, there seems to be substantial AA differences between fractions.[20,21] In summary, most data indicate there are no major differences in AA distribution between the whole protein and the RUP fraction except for animal-based protein meals or those products that have been damaged, by heat or silages that have undergone extensive protein hydrolysis and/or which have been subject to aeration and secondary fermentation.

Endogenous Protein

The third source of duodenal AA flow is AA from endogenous secretion.[7] Endogenous protein includes salivary, gastric, pancreatic and bile secretions, and mucus and sloughed cells.[22] The amount of endogenous protein is currently thought to be related to the dry matter intake (DMI), although estimates of endogenous protein vary significantly (from −0.85 at low intakes to 8.5 g N/kg DMI at high intake[23]). There is only one study that has directly measured the AA content of pre-duodenal endogenous protein in cattle.[24] Because of limited data, some modelers ignore the AA contribution of endogenous protein to duodenal flow and consider that any AA from endogenous protein is part of the maintenance requirement.

- Endogenous protein contribution is estimated between 1%[8] and 15%[25] of total duodenal AA flow and everywhere in between.[10]
- Endogenous protein secretion in the duodenal flow does not represent a net supply because these AA have already been absorbed.

Protein in the Diet

The true protein content of the dietary CP depends on the type of feed. In refined protein meals, there is a high amount of true protein, typically greater than 88%. For forages other than corn silage, there is a high percentage of NPN, typically about 40% to 45% for grasses and up to 88% for alfalfa silages. Legumes usually contain more NPN than true protein[19]; however, this does not normally present a problem because it is considered part of the degradable protein and, if matched with sufficient carbohydrate, makes for efficient production of bacterial protein.

The NPN sources found in feeds include the following:

- Free AA
- Urea
- Ammonia
- Amines
- Nitrates and nitrites
- Small peptides.

Depending on the microbial species present and the amount of fermentable organic matter, all NPN can contribute to AA synthesis.

- The AA composition of feed is genetically determined, and, therefore, tends to be conserved.

However, the genetically determined AA composition of the intact protein can be modified by processing (particularly heating), hydrolysis (such as occurs in silages or wet storage), and contamination by bacteria or mold (as happens under poor storage conditions). Heated products (such as blood meal, roasted soy beans, and dry distillers grain), byproduct feeds (ie, cookie meal and bakery waste), as well as poorly fermented silages are products whose AA content and availability can vary greatly[26] and should be tested for degradability, digestibility, and AA content.

Transformation of Dietary Protein in the Rumen

There are 3 fates for dietary CP once it reaches the rumen[7]:

- NPN fraction is quickly converted to rumen ammonia
- Degradable true protein (RDP) is fermented by some species of bacteria to produce CO_2, volatile fatty acids, ammonia, peptides, and free AA
- RUP fraction passes from the rumen into the omasum.

Recent studies[27,28] suggest that more peptide and free AA pass from the rumen to the omasum and perhaps to the small intestine than was previously estimated because these pass quickly with the liquid fraction. Excess ammonia can be absorbed directly from the rumen[12] or from the small intestine (33%–50% of ammonia absorption).[29]

Ammonia absorbed into portal blood flows to the liver where it is detoxified into urea. Urea produced by the liver is partly reintroduced into the gut, including the rumen, via saliva or directly from arterial blood through the gut wall, apparently as salvage mechanisms for N, or is removed by the kidneys to be excreted in urine.[23,30] Urine nitrogen is the primary source of ammonia emitted from manure.[31] The proportion of the urea produced, which is recycled to the rumen, is reduced as MP supply is increased[32] and as N is consumption is increased.[33]

Supply Summary

Despite all the factors affecting the fate of dietary protein in the rumen and sometimes contradictory research, the newer computer models have been able to capture the complexity of rumen metabolism and produce adequate estimates of MCP, RUP, and EAA flow to the small intestine across a wide range of diet types.[17]

POSTRUMEN AMINO ACID METABOLISM

Although there have been a limited number of studies on postruminal AA metabolism of the milking cow, and while this is still a "work in progress," this research promises to enhance the understanding of AA utilization toward anabolic functions, such as milk protein synthesis. A thorough understanding of AA metabolism will allow the updating of models to balance dairy rations for protein and AA and allow reduced N intake without penalizing milk yield. Because these models will be based on dairy cow physiology, they will therefore be robust in operation, especially in response to constantly changing feed ingredient composition.

Protein Digestion/Amino Acid Absorption

True gastric digestion of proteins that pass from the rumen begins in the abomasum with the addition of hydrochloric acid and gastric enzymes to initiate hydrolysis.[34] When the digesta reaches the small intestine, it is buffered back to near neutral pH and both pancreatic and intestinal digestive enzymes are added.

Ruminant digestion in the small intestine is analogous to that in the nonruminant, with pancreatic trypsin, chymotrypsin, and elastase beginning the breakdown, and carboxypeptidases A and B completing the intestinal digestion.[34]

The AA must be absorbed from the small intestine, principally from the jejunum by specific binding proteins.[35] Although limited research does show some uptake of AA by rumen tissue and/or the deaminated form of AA, this does not seem to be a significant source of blood AA.[36]

Assuming no growth of the gastrointestinal tissue (GIT), AAs removed, on a net basis, by the GIT have 2 major fates. A portion, which includes all AAs, is used directly for the synthesis of endogenous secretions; those AAs not digested and reabsorbed are excreted in the feces (fecal metabolic nitrogen). Another fraction that includes only some AA, most particularly the branched-chain AA and the NEAA, are catabolized by the GIT.[37] This catabolism seems to be blood concentration–dependent as more branched-chain AA are removed with higher concentrations.[6] Although some AAs used by the intestinal tissue originate from the intestinal lumen from protein digestion, most of the AAs used by the GIT originate from the arterial supply.[38]

Intestinal Amino Acid Digestibility

The digestibility of the individual AA that passes to the small intestine is another critical consideration. Globally, the digestibility of all AAs in protein that reaches the duodenum is approximately 80%.[39] Some models use this average, whereas other models use a coefficient of digestibility different for each feed ingredient, based on estimates made using the mobile bag technique.[40] This technique, however, provides rather wide estimates of AA digestion. Furthermore, it is evident that this varies considerably with both the protein source and the individual AA.[17,19] The digestibility of microbial true protein is also currently estimated at 80% by most of the models, but data are scarce on this important parameter.

Hepatic Metabolism

The liver plays a role in the regulation of plasma AA concentrations. Whether the liver is the primary regulator or if it is only responding to blood concentrations is not defined at present. The liver serves as a major site of both deamination of excess AA and gluconeogenesis mainly from NEAA, as well as a site of production of required NEAA, although all tissues can synthesize NEAA. The nature of the regulation or the signals that control the removal of AA from the liver are not understood at this time. Furthermore, data suggest that, in high-producing dairy cows, branched-chain AA and Lys are barely removed on a net basis, whereas His, Met, and Phe show the highest liver removal rate for the EAA.[41,42]

Mammary Metabolism

Most of the net supply of AA in the dairy cow is used by the mammary gland for protein secretion into milk. It is not unusual for cows to secrete more than 1.5 kg of protein in milk per day. Much new information has been developed regarding the use of AA for milk protein synthesis.

The direct source of milk protein AA is the free AA in blood arterial supply. These AAs are taken up by specific binding proteins, which are the same or analogous to those of the intestine.[43] Whether small peptides can be taken up as suggested by Bequette and colleagues[44] is still unproven.

It has long been known that milk protein synthesis is under the control of various hormones, including somatotropin, prolactin, insulin, and the locally produced insulin-like growth factors.[5] Recently, it has been observed that protein elongation is under the local control of the mammalian target of rapamycin (mTor) as part of protein transcription and subsequent activation of proteins 4E-BP1 and S6K1.[6,45] This complex has been shown to be activated by increased concentrations of Leu within the mammary cell, which led to suggestions that increasing Leu supply could result in increased milk protein production.[45]

It had been assumed that the percentage of AA in blood taken up by the mammary gland was constant, leading to the speculation that blood flow through the mammary gland was also constant. Both of these assumptions have been shown to be incorrect.

In a classic study, Bequette and colleagues[46] found that when blood His concentration was low, mammary blood flow increased as did the rate of extraction relative to supply of His, effectively decreasing the negative impact of low His arterial concentration on His supply and mitigating the impact on milk protein synthesis. Also, from a literature study, it was confirmed that although milk protein yield increased as duodenal flow of AA increased, there was a decreased efficiency of AA utilization that tended to plateau,[47] proving that AA secretion into milk protein was not a constant fraction of supply.

It has been reported in both swine[48] and dairy cows[39] that when plasma concentrations of EAA are increased, the mammary gland will take up greater quantities of these AAs in preference to NEAA. The clear implication is that the gland uses the EAA to produce NEAA that are nevertheless vital for milk protein production. This process would seem to be an unusual biological adaption as AA cannot be stored and energy is required for AA recycling and resynthesis, but this may offer flexibility in terms of energy source to the mammary gland.

- From these studies, it appears the mammary gland has the ability to control the use of AA by the amount and perhaps the pattern of AA in the blood.
- Whether this control is external or internal to the mammary gland is unknown.

Fates of Amino Acids in the Cow

Integration of all the previously described factors will lead to calculations such as those prepared by Lapierre and colleagues[39] as presented in **Table 2**. Presented is the flow of key EAA through the digestive tract. Although in reality these are calculations of what was observed from one experiment, the best use of these calculations is to develop statistical relationships to define requirements.

Table 2
Flow of selected essential AAs (g/d) at different sites of measurement in dairy cows

	Amino Acids					
Site	**His**	**Ile**	**Leu**	**Lys**	**Met**	**Val**
Duodenum	53	120	189	144	55	133
Endogenous duodenal[a]	15	19	20	30	6	25
Net duodenal	39	101	169	114	49	108
Ileal	24	38	61	37	19	55
Apparent ileal digestible[b]	30	82	128	107	36	78
Endogenous ileal[c]	7	11	14	16	4	15
From undigested endogenous duo	5	6	6	9	2	8
From nonreabsorbed endogenous from small intestine	3	5	8	7	3	8
True ileal digestible[d]	32	87	136	114	39	85
True ileal digestible from net supply[e]	22	73	122	93	35	68
Available, accounting for endogenous loss[f]	15	63	108	77	30	53
Portal absorption	22	51	80	60	24	40
Milk	15	33	54	45	15	37
Milk as % of duodenal flow	28	28	29	31	27	28
Milk as % of available	100	52	50	58	50	70

[a] Assuming 4.3 g of N per kg DMI and AA composition of abomasal isolate.[24]
[b] Duodenal–ileal, scurf protein, and endogenous urinary secretion.
[c] Assuming 28% of ileal CP flow, 1/2 from undigested.
[d] Apparent digestible + endogenous ileal from small intestine.
[e] True digestible − endogenous duodenal − endogenous ileal from undigested preduodenal endogenous.
[f] True ileal digestible from net supply − endogenous ileal.

Adapted from Lapierre H, Pacheco D, Bethiaume R, et al. What is the true supply of amino acids for a dairy cow? J Dairy Sci 2006;89(E Suppl):E1–14.

In particular, these calculations show 3 important traits of AA use by lactating cows:

- Conversion of duodenal AA into milk protein ~ 30%
- The true ileal digestible AA is only about 70% of that isolated at the duodenum
- Conversion of truly available AA into milk can range from 40% to 100%.

AMINO ACID REQUIREMENTS

The most surprising of all aspects of balancing dairy rations for AA is that actual requirements have not been clearly defined. It is this fact that has caused working nutritionists to question the value of AA balance for dairy cattle. In classical nutrition, requirements are established for various biological processes. These include the following:

- *Maintenance* (ie, AA needed to be replaced in already constructed proteins and excreted as metabolic fecal protein, scurf protein, and endogenous urinary secretion)
- *Growth* (ie, AA required for skeletal muscle and bone accretion)
- *Lactation* (ie, AA required for the production of milk protein)
- *Reproduction* (ie, AA required for the growth of the placenta and fetus).

There is no evidence that on a tissue level the AA requirement for maintenance is different between dairy cattle and other mammalian species. Likewise, the AA requirements for growth and fetal growth have been well investigated in several species, and only minor differences between species have been observed. The large unknowns are the AA requirement for lactation and AA contents of metabolic fecal protein.

Determining Amino Acid Requirements for Lactation

Methods for determining lactation requirements could be

- To determine the amount of AAs that are secreted in milk protein, then make assumptions about digestibility and efficiency of utilization of AA.
- To measure the uptake of AA by the mammary gland compared with the amount of AA in the secreted milk protein.
- To assume that there is an "ideal protein" generally considered to have an AA composition like casein or MCP.

For Method 1, summing these variables provide estimates of each AA and MP needed for lactation. This method is simple, but there is no way to evaluate the accuracy of assumptions regarding digestibility and efficiency.

For Method 2, estimates for AA uptake versus output for various EAA are presented in **Table 3**. The uptake-to-output ratio has been suggested to represent the efficiency of use of AA[49] and is used in conjunction with milk protein AA composition to arrive at AA requirements. On average, some EAA are taken up in about the same ratio as they are exported (His, Met, and Phe + tyrosine).[50] Others (Arg, Leu, and Lys) are taken up greatly in excess of what is exported as protein, while the other EAA are taken up in somewhat intermediate quantities. Although the thinking behind this method is dated, it is still used by several models.

Arg is taken up in greatest quantity compared with output and is one reason some models have a large Arg requirement. The question is, does this uptake reflect requirements for synthesis of NEAA or regulatory proteins or is this simply "luxury consumption"? This model is subject to the same errors as the technique above.

Table 3
Mean ratio of uptake (U) of essential AAs across the mammary gland in relation to output (O) in milk protein

Variable	Mean Ratio	Standard Deviation	Minimum	Maximum
Milk true protein yield, g/d	794	155	370	1076
Metabolizable protein, g/d	1794	485	747	3619
Arg U:O[a]	2.45	0.60	0.88	4.18
His U:O	1.08	0.25	0.46	1.80
Ile U:O	1.41	0.20	1.01	1.96
Leu U:O	1.31	0.24	0.98	2.37
Lys U:O	1.33	0.25	0.60	2.09
Met U:O	0.96	0.11	0.59	1.18
Phe U:O	1.07	0.08	0.82	1.29
Thr U:O	1.19	0.18	0.87	1.58
Val U:O	1.49	0.27	0.85	2.22
Mammary plasma flow, L/d	14,160	2784	9384	23,976

[a] U:O = mammary AA uptake/AA secreted in milk protein.
From Lapierre H, Lobley GE, Doepel L, et al. Triennial lactation symposium: mammary metabolism of amino acids in dairy cows. J Anim Sci 2012;90:1708–21.

For Method 3, the ideal protein is fed to fulfill the MP requirement. The AA requirements are determined as the MP × the percentage of each AA in the ideal protein. This technique is also vulnerable to errors in the assumptions of digestion and transfer for MP as well as to the lack of knowledge of the exact MP requirement and whether the AA distribution affects the MP requirement.

Thus, although firm AA requirements have not been established, ranges of required EAA can be provided. It is assumptions of authors of models made from rather limited data that that produce differences in model requirements. In fact, there is speculation that given all the partial efficiencies of extraction and mammary blood flow that make up EAA requirements for lactation, it may be impossible to set "exact" requirements.[50]

Metabolizable Protein Requirement

Unfortunately, there is disagreement among models regarding MP requirements. As defined,[7] the MP requirement signifies the total supply of EAA and NEAA that a cow needs to support a defined level of production. Two meta-analysis studies[17,51] found that the NRC MP requirements[7] were not fulfilled in about one-third of the studies that were summarized for their meta-analysis, suggesting that the NRC MP requirements were too high. The unfulfilled MP requirements may also reflect the fact that NRC does not take into account the AA balance of the MP when computing requirements. The AminoCow model, which has significantly lower MP requirements,[51] assumes that MP has the exact amount of EAA that is "required" by the cow.[26]

Some of these differences in MP requirement may be due to different assumptions regarding the effects of AA composition on the MP needed to maintain production.

Another factor is the need for AA to contribute to gluconeogenesis. Bell[52] suggested that for the developing fetus and for cows in very early lactation, greater than 50% of the glucose is due to the conversion of AA. Thus, a high demand for use as a glucose precursor might need to be integrated into the AA and MP requirements at various stages, and probably in relation with energy supply.

It has been suggested that AA requirements should be expressed as grams per day on a factorial basis. In a recent study,[53] it was found that both milk protein yield and milk protein percentage were better related to grams of duodenal AA flow per day than for AA as a percentage of MP.

Nutritional programs do vary in their requirements (**Table 4**). Because of the large differences for some AA and MP, it is easy to think that one or more models are "wrong." The differences are a reflection of the way authors have looked at the data and of assumptions they have made in the development of their models. Because estimates of protein and EAA duodenal flows are close to measurements (**Table 5**), it appears the differences are largely due to the assumptions regarding postruminal metabolism. In fact, it is certain that all models are "wrong," but by using them and challenging them meaningful requirements may be developed.

Limiting Amino Acids

On a practical basis, to determine a limiting AA, there needs to be a response that can be measured as this AA is added. For lactation studies, milk protein yield is the appropriate response for AA limitation, utilization, and AA efficiency. The yield of milk protein represents both a volume and a percentage function. As pointed out,[51] milk protein percentage can increase with no increase in AA utilization for lactation if milk production is decreased; conversely, if yield is increased, but percentage milk protein decreased sharply, there may also be no change in AA utilization.

Since the pioneering research of Rulquin and coworkers[54,55] and Schwab and coworkers[56,57] as well as the publication of NRC 2001, it has been fashionable to

Table 4
Requirement estimates for MP and metabolizable AAs by various nutrition programs

Requirement[a]	Nutrition Program			
	NRC[b]	AC[c]	CPM[d]	CNCPS[e]
g/d				
MP	2784	2047	2266	2759
Arg	—	78	136	167
His	—	57	44	52
Ile	—	111	120	129
Leu	—	200	185	206
Lys	200[f]	168	131	150
Met	67[g]	55	40	45
Phe	—	98	72	83
Thr	—	97	71	130
Trp	—	30	24	30
Val	—	129	133	146
Requirement, % MP				
Arg	—	3.81	6.00	6.05
His	—	3.03	1.94	1.88
Ile	—	5.42	5.30	4.68
Leu	—	9.77	8.16	7.47
Lys	7.2	8.21	5.78	5.44
Met	2.4	2.69	1.77	1.63
Phe	—	4.79	3.18	3.01
Thr	—	4.74	3.13	4.71
Trp	—	1.47	1.06	1.09
Val	—	6.30	5.87	5.29
Total EAA		50.23	42.19	41.25

[a] For this comparison it is assumed that the cow is a Holstein, 3rd Lactation, weight 650 kg, with a body score of 2.75 and an average daily gain of 136 g per day while producing 41 kg of milk with a 3.60% butter fat test and a 3.10% true milk protein at 180 days in milk.
[b] Data from NRC is National Research Council model.
[c] AC is AminoCow, Evonik Industries, Hanau, Germany.
[d] CPM is Cornell-Penn-Minor Model version 3.
[e] CNCPS is Cornell Net Carbohydrate-Protein System version 6.1.54.
[f] Calculated as NRC MP requirement × .072.
[g] Calculated as MP requirement × .024.

concentrate only on Lys and Met as limiting AA on North American–type diets with His as a limiting AA on grass silage diets.[58] Since then, it has been proven that His can be a limiting AA in North American diets, especially in diets with a low protein supply because MCP contributes more to total MP.[3] Because of obligate use by intestinal tissue as energy sources, the branched-chain AAs (Ile, Leu, and Val) have also been suggested as limiting at high levels of milk production. Less often Arg and glutamine have been proposed to be limiting. Much summarized research[51] has shown that the addition of rumen protected Met results in more production of milk protein, more or less confirming the supposition that Met is often a limiting AA in North American–type diets.

Less convincing is the effect of Lys in established lactation. Robinson[59] summarized studies where dietary Lys was increased and observed no effects. In other studies[60,61]

Table 5
Simplified comparison of commercially available models to predict protein and AA flows

Item	Observed Mean	Observed SE	AC Mean	AC SE	AC % Obs.[a]	AMTS Mean	AMTS SE	AMTS % Obs.	CPM Mean	CPM SE	CPM % Obs.	NRC Mean	NRC SE	NRC % Obs.
CP	3027	790	2945	769	97.3	3026	638	100	3148	633	104	2951	708	97.5
MCP[b]	1610	407	1605	499	99.7	1678	314	104.2	2050	415	127.3	1573	338	97.7
RUP	1480	614	1368	372	92.4	1348	409	91.1	1126	315	76.1	1415	416	95.6
Arg	122	38	123	33	100.8	152	37	124.6	160	38	131.1	116	28	95.1
His	61	20	59	18	96.7	66	18	108.2	69	20	113.1	56	16	91.8
Ile	119	36	127	34	106.7	126	28	105.9	134	30	112.6	120	27	100.8
Leu	230	79	220	64	95.7	219	60	95.2	224	61	97.4	226	62	98.3
Lys	157	48	161	45	102.5	164	40	104.5	178	43	113.4	160	38	101.9
Met	47	16	48	13	102.1	53	11	112.8	59	13	125.5	47	11	100
Phe	129	38	128	34	99.2	134	33	103.9	140	34	108.5	126	31	97.7
Thr	123	34	124	32	100.8	120	28	97.6	127	29	103.3	120	27	97.6
Val	141	45	145	37	102.8	147	36	104.3	155	38	109.9	138	32	97.9

Abbreviations: AC, AminoCow version 3.5.2; AMTS, Argricultural Modeling and Training Systems LLC, version 2.0.15; CPM, Cornell-Penn-Miner Dairy, version 3.01; NRC, National Research Council (2001). After Pacheco, Patton, Parys et al.[17]

[a] Predicted value as a percentage of observed value.
[b] Microbial crude protein.

in which Lys was deleted from a mixture of infused AA, production of milk and milk protein was reduced in the Lys-deficient infusion, confirming the importance given to Lys by NRC 2001. In contrast, Patton[51] could find no relationship between Lys supply and milk protein response to Met. Thus, the exact relation of Lys to AA deficiencies has yet to be established. However, increased Lys supply does appear important in very early lactation,[58,62] a time when microbial synthesis is reduced because of lower DMI, to drive output of both milk and milk protein.

Although His has long been established as a limiting AA on grass diets, this may be more related to diets with a high contribution of MCP relative to total MP supply (>70% from the authors' data) regardless of diet type.[2] When His was added to low MP diets, improved DMI and milk production without changing milk protein percentage were observed.[3] It has been demonstrated that blood His concentration is greatly reduced on low protein diets.[63] Thus, because of low concentration in MCP, His has the potential to be limiting on reduced MP diets.

Despite speculation based on mTor studies, addition or deletion of Leu to diets has resulted in no changes in milk protein yield.[60,64] Studies with branched-chain EAA also have been disappointing, generally having no effect on milk protein production.[60,64,65] It appears well established that Arg is not greatly limiting, because both a deletion[66] and an infusion experiment[65] have shown no response to Arg.

Studies with the other AA (Ile, Phe, Thr, Trp, Val, glutamine, and cysteine) have been inconclusive as to their potential to be limiting. However, any AA has the potential to be limiting depending on the amount and type of RUP and proportion of MCP.

In summary, limiting AA in typical North American diets appears to be as follows:

- Met—still the most likely to be limiting
- His—may be the most limiting on low MP diets
- Lys—appears to have good efficacy in early lactation; supplement studies in established lactation are disappointing.

THE MEANING AND PRACTICAL USE OF MILK UREA NITROGEN

One of the most active areas of research over the last decade has been the effect of excess protein on milk urea nitrogen (MUN). Whether from rumen ammonia or AA in RUP, excess protein results in higher urea production.[33] Higher urea production results in the loss of N in the urine, not only wasting an expensive resource (protein) but also causing greater environmental pollution.[67] Monitoring of MUN offers the potential to increase protein efficiency and to decrease feed costs.[68]

Because ammonia is toxic, it must be removed from the blood and converted to urea by the liver. The kidneys then filter urea into the urine. There is an energy cost to ureagenesis that must be borne by the animal.[69] Because urea is a small molecule and readily diffusible, blood urea nitrogen (BUN) or plasma urea nitrogen (PUN) is in rough equilibrium with MUN.[67] Studies indicate that MUN is related to BUN and PUN with correlations between 84% and 98%.[70] Equations for conversion of BUN or PUN have been proposed with these be most widely used:

$$MUN \text{ mg/dL} = 0.620 \times BUN \text{ mg/dL} + 4.75^{71}$$

$$MUN \text{ mg/dL} = 1.176 \times PUN \text{ mg/dL} - 3.76^{72}$$

Likewise, milk urea (MU) or MUN expressed as millimole per liter can be converted to milligram per deciliter by the following formula:

MUN mg/dL = 2.8 × MU mmol/L

MUN mg/dL = 5.6 × MUN mmol/L

Normal Milk Urea Nitrogen Values

Normal mean MUN values range from 10 to 15 mg/dL for herds in the United States, while individual cows within herds can range from 5 to 25 mg/dL. Herds on high protein pastures will often exhibit MUN from 17 to 22 mg/dL[73,74] without apparent loss of production, although another study reported loss of production at 17 mg/dL.[75] This wide range both across and within herds suggests that there are many factors that influence MUN and that there may be subpopulations within herds that are affected differently by the ration consumed.

Reproductive Concerns

Many practitioners are concerned about BUN or MUN for previously reported effects on reproductive efficiency.[76,77] However, more recent studies using more sophisticated statistical analyses have found little relationship of MUN to reproductive efficiency.[78,79] These authors found that MUN was confounded with loss of body condition in early lactation and insufficient energy in other stages of lactation. Guo and colleagues[80] found that MUN had no effect on conception rate across herds, but within a herd, a 10 mg/dL increase in MUN resulted in 2% to 4% loss in conception rate. Thus, although it may have an effect on reproduction, high MUN levels do not appear to be a large cause of reproductive failure; rather, high MUN levels may coincide with other factors that have a greater direct impact on reproductive efficiency.

Factors Affecting Milk Urea Nitrogen

Excess CP intake is largely responsible for high MUN,[67] with a 1% decrease in CP resulting in 1.1 mg/dL decrease in MUN. In addition, there are a multitude of other factors that can affect MUN positively, including body weight (BW), yield of fat corrected milk, DMI, and days in milk (DIM).[71] Breed differences are significant,[81] although breed effects become insignificant when BW enters the equation. Also, there are no effects of parity if BW is considered.[82] The effect of DIM is generally such that MUN is higher in the first 25 DIM and then drops to its lowest levels after peak lactation. After this, MUN tends to creep up as lactation progresses. Season also has an effect as MUN rises and falls with the mean monthly temperature.[83] Time of milking in relation to time of feeding and water intake and amount of urine production are other factors that are proposed as important in MUN concentration.[68] Unfortunately, MUN is sensitive to adjustments in analytical equipment and differences in equipment as well as changes in equipment calibration. Although within a given machine comparisons are perfectly valid, it is more problematic to compare values between machines and laboratories (Hristov and colleagues, unpublished data).

Ration Factors

As stated, protein intake in relation to milk output is the largest determinate, and by far the most important nutritional determinate of MUN. There is a small and inconsistent effect depending on the amount of RDP,[33,82] but if RDP is fed in excess, high MUN results. However, the same will occur with excess RUP. It has been suggested that protein balanced for AA (rather than CP, RDP, and RUP) lowers MUN.[72,84] Increasing readily digestible carbohydrates in the diet has been shown to decrease MUN.[85–87] It has been shown that corn can be more effective at reducing MUN than barley,[20] presumably because of a longer fermentation time allowing capture of more ammonia N by rumen bacteria, although grain processing may have a greater effect than grain type. High sodium diets (13.5 g of Na/kg of dry matter [DM]) lowered MUN in milk by 1.7 mg/dL, but without decreasing urinary urea excretion[83] and may be a reflection of increased water intake and corresponding increased urine volume.

Recommended Milk Urea Nitrogen Levels

Recommendations for acceptable MUN levels are difficult to obtain, but they do seem to center around 11 mg/dL. Kalsheur and colleagues[88] found that RDP had to be 9.7% of DM and that MUN had to be less than 11.6 mg/dL before production declined. Nousiainen and colleagues[89] suggested that an MUN of 11.7 mg/dL reflected sufficient degradable protein. However, as they point out, this did not account for ruminally recycled N; therefore, MUN of 9 to 10 could be adequate. Data from Cyriac and colleagues[90] suggest RDP at 8.8% of DM and MUN at 12.4 mg/dL as the point at which milk yield begins to suffer. Although these recommendations differ slightly because of differences in nutritional balance, they do seem to indicate that with adequately balanced fiber, NFC, and AA, high milk production (>40 kg per head per day) can be obtained with CP levels near 15% to 16%, RDP levels around 9.0% to 10% of DM, with MUN in the 9 to 12 mg/dL range.

Use of Milk Urea Nitrogen Levels

Because of all the influencing factors described above, it has been suggested that MUN be monitored on a bulk tank basis and a baseline for the herd be established,[91] suggesting that changes in MUN are the most important factor to monitor. Although strictly correct, if MUN values are to be used to evaluate protein efficiency, more precise use of MUN should be encouraged. It must be recognized that MUN testing and interpretation as well as average herd MUN values have decreased during the past 5 years as nutritionists have adopted the use of MP and AA balance, as well as the pressure exerted by producers to lower ration cost as protein prices have soared.

In practice, MUN is monitored in groups of cows, but only after balancing the MP and EAA for each group, which requires first agreeing on goal MUN and second evaluating MUN for groups of cows across the lactation. The authors recommend examining groups of cows as follows:

Group	Range of MUN Recommended (mg/dL)	Acceptable (mg/dL)
Herd	10–12	9–13
Group 1 = 0–30 DIM	14–15	14–16.5
Group 2 = 31–60 DIM	10–11	9–12
Group 3 = 61–180 DIM	10–12	9–12
Group 4 = 181–270 DIM	10–12	9–13
Group 5 >271 DIM	10–13	9–14

The acceptable range depends on many factors including the feeding strategy. For herds fed a single total mixed ration (TMR), it has been found that the MUN runs 1.0 to 1.3 mg/dL higher. For herds not feeding a separate fresh group, it is found that during the first 10 days MUN trends 2–2.5 mg/dL higher than goal. The authors suspect this is from greater mobilization of body reserves, although overfeeding RDP is certainly a possibility. Likewise, for herds with a wide difference of BW within groups, it has been found that the MUN averages 0.25 to 0.50 mg/dL higher than typical.

Determining these numbers is relatively straightforward where there is test day data for individual cows. The caveat is that 7 of 10 cows should show the same trend (ie, higher or lower). That also means that there should be a minimum of 10 cows per group. For herds without monthly testing (generally larger herds) where the only data are monthly or daily bulk tank results, as long as the results are within the acceptable ranges and production consistent with nutritional balance, no further action need be taken. If the MUN are greater than the acceptable range, and MP and RDP are in balance, the first option is to increase starch and sugar in the diet. Often this results not only in lower MUN but also in greater milk production as well. If MUN are lower, more RDP is added and it is evaluated whether more milk is seen. If only the MUN goes up without additional milk yield, then previous RDP levels are reverted to. Obviously the challenge is to evaluate whether milk production goes up or not without individual tests of milk yield and MUN, but to the extent that a production trend is convincing, with the use of the above strategy. If a single TMR is fed, the only remedy is to lower or increase the CP depending on the situation.

If either the levels of peak milk production or the persistency of lactation are not satisfactory, then blood tests are done for BUN in groups of 10 cows to determine if poor protein utilization in a particular group or groups is contributing to this problem. The authors like to take 2 sets of samples within the same week at approximately the same time in relation to feeding and milking, adding the same precaution that at least 7 from 10 show the same trend.

Finally, and perhaps most importantly, MUN is a tool to help diagnose ration problems. It is not a replacement for nutritional knowledge and ration balance.

PRACTICAL APPLICATION

Obviously, the protein and AA nutrition of dairy cattle are too complicated to adequately meet the needs of the cow without the use of a model that takes into account the various fates of ingested protein, MCP, and endogenous protein and integrates this all into the cow metabolism. The well-known phrase, "All models are bad, but some are useful," applies here. Fortunately, most models at the disposal of the nutritionists are relatively accurate at predicting the duodenal flow of CP and individual AA[17] (see **Table 5** for a comparison of some models). This acceptable accuracy can be used to formulate more productive, economical, and less environmentally damaging rations. However, to do this will take work and dedication on the part of the user.

The authors recommend the following steps for formulating AA balanced rations:

- Commit to balancing all rations for MP and AA. CP is a term whose use in setting requirements has passed into history.
- Choose a model and learn to use it. The assumptions of the model should be sufficiently clear so that the user can understand what the model calculates and how the model calculates it. Likewise, there should be studies that validate the model. Although it may be preferable if studies are published in refereed journals, recommendations from friends and peers are also valuable.
- Collect the information that the model requires to produce accurate results. Do not assume all cow groups weigh the same. Do not assume that the default values will be sufficient for your feeds. Know what tests to request from the feed laboratory to maximize the performance of your chosen model.
- Measure DMI. Because DMI has such a huge effect on MCP and RUP, it is critical that actual DMI be used. In the work of Pacheco and colleagues,[17] the best model predicted the DMI within 1.6 kg only 60% of the time.

- Optimize MCP. The key to economic production of milk and milk protein is the maximization of NDF digestion coupled with optimization of nonfiber carbohydrate digestion. Because MCP increases marginally with each increment of NDF, NFC, and RDP, it is economically unwise to "maximize" MCP. The only way to optimize MCP is to rigorously track feed costs and to monitor the difference in income over feed costs that result from increasing MCP versus decreasing MCP and adding RUP and rumen protected EAA to meet model requirements.
- Meet projected AA deficiencies on a gram basis with either RUP or rumen-protected AA. The debate regarding setting the requirements as grams versus ratios will go on for some time. Ratios of one EAA versus another, percentages of DM, or percentage of MP might be useful guides, but cows eat pounds and grams of nutrients. When satisfying program requirements for EAA, it is recommended that they be met as grams per day.
- Believe in the cow. If the cows are producing a given quantity of milk and the model estimates they are deficient by X g of MP or a given AA is deficient by Y g, then it is obvious that the cow is receiving sufficient nutrients to produce this milk and milk protein. Body condition should be monitored to make sure that the nutrients are not coming from mobilization of body reserves. Given no body condition mobilization, in most cases, models will predict the correct flow within a reasonable margin of error if the correct model inputs have been entered. Although model inputs should be checked, what is plain is that the cow is consuming sufficient nutrients to produce the milk that she is making. What should be suspected is the requirements of the model are not correct. At least mentally, adjust the model with this in mind.
- Monitor the situation. If MP is lowered, or if AAs are added, check the response, not only the immediate response, but longer term as well. Check body condition and reproductive efficiency as well as production of milk and milk protein. Farmers and nutritionists often report both improved over the longer term with AA balance.

Experience indicates that with stable forages, production of greater than 41 kg of milk with greater than 3.15% true milk protein are possible with 15.0% to 16% CP in the ration when AA are balanced. When forages are of variable quality, the CP content of the ration may need to be increased to insure sufficient MP at all times. Maintaining sufficient energy is always critical for optimizing both milk yield and MCP production.

Like so many of the advancements in dairy nutrition, advances in AA balance will come from the field. Using AA balance and sharing results with colleagues are the best way to work out the best balance for your chosen model with your clients.

ACKNOWLEDGMENTS

The authors would like to express their appreciation to Dr Claudia Parys of Evonik Industries for supplying the AA analyses of feeds and to Dr Tom Overton of Cornell University for simulations in the CNCPS model.

REFERENCES

1. Benefield BC, Patton RA, Stevenson MJ, et al. Evaluation of rumen-protected methionine sources and period length. J Dairy Sci 2009;92:4448–55.
2. Broderick GA, Stevenson MJ, Patton RA, et al. Effect of supplementing rumen-protected methionine on production and nitrogen excretion in lactating dairy cows. J Dairy Sci 2008;91:1092–102.

3. Lee C, Hristov AN, Cassidy TW, et al. Rumen-protected lysine, methionine, and histidine increase milk protein yield in dairy cows fed a metabolizable protein-deficient diet. J Dairy Sci 2012;95:6042–56.

4. Broderick GA, Stevenson MJ, Patton RA. Effect of dietary protein concentration and degradability on response to rumen-protected methionine in lactating cows. J Dairy Sci 2009;92:2719–26.

5. Lee C, Hristov AN, Heyler KS, et al. Effects of metabolizable protein supply and amino acid supplementation on nitrogen utilization, milk production, and ammonia emissions from manure in dairy cows. J Dairy Sci 2012;95:5253–68.

6. Lei J, Feng D, Shang Y, et al. Nutritional and regulatory role of branched-chain amino acids in lactation. Front Biosci 2012;17:2725–39.

7. National Research Council. Protein and amino acids. In: Nutrient requirements of dairy cattle seventh revised edition. Washington, DC: National Academy Press; 2001. p. 43–104.

8. Sniffen CJ, O'Connor JD, Van Soest PJ, et al. A net carbohydrate and protein system for evaluating cattle diets: II. Carbohydrate and protein availability. J Anim Sci 1992;70:3562–77.

9. Hoover WH, Stokes SR. Balancing carbohydrates and proteins for optimum rumen microbial yield. J Dairy Sci 1991;74:3630–44.

10. Shabi Z, Tagari H, Murphy MR, et al. Partitioning of amino acids flowing to the abomasum into feed, bacterial, protozoal and endogenous fractions. J Dairy Sci 2000;83:2326–34.

11. Firkins JL, Yu Z, Morrison M. Ruminal nitrogen metabolism: perspectives for integration of microbiology and nutrition for dairy. J Dairy Sci 2007;90(E Suppl):E1–16.

12. Reynolds CK, Kristensen NB. Nitrogen recycling through the gut and the nitrogen economy of ruminants: an asynchronous symbiosis. J Anim Sci 2007;86(E Suppl):E293–305.

13. Hall MB. Dietary starch source and protein degradability in diets containing sucrose: effects on ruminal measures and proposed mechanism for degradable protein effects. J Dairy Sci 2013;96:7093–109.

14. DePeters EJ, Cant JP. Nutritional factors influencing the nitrogen composition of bovine milk: a review. J Dairy Sci 1992;75:2043–70.

15. Clark JH, Klusmeyer TH, Cameron MR. Microbial protein synthesis and flows of nitrogen fractions to the duodenum of dairy cows. J Dairy Sci 1992;75:2304–23.

16. Dhiman TR, Korevaar AC, Satter LS. Particle size of roasted soybeans and the effect on milk production of dairy cows. J Dairy Sci 1997;80:1722–7.

17. Pacheco D, Patton RA, Parys C, et al. Ability of commercially available dairy ration programs to predict duodenal flows of protein and essential amino acids in dairy cows. J Dairy Sci 2012;95:937–63.

18. Boucher SE, Calsamiglia S, Parson CM, et al. In vitro digestibility of individual amino acids in rumen-undegraded protein: the modified three-step procedure and the immobilized digestive assay. J Dairy Sci 2009;92:3939–50.

19. Edmunds B, Sudekum KH, Bennett R, et al. The amino acid composition of rumen-undegradable protein: a comparison between forages. J Dairy Sci 2013;96:4568–77.

20. Boucher SE, Calsamiglia S, Parson CM, et al. Intestinal digestibility of amino acids in rumen undegradable protein estimated using a precision-fed cecectomized rooster bioassay: I. Soybean meal and SoyPlus. J Dairy Sci 2009;92:4489–98.

21. Boucher SE, Calsamiglia S, Parson CM, et al. Intestinal digestibility of amino acids in rumen undegradable protein estimated using a precision-fed

cecectomized rooster bioassay: II. Distillers dried grains with solubles and fish meal. J Dairy Sci 2009;92:6056–67.

22. Tamminga S, Schulze H, Van Bruchem J, et al. The nutritional significance of endogenous N-Losses along the gastro-intestinal tract of farm animals. Arch Anim Nutr 1995;48:9–22.

23. Marini JC, Fox DG, Murphy MR. Nitrogen transaction along the gastrointestinal tract of cattle: a meta-analytical approach. J Anim Sci 2008;86:660–79.

24. Ørskov ER, McLeod NA, Kyle DJ. Flow of nitrogen from the rumen and abomasum in cattle and sheep given protein-free nutrients by intragastric infusion. Br J Nutr 1986;1986(56):241–8.

25. Ouellet DR, Berthiaume R, Holtrop G, et al. Effect of method of conservation of timothy on endogenous nitrogen flows in lactating dairy cows. J Dairy Sci 2010; 93:4252–61.

26. Evonik Degussa Industries GmBH. Philosophy of AminoCow. In: Patton RA, editor. AminoCow version 3.5.2. Hanau (Germany): Evonik Industries; 2007. p. 11–2.

27. Choi CW, Vanhatalo A, Ahvenjarvi S, et al. Effects of several protein supplements on flow of soluble non-ammonia nitrogen from the forestomach and milk production in dairy cows. Anim Feed Sci Technol 2002;102:15–33.

28. Reynal SM, Ipharraguerre IR, Lineiro M, et al. Omasal flow of soluble proteins, peptides, and free amino acids in dairy cows fed diets supplemented with proteins of varying ruminal degradabilities. J Dairy Sci 2006;90:1887–903.

29. Rémond D, Bernard L, Chauveau B, et al. Digestion and nutrient fluxes across the rumen, and the mesenteric- and portal-drained viscera in sheep fed with fresh forage twice daily: net balance and dynamic aspects. Br J Nutr 2003;89:649–66.

30. Lapierre H, Lobley GE. Nitrogen recycling in the ruminant: a review. J Dairy Sci 2001;84(E Suppl):E223–36.

31. Lee C, Hristov AN, Cassidy T, et al. Nitrogen isotope fractionation and origin of ammonia nitrogen volatilized from cattle manure in simulated storage. Atmosphere 2011;2:256–70.

32. Raggio G, Pacheco D, Berthiaume R, et al. Effect of level of metabolizable protein on splanchnic flux of amino acids in lactating dairy cows. J Dairy Sci 2004; 87:3461–72.

33. Roseler DK, Ferguson JD, Sniffen CJ, et al. Dietary protein degradability effects on plasma and milk urea nitrogen and milk nonprotein nitrogen in Holstein cows. J Dairy Sci 1993;76:525–34.

34. Harmon DL. Nutritional regulation of postruminal digestive enzymes in ruminants. J Dairy Sci 1993;76:2102–11.

35. Baumrucker CR, Guerino F, Huntington GB. Transport of nitrogenous compounds by the ruminant gastrointestinal tract. In: Friedman EM, editor. Absorption and utilization of amino acids, vol. 3. Boca Raton (FL): CRC Press; 1989. p. 159–72.

36. Rémond D, Bernard L, Poncet C. Amino acid flux in ruminal and gastric veins of sheep: effects of ruminal and omasal injections of free amino acids and carnosine. J Anim Sci 2000;78:158–66.

37. Lapierre H, Blouin JP, Bernier JF, et al. Effect of supply of metabolizable protein on whole body and splanchnic leucine metabolism in lactating dairy cows. J Dairy Sci 2002;85:2631–41.

38. MacRae JC, Bruce LA, Brown DS, et al. Amino acid use by the gastrointestinal tract of sheep given Lucerne forage. Am J Physiol 1997;273:G1200–7.

39. Lapierre H, Pacheco D, Bethiaume R, et al. What is the true supply of amino acids for a dairy cow? J Dairy Sci 2006;89(E Suppl):E1–14.

40. Hvelplund T, Weisbjerg MR. In situ techniques for the estimation of protein degradability and post rumen availability. In: Givens DI, Owen E, Axford RF, et al, editors. Forage evaluation in ruminant nutrition. London: CABI Publishing; 2000. p. 233–58.

41. Wray-Cahen D, Metcalf JA, Backwell FR, et al. Hepatic response to increased exogenous supply of plasma amino acids by infusion into the mesenteric vein of Holstein-Friesian cows in late lactation. Br J Nutr 1997;78:913–30.

42. Hanigan MD. Quantitative aspects of ruminant splanchnic metabolism as related to predicting animal performance. Anim Sci 2005;80:23–92.

43. Baumrucker CR. Amino acid transport systems in bovine mammary tissue. J Dairy Sci 1985;68:3436–51.

44. Bequette BJ, Backwell FR, Kyle CE, et al. Vascular sources of phenylalanine, tyrosine, lysine, and methionine for casein synthesis in lactating goats. J Dairy Sci 1999;82:362–77.

45. Cant JP, Purdie NG, Burgos SA, et al. Manipulation of milk synthesis with amino acids. Proceeding of the 45th Eastern Nutrition Conference May 13-14. Quebec City (Canada): Animal Nutrition Association. of Canada; 2009. p. 1–8.

46. Bequette BJ, Hanigan MD, Calder AG, et al. Amino acid exchange by the mammary gland of lactating goats when histidine limits milk production. J Dairy Sci 2000;83:765–75.

47. Doepel L, Pacheco D, Kennelly JJ, et al. Milk protein synthesis as a function of amino acid supply. J Dairy Sci 2004;87:1279–97.

48. Trottier NL, Shipley CF, Easter RA. Plasma amino acid uptake by the mammary gland of the lactating sow. J Anim Sci 1997;75:1266–78.

49. Fox DG, Tedeschi LO, Tylutki TP, et al. The Cornell Net Carbohydrate and Protein System model for evaluating herd nutrition and nutrient excretion. Anim Feed Sci Technol 2004;112:29–78.

50. Lapierre H, Lobley GE, Doepel L, et al. Triennial Lactation Symposium: mammary metabolism of amino acids in dairy cows. J Anim Sci 2012;90: 1708–21.

51. Patton RA. Effect of rumen-protected methionine on feed intake, milk production, true milk protein concentration, and true milk protein yield, and the factors that influence these effects: a meta-analysis. J Dairy Sci 2010;93:2105–18.

52. Bell AW. Regulation of organic nutrient metabolism during transition from late pregnancy to early lactation. J Anim Sci 1995;73:2804–19.

53. Patton RA, Lapierre H, Parys C. Relationships between circulating plasma amino acid concentrations and milk protein production in lactating dairy cows [abstract T95]. J Dairy Sci 2013;96(Suppl 1).

54. Rulquin H, Pisulewski PM, Vérité R, et al. Milk production and composition as a function of postruminal lysine and methionine supply: a nutrient-response approach. Livest Prod Sci 1993;37:69–90.

55. Rulquin H, Vérité R. Amino acid nutrition of dairy cows: production effects and animal requirements. In: Garnsworthy PC, Cole DJ, editors. Recent advances in animal nutrition. Nottingham, United Kingdom: Nottingham University Press; 1993. p. 55–77.

56. Schwab CG, Bozak CK, Whitehouse NL, et al. Amino acid limitation and flow to the duodenum at four stages of lactation. 1. Sequence of lysine and methionine limitation. J Dairy Sci 1992;75:3486–502.

57. Schwab CG, Bozak CK, Whitehouse NL, et al. Amino acid limitation and flow to the duodenum at four stages of lactation. 2. Extent of lysine limitation. J Dairy Sci 1992;75:3503–18.

58. Vanhatalo A, Huhtanen P, Toivonen V, et al. Response of dairy cows fed grass silage diets to abomasal infusions of histidine alone or in combination with lysine and methionine. J Dairy Sci 1999;82:2674–85.
59. Robinson PH. Impacts of manipulating ration metabolizable lysine and methionine levels on the performance of lactating dairy cows: a systematic review of the literature. Livest Sci 2010;127:115–26.
60. Weeks TL, Luimes PH, Cant JP. Responses to amino acid imbalances and deficiencies in lactating dairy cows. J Dairy Sci 2006;89:2177–87.
61. Lapierre H, Doepel L, Milne E, et al. Responses in mammary and splanchnic metabolism to altered lysine supply in dairy cows. Animal 2009;3:360–71.
62. Robinson PH, Swanepoel N, Shinzato I, et al. Productive responses of lactating dairy cattle to supplementing high levels of ruminally protected lysine using a rumen protection technology. Anim Feed Sci Technol 2011;168:30–41.
63. Ouellet DR, Valkeners D, Lapierre H. Effects of metabolizable protein supply on N efficiency: plasma amino acid concentrations in dairy cows. In: Oltjen JW, Kebreab E, Lapierre H, editors. Energy and protein metabolism and nutrition in sustainable animal production EAAP publication no 134. The Netherlands: Wageningen Academic Publishers; 2013. p. 453–4.
64. Appuhamy JA, Knapp JR, Becvar O, et al. Effects of jugular-infused lysine, methionine and branched-chain amino acids on milk protein synthesis in high-producing dairy cows. J Dairy Sci 2011;94:1952–60.
65. Haque MN, Rulquin H, Lemosquet S. Milk protein response in dairy cows to changes in postruminal supplies of arginine, isoleucine and valine. J Dairy Sci 2013;96:420–30.
66. Doepel L, Lapierre H. Deletion of arginine from an abomasal infusion of amino acids does not decrease milk protein yield in Holstein cows. J Dairy Sci 2011; 94:864–73.
67. Jonker JS, Kohn RA, Erdman RA. Using milk urea nitrogen to predict nitrogen excretion and utilization efficiency in lactating dairy cows. J Dairy Sci 1998;81:2681–92.
68. Kauffman AJ, St-Pierre NR. The relationship of milk urea nitrogen to urine nitrogen excretion in Holstein and Jersey cows. J Dairy Sci 2001;84:2284–94.
69. Milano GD, Hotston-Moore A, Lobley GE. Influence of hepatic ammonia removal on ureagenesis, amino acid utilization and energy metabolism in the ovine liver. Br J Nutr 2000;83:307–15.
70. Rodriguez LA, Stallings CC, Herbein JH, et al. Diurnal variation in milk and plasma urea nitrogen in Holstein and Jersey cows in response to degradable dietary protein and added fat. J Dairy Sci 1997;80:3368–76.
71. Broderick GA, Clayton MK. A statistical evaluation of animal and nutritional factors influencing concentrations of milk urea nitrogen. J Dairy Sci 1997;80:2964–71.
72. Baker L, Ferguson JD, Chalupa W. Responses in urea and true protein of milk to different protein feeding schemes for dairy cows. J Dairy Sci 1995;78:2424–34.
73. Smith JF, Beaumont S, Hagemann L, et al. Relationship between bulk milk urea nitrogen and reproductive performance of New Zealand dairy herds. Proc New Zeal Soc Anim Prod 2001;61:192–4.
74. Van der Merwe BJ, Dugmore J, Walsh KP. The effect of monensin on milk production, milk urea nitrogen and body condition score of grazing dairy cows. S Afr J Anim Sci 2001;31:49–55.
75. Bahrami-Yekdangi H, Khorvash M, Ghorbani GR, et al. Effects of decreasing metabolizable protein and rumen-undegradable protein on milk production and composition and blood metabolites of Holstein dairy cows in early lactation. J Dairy Sci 2014;97:3042–52.

76. Canfield RW, Sniffen CJ, Butler WR. Effects of excess degradable protein on postpartum reproduction and energy balance in dairy cattle. J Dairy Sci 1990; 73:2342–9.
77. Butler WR, Calaman JJ, Beam SW. Plasma and milk urea nitrogen in relation to pregnancy rate in lactating dairy cattle. J Anim Sci 1996;74:858–65.
78. Godden SM, Kelton DF, Lissemore KD, et al. Milk urea testing as a tool to monitor reproductive performance in Ontario dairy herds. J Dairy Sci 2001;84: 1387–406.
79. Mitchell RG, Rogers GW, Dechow CD, et al. Milk urea nitrogen concentration: heritability and genetic correlations with reproductive performance and disease. J Dairy Sci 2005;88:4434–40.
80. Guo K, Russek-Cohen E, Varner MA, et al. Effects of milk urea nitrogen and other factors on probability of conception of dairy cows. J Dairy Sci 2004;87: 1878–85.
81. Spek JW, Bannink A, Gort G, et al. Interaction between dietary content of protein and sodium chloride on milk urea concentration, urinary urea excretion, renal recycling of urea, and urea transfer to the gastrointestinal tract in dairy cows. J Dairy Sci 2013;96:5734–45.
82. Davidson S, Hopkins BA, Diaz DE, et al. Effect of amounts and degradability of dietary protein on lactation, nitrogen utilization, and excretion in early lactation Holstein cows. J Dairy Sci 2003;86:1681–9.
83. Fatehi F, Xali A, Honarvar M, et al. Review of the relationship between milk urea nitrogen and days in milk, parity, monthly temperature mean in Iranian Holstein cows. J Dairy Sci 2011;95:5156–63.
84. Kröber TF, Külling DR, Menzi H, et al. Quantitative effects of feed protein reduction and methionine on nitrogen use by cows and nitrogen emission from slurry. J Dairy Sci 2000;83:2941–51.
85. Hristov AN, Ropp JK. Effect of dietary carbohydrate composition and availability on utilization of ruminal ammonia nitrogen for milk protein synthesis in dairy cows. J Dairy Sci 2003;86:2416–27.
86. Agle M, Hirstov AN, Zaman S, et al. The effects of ruminally degraded protein on rumen fermentation and ammonia losses from manure in dairy cows. J Dairy Sci 2009;93:1625–37.
87. Foley AE, Hristov AN, Melgar A, et al. Effect of barley and its amylopectin content on ruminal fermentation and nitrogen utilization in lactating dairy cows. J Dairy Sci 2006;89:4321–35.
88. Kalsheur KF, Baldwin RL VI, Glenn BP, et al. Milk production of dairy cows fed differing concentrations of rumen-degradable protein. J Dairy Sci 2006;89: 249–59.
89. Nousiainen JK, Shingfield J, Huhtanen P. Evaluation of milk urea nitrogen as a diagnostic of protein feeding. J Dairy Sci 2004;7:386–98.
90. Cyriac J, Rius AG, McGilliard ML, et al. Lactation performance of mid-lactation dairy cows fed ruminally degradable protein at concentrations lower than national research council recommendations. J Dairy Sci 2008;91:4704–13.
91. Bucholtz H, Johnson T. Use of milk urea nitrogen in herd management. Proceedings of 2007 Tri-State Dairy Nutrition Conference. Eastridge ML, editor. Ohio (Columbus): The Ohio State University; 2007. p. 63–7.
92. Ibrahim EA, Ingalls JR. Microbial protein biosynthesis in the rumen. J Dairy Sci 1972;55:971–8.

Lipid Feeding and Milk Fat Depression

Thomas C. Jenkins, MSc, PhD[a],*, Kevin J. Harvatine, MSc, PhD[b]

KEYWORDS

- Dietary lipids • Rumen • Biohydrogenation • Milk fat depression
- Conjugated linoleic acid

KEY POINTS

- Diets fed to cattle contain mostly unsaturated fatty acids supplied in grains and forages, by-products, and fat supplements.
- Lipid intake by dairy cattle must be restricted to prevent alterations of microbial populations in the rumen that can negatively affect the yield of milk and components.
- Unsaturated fatty acids consumed by cattle are extensively metabolized by microorganisms in the rumen in a process called biohydrogenation, yielding stearic acid as the end product plus a multitude of bioactive intermediates.
- Intermediates of biohydrogenation include a variety of conjugated linoleic acid (CLA) and *trans*-monoenoic acid isomers. Production of bioactive CLA isomers by rumen microorganisms is controlled by interactions among several dietary risk factors.
- Three specific CLA intermediates of biohydrogenation have been shown to cause milk fat depression in dairy cattle through coordinated suppression of mammary lipogenic genes by a transcription factor that is a central regulator of lipid synthesis.

FEED LIPIDS
Key Definitions and Nomenclature

- Ether extract: The fraction of feed extracted by organic solvents that includes nonlipid contaminants (such as pigments, water, and sugars), non–glycerol-based lipids (such as alkanes and waxes), and glycerol-based lipids (such as triglycerides, glycolipids, and phospholipids).
- Fatty acids: Chains of carbons that end in an acid or carboxyl group. In cereal grains and forages, the predominant fatty acids vary in length from 12 to 18 carbons.

The authors have nothing to disclose.
[a] Department of Animal & Veterinary Sciences, Clemson University, 117 Poole Agricultural Center, Clemson, SC 29634, USA; [b] Department of Animal Sciences, Penn State University, 301 Henning Building, University Park, State College, PA 16802, USA
* Corresponding author.
E-mail address: tjnkns@clemson.edu

Vet Clin Food Anim 30 (2014) 623–642
http://dx.doi.org/10.1016/j.cvfa.2014.07.006
0749-0720/14/$ – see front matter
vetfood.theclinics.com

- Fatty acid abbreviations: Because of the large number of fatty acids found in plant and body tissues, it is often difficult to remember all their names. It is common to simply refer to a fatty acid by the abbreviation "# carbons:# double bonds."
- Saturated fatty acids: Have no double bonds in the fatty acyl chain, such as C16:0 (palmitic acid) or C18:0 (stearic acid).
- Monounsaturated fatty acids: Have a single double bond somewhere in the fatty acyl chain, such as C16:1 (palmitoleic acid) or C18:1 (oleic acid).
- Polyunsaturated fatty acids (PUFA): Have more than 1 double bond in the fatty acyl chain, such as C18:2 (linoleic acid) or C18:3 (linolenic acid).

Lipid Components

Lipids are generally defined as organic compounds that are relatively insoluble in water but soluble in organic solvents.[1] A simple classification divides lipids into glycerol-based and non–glycerol-based components. Nonglycerol lipids include waxes and cutin, which provide an indigestible, impervious barrier on the exterior plant surface to reduce water loss and provide protection against plant pathogens and toxins. Surface lipids also inhibit plant digestion by ruminants because they limit bacterial penetration into the inner plant structures where most of the digestible nutrients are located. Disruption of this barrier by chewing or processing (eg, grinding or chopping) greatly increases bacterial access and rates of nutrient digestion.

The glycerol-based lipids contain fatty acids bound to a glycerol backbone. The value of fats and oils as animal feed ingredients is based on their fatty acid content and fatty acid composition. Content refers to the total concentration (% dry matter [DM]) of fatty acids in a lipid supplement, and composition (% total fatty acids) refers to the mixture of individual fatty acids that make up the lipid supplement. The most important glycerol-based lipids found in animal feed include triglycerides, phospholipids, and galactolipids (**Table 1**).

Fatty Acids

Fatty acids are chains of carbons that end in an acid group, or carboxyl group as it is referred to in biochemistry. An example of a common fatty acid is stearic acid, with 18 carbons and no double bonds. Fatty acids, such as stearic acid, are referred to as saturated because all the carbons are holding the maximum number of hydrogens possible, so the fatty acid is "saturated" with hydrogen. Stearic acid is low in plant oils but is present in higher amounts in animal fats, particularly in fats obtained from ruminant species such as beef tallow.

Oleic acid and linoleic acid are examples of unsaturated fatty acids containing 1 or more double bonds (**Fig. 1**). Oleic acid has a single double bond between carbons 9 and 10, and is referred to as a monounsaturated fatty acid. Linoleic acid is a PUFA

Table 1			
Glycerol-based lipids in animal feed ingredients			
Lipid	Components	Source	Fatty Acids (g/100 g)[a]
Triglyceride	Glycerol, 3 FA[b]	Cereal seeds	95
Galactolipids	Glycerol, 2 FA, sugar	Forages	56
Phospholipids	Glycerol, 2 FA, P, N	Plant membrane lipids	72[c]

[a] Calculated for a pure compound containing only oleic acid.
[b] Fatty acids.
[c] Assuming the phospholipid consisted only of lecithin or phosphatidylcholine.

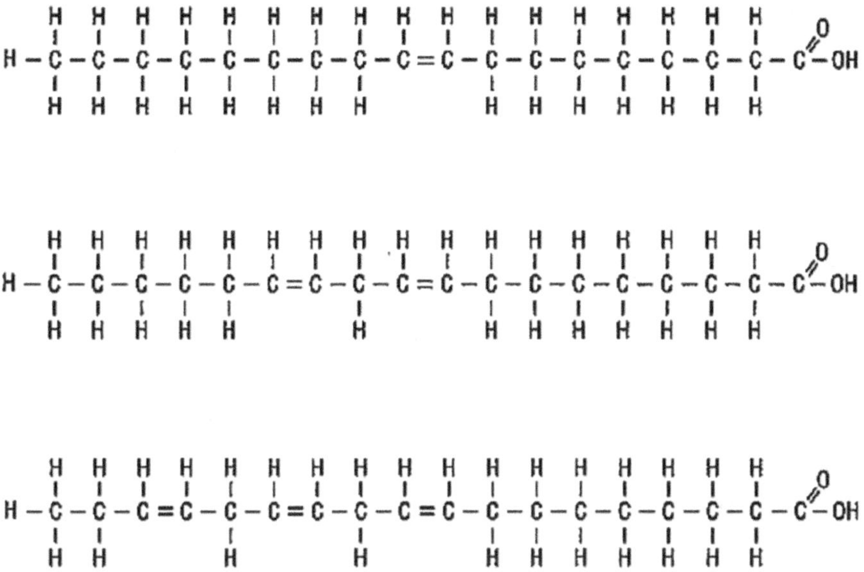

Fig. 1. Structures of the 3 primary unsaturated fatty acids consumed by cattle: oleic acid (*top*), linoleic acid (*middle*), and α-linolenic acid (*bottom*).

containing 2 double bonds, between carbons 9 and 10 and between carbons 12 and 13. Oleic acid is the predominant fatty acid in animal fats and some plant oils, such as canola oil (**Table 2**). Linoleic acid is the predominant fatty acid in many plant oils, including cottonseed oil, soybean oil, and corn oil. Linolenic acid, with 3 double bonds, is the primary fatty acid in most pasture species and in linseed oil from flax.

Table 2
Nomenclature, structural features, and example sources of common fatty acids found in animal feed

| | | Double-Bond Geometry/Location | | |
Abbreviation[a]	Name	Double-Bond Location[b]	ω Double-Bond Designation[c]	Fat/Oil Sources
C14:0	Myristic	NA		Animal fats
C16:0	Palmitic	NA		Animal fats
C18:0	Stearic	NA		Animal fats
C18:1	Oleic	c9	ω9	Canola
C18:2	Linoleic	c9c12	ω6	Corn, soybean
C18:3	Linolenic	c9c12c15	ω3	Linseed
C20:5	EPA	c5c8c11c14c17	ω3	Fish
C22:6	DHA	c4c7c10c13c16c19	ω3	Fish

[a] Number of carbons:number of double bonds.
[b] *cis* (c) followed by carbon position of double bond using the acid carbon (carbon 1) as reference. NA, not applicable because no double bonds are present.
[c] Omega (ω) position refers to number of carbons from the methyl end of fatty acyl chain to the first double bond.

Sources of Lipid Intake by Cattle

Grain and forage lipids

The fatty acid content of most cereal seeds and forages typically ranges from 1.0% to 3.0% DM, with most fatty acids classified as unsaturated (predominately oleic, linoleic, and α-linolenic acids). Among the unsaturated fatty acids, linolenic acid is the predominant fatty acid in most forage species, followed by linoleic acid.[2] In the cereal seeds, fatty acids are composed mainly of linoleic acid followed by oleic acid.

Fatty acid concentrations in some pasture can exceed 5.0% of DM, depending on plant species, stage of maturity, environment, and so forth. Fatty acid content of annual ryegrass pasture that was clipped in the field, immediately immersed in liquid nitrogen, and then freeze-dried contained as much as 6.8% DM as total fatty acids.[3] Cattle grazing some species of immature pasture, in effect, may be consuming a high-fat diet. Much lower concentrations are usually seen in hay and silage prepared from the same plant species, partially owing to loss of plant leaves whereby chloroplast lipid is concentrated but also because of plant metabolism of fat present as stored energy. Considerable variation in total fatty acid content has been reported in grass and corn silage samples (**Table 3**). Although the magnitude of the difference in fatty acid concentration is small in forages and cereal grains, they have a large impact as they make up most of the diet.

Plant maturity has a definite impact on both fatty acid content and fatty acid composition. Fatty acid content (% DM) generally is highest in the spring and fall seasons and lowest in the summer months. For example, fresh perennial ryegrass contained 3.2% DM total fatty acids during primary growth in May, but only 1.2% DM total fatty acids at the beginning of second regrowth.[4] Linolenic acid follows a similar seasonal pattern.[4] As linolenic acid declines over the summer months, the concentration of palmitic and linoleic acid increases.

Fatty acids can be released from glycerol in plant tissue through the action of plant-based lipases. Plant lipases were shown to release free fatty acids from damaged tissue after cutting,[5] and can continue to function in dried forage containing as little as 5% to 10% moisture.[6] Plant matter containing a high content of free fatty acids increases the risk of fermentation problems in the rumen of cattle and sheep.

Fat supplements

A useful way to categorize fat supplements for dairy rations is based on how they affect ruminal fermentation and digestion. One group includes fats that were specifically designed to avoid digestibility problems, such as calcium salts of fatty acids and hydrogenated fats. These fats are available commercially and have the added advantage of being dry fats that are easily transported and mixed with other feed ingredients. This group is best referred to as "rumen-inert" fats, to emphasize that they have little, if any, negative effects on fiber digestion in the rumen. The rumen-inert fats are also often referred to as bypass fats.

Table 3		
Range of total fatty acids (FA) in grass and corn silage samples		
FA (% Dry Matter)	**Grass Silage**	**Corn Silage**
Mean	1.9	2.0
Minimum	0.8	1.2
Maximum	3.3	3.5

Data from Khan NA, Cone JW, Fievez V, et al. Causes of variation in fatty acid content and composition in grass and maize silages. Anim Feed Sci Tech 2012;174:36–45.

The second group of fat supplements includes the unaltered extracts from plant and animal sources that can cause digestion problems in dairy cattle to varying degrees. Included in this group are fats of animal origin (tallow, grease, and so forth), plant oils (soybean oil, canola oil, and so forth), whole oilseeds (cottonseeds, soybeans, and so forth), and high-fat by-products such as residues from food-processing plants. These fats are referred to here as rumen-active to identify their potential to cause significant microbial and fermentation shifts in the rumen.

The distinction between the two groups is not always clear. At normal levels of supplementation some unprotected fats, such as tallow, are fed to dairy cows without evidence of consistent problems with fiber digestion. Even whole oilseeds help to lessen the severity of digestion problems by encapsulation of antimicrobial fatty acids within their hard outer seed coat. Disruption of the outer seed coat exposes the oil to the microbial population, and increases the risk for fermentation problems and microbial shifts. The seed coat can be broken by chewing and rumination, or through a variety of processing techniques such as extrusion or grinding. Roasting of cottonseed was reported to reduce biohydrogenation.[7] Classification according to ruminal digestion is better defined at high levels of supplementation, whereby the frequency of digestibility problems for tallow and oilseeds is much greater than for the rumen-inert fats.

Other rumen-active fats in high use are various corn coproducts from the fermentation industry. Fermentation of corn mash produces ethanol, which is distilled to remove the ethanol and centrifuged to remove as much excess liquid as possible. The liquid fraction can be dehydrated to produce condensed solubles, and the solid fraction may be sold directly as wet distillers grains or dehydrated to produce dried distillers grains. The condensed soluble can be blended with the distillers grains to produce wet distillers grains + soluble (WDGS) or dried distillers grains + soluble (DDGS). The resulting corn-processing procedures leave by-products high in protein and energy, including a high fat content (**Table 4**). Importantly the unsaturated fatty acids are rapidly available in the rumen and are at higher risk for disruption of rumen fermentation. In addition, large variation in the fat concentration can occur between production facilities and runs within some facilities. More recently lowering the oil content has become common, making low-fat distillers products available as animal feed and reducing the risk of disturbance of rumen fermentation.

Uses and Benefits of Fat Supplements

Adding fat to dairy rations can affect the productive efficiency of dairy cows through a combination of caloric and noncaloric effects (**Table 5**). Caloric effects are attributable

Table 4
Nutrient composition of corn coproducts

Nutrient	WDG	MDGS	DDG	DDGS
DM (%)	25–35	50	88–90	88–90
CP (%)	30–35	30–35	25–35	25–32
Fat (%)	8–12	8–12	8–10	8–10
NDF (%)	30–50	30–50	40–45	39–45
TDN (%)	70–110	70–110	77–88	85–90

Abbreviations: DDG, distillers dried grains; DDGS, distillers dried grains + soluble; MDGS, modified distillers grains + soluble; WDG, wet distillers grains.

Adapted from Tjardes K, Wright C. Feeding corn distillers coproducts to beef cattle. Extension Extra. Brookings (SD): South Dakota State University; 2002. Available at: http://www.extension.umn. edu/agriculture/beef/components/docs/feeding_corn_distillers_grains_to_beef_cattle_sdsu.pdf.

Table 5 Use and benefits of fat supplements	
Fat Use	**Benefits**
Increase diet energy density	Increase meat and milk production, increase body condition
Reduce dustiness and particle separation of mixed feeds	Improve feed handling and safety
Alter fatty acid profile of meat and milk	Conform to published nutritional guidelines for humans and enhance consumption of animal food products
Enhance tissue delivery of unsaturated fatty acids	Enhance metabolic and physiologic functioning such as improved reproductive performance and immunity
Increase milk fat	Increased milk components

to greater energy content and energetic efficiency of lipid in comparison with carbohydrate or protein, with the overall benefit being increased milk production. Noncaloric effects are benefits of added fat that are not directly attributable to its energy content or increased milk production. Examples of noncaloric effects include improved reproductive performance and altered fatty acid profile of milk.

The noncaloric benefits of fat supplements are directed at maintaining an adequate tissue supply of 2 unsaturated fatty acids: linoleic and linolenic acids. Linoleic and linolenic acids are regarded as essential because they are required for normal cell function but cannot be synthesized in amounts needed by body tissues. A typical total mixed ration (TMR) of grains and forages generally contains adequate essential fatty acids to meet the needs of the animal. However, most of the dietary essential fatty acids are transformed by microorganisms through biohydrogenation. As an example of increasing the rumen output of essential fatty acids, feeding fat to lactating dairy cows has improved reproductive performance in some studies.[8]

FAT METABOLISM IN THE RUMEN
Key Definitions and Nomenclature

- Lipolysis: Hydrolysis of fatty acids from glycerol by lipases produced either by plants or by microbial lipases produced in the rumen.
- Biohydrogenation (BH): Conversion of unsaturated fatty acids to more saturated end products by microorganisms in the rumen, resulting in formation of *trans* fatty acids as intermediates.
- Conjugated linoleic acid (CLA): The first intermediate in BH, whereby microbial isomerases move double bonds in plant unsaturated fatty acids closer together. More than 20 CLA isomers are produced in the rumen, the most recognized being *cis*-9, *trans*-11 18:2.
- CLA_{MFI}: The 3 CLA isomers produced in the rumen shown in research studies to inhibit milk fat synthesis.
- *Trans*-18:1: The intermediate of BH formed following the elimination of a double bond in CLA.

Lipolysis and Biohydrogenation in the Rumen

Food consumed by ruminants first passes through the rumen, where countless numbers of bacteria, protozoa, and fungi ferment the feed, releasing end products that are used by the host animal for maintenance and growth of body tissues. The microbial population in the rumen also is responsible for extensive transformation of dietary lipid. Lipid transformations include lipolysis to release free fatty acids from glycerol-based plant lipids, and BH to convert unsaturated fatty acids in plant matter to more saturated lipid end products.

Lipids entering the rumen are first transformed by microbial lipases in a process called lipolysis. The microbial lipases hydrolyze the ester linkages in glycerol-based lipids, causing release of fatty acids and glycerol. The glycerol produced is fermented, yielding mostly volatile fatty acids (VFA). Microbes have a high capacity for lipolysis, and the rate of lipolysis predominantly depends on the availability of esterified fatty acids and their release from feed particles.

The BH of linoleic acid in the rumen (**Fig. 2**) begins with its conversion to CLA. In this initial step, the number of double bonds remains the same but one of the double bonds is shifted to a new position by microbial enzymes. Normally the double bonds in linoleic acid are separated by 2 single bonds, but in CLA the double bonds are only separated by a single bond. Many types of CLA are produced in the rumen of dairy cows,[9] but a common CLA produced from BH of linoleic acid under normal rumen conditions is *cis*-9, *trans*-11 C18:2 (rumenic acid). Under altered conditions a large number of different CLA isomers are synthesized.

As BH progresses, double bonds in the CLA intermediates are then hydrogenated further to *trans* fatty acids having only 1 double bond. A final hydrogenation step by the ruminal microbes eliminates the last double bond, yielding stearic acid as the end product. *Trans* double bonds only differ from *cis* double bonds in the placement of the hydrogens (**Fig. 3**). The hydrogens are located on opposite sides of the double bond for *trans* fatty acids, but on the same side of the double bond for *cis* fatty acids. Although the difference in structure between *trans* and *cis* fatty acids appears to be small, it causes significant differences in their physical and metabolic properties. In cows on a typical forage diet, the major *trans* C18:1 present in ruminal contents is *trans*-11 C18: 1 (vaccenic acid).

The rate of rumen BH and the pathways used depend highly on the microbial population, which is influenced by diet composition and rumen environment. For example,

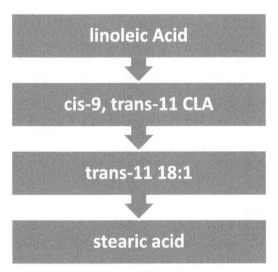

Fig. 2. Major steps in the biohydrogenation of linoleic acid to stearic acid by microorganisms in the rumen.

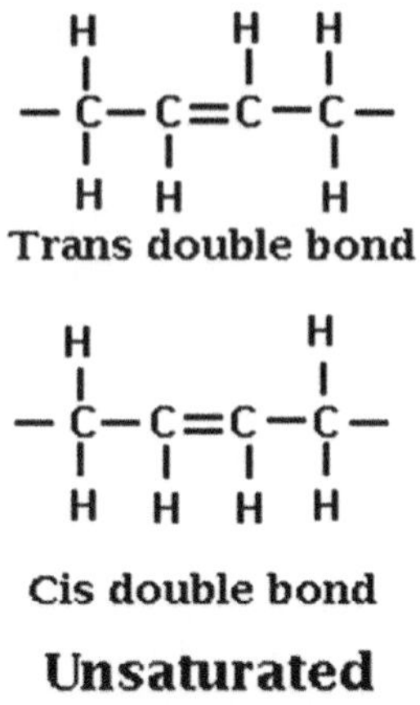

Trans double bond

Cis double bond

Unsaturated

Fig. 3. Structural differences between *cis* and *trans* fatty acids.

increasing unsaturated fatty acids and diet fermentability slow the normal BH pathway and shift BH to alternative pathways.

Key Points About Biohydrogenation in the Rumen

- BH is a microbial pathway designed to reduce unsaturation of lipids found within plant matter, and is likely an evolutionary adaptation to protect the microbial population from antimicrobial effects of unsaturated fatty acids. The resulting *trans* and saturated fatty acids are also preferentially incorporated into microbial phospholipid membranes, as microbial membranes are high in saturated and *trans* fatty acids and low in unsaturated fatty acids.
- The major intermediates of BH include an array of *trans*-C18:1 and conjugated linoleic acid isomers, but most published pathways have traditionally ignored most minor intermediates and present only a superficial view of BH because of the complexity of the analysis.
- The rates and predominant pathways of BH depend on the diet and rumen environment.
- Increasing dietary unsaturated fatty acids challenges the capacity of BH pathways and increases accumulation of bioactive intermediates in the rumen. Fatty acids originate from intake of forages and grains, oilseeds, by-products, and fat supplements.
- The impacts of BH on animal performance include protection of ruminal fermentation from antimicrobial effects of unsaturated fatty acids, loss of dietary ω fatty acids needed for optimal reproduction and immune function, and accumulation of conjugated intermediates with physiologic activity, such as the *trans*-10, *cis*-12 isomer that inhibits mammary lipogenesis and causes milk fat depression (MFD).

MILK FAT DEPRESSION
Previous Theories on Etiology

MFD has been investigated for well over a century and has a rich history of different theories. Identification of the causative factor linking changes in the diet to changes in milk fat synthesis was complicated by complex environmental conditions in the rumen during MFD. One of the earliest theories proposed that a limitation in fatty acid absorption resulted in MFD,[10] which was quickly disproved, as MFD also occurs when feeding diets high in fat. Recently, it was reported that abomasal fatty acid infusion could not overcome the effects of *trans*-10, *cis*-12 CLA, one of the bioactive CLA isomers that reduces milk fat synthesis.[11] Other theories focused on changes in rumen VFA synthesis and their impact on metabolism. Changes in rumen fermentation during MFD typically decrease the acetate to propionate molar ratio.[12] The low acetate to propionate ratio formed the basis for a widely known theory proposing that inadequate acetate supply was limiting milk fat synthesis. However, the reduced ratio of acetate to propionate with highly fermentable diets is predominantly due to increased ruminal production of propionate,[12,13] and ruminal infusion of acetate to cows during MFD had only a marginal impact on milk fat yield.[14]

Increased absorption of propionate was then proposed as the cause of MFD. The theory was that increased propionate resulted in increased plasma glucose, which stimulated insulin secretion. Increased insulin then would increase adipose tissue lipogenesis and decrease lipolysis (mobilization of body fat stores). However, direct testing by propionate, glucose, or insulin infusion resulted in milk fat reductions of less than 15% in well-fed cows. Infusion of insulin in cows in negative energy balance using hyperinsulinemic-euglycemic clamps resulted in a 35% decrease in milk fat yield, whereas well-fed cows averaged a 5% reduction.[15–17] However, the decrease in milk fat during insulin clamps was due to a decrease in preformed fatty acids originating from the diet and adipose tissue, whereas classic diet-induced MFD is characterized by a substantial decrease in de novo synthesized fatty acids. Lastly, reduced ruminal synthesis of vitamin B_{12} was also proposed as a possible mechanism of MFD. Vitamin B_{12} deficiency may result in increased circulating methylmalonyl-CoA, which is a competitive inhibitor fatty acid synthase, resulting in a reduction in de novo synthesis of fatty acids. However, supplementation of B_{12} failed to alleviate diet-induced MFD. Overall, several decades of research has tested numerous theories based on substrate limitations, and has found little to no evidence in their support.[13,18,19]

The Biohydrogenation Theory of Milk Fat Depression

The BH theory links MFD with the formation of specific CLA isomers produced from the BH of PUFA in the diet. Lipids in feed are metabolized by the rumen microbial population, which leads to the formation of bioactive CLA that affect living cells and tissue. Microorganisms in the rumen produce more than 20 types of known CLA isomers, 3 of which have been shown to cause MFD, subsequently referred to as CLA_{MFI}, because these CLA act as milk fat inhibitors. One of the most studied CLA_{MFI} is *trans*-10, *cis*-12 18:2. The CLA_{MFI} produced in the rumen travel via the blood to the mammary gland, where they inhibit the synthesis of milk fat by impairing the production of several enzymes essential for fat synthesis in the mammary gland. CLA_{MFI} are also present in cows that produce acceptable milk fat levels, but at concentrations too low to cause MFD.

Overproduction of CLA_{MFI} is triggered by nutrition-driven changes in the rumen. Formation of the CLA isomers causing MFD has been associated with several dietary risk factors including excessive unsaturated fat intake, high-grain diets, and low rumen pH. Substrates for BH include both linoleic and linolenic acids[20,21] found in nearly all plant-based components of dairy diets. The bottom line is that the type of feed the cow consumes affects rumen conditions, which in turn affects the amount and type of CLA produced. Because CLA_{MFI} overproduction in the rumen leads to MFD, excess CLA_{MFI} and, therefore, MFD can be controlled by paying close attention to several key nutritional risks.

Changes in the ruminal environment initiated through the diet can lead to a microbial population shift that is accompanied by a change in the type of CLA produced (**Fig. 4**). For example, low rumen pH can be a key factor contributing to a microbial shift and changes in the type of CLA produced. Dropping pH in continuous cultures of mixed ruminal microorganisms caused an increase in the concentration of *trans*-10, *cis*-12 CLA but no change in *cis*-9, *trans*-11 CLA.[22] Qiu and colleagues[23] reported that reduced ruminal pH can affect microbial populations, especially cellulolytic bacteria. Total cellulolytic bacteria numbers were reduced, accompanied by reduced acetate to propionate ratio and altered BH when pH was low.

The BH theory was directly demonstrated by the abomasal infusion of pure preparations of the normal CLA intermediate (*cis*-9, *trans*-11 CLA) and one of the major alternative (*trans*-10, *cis*-12) intermediates.[24] The *trans*-10, *cis*-12 CLA rapidly decreased milk fat yield over the course of 2 to 4 days, and recapitulates all postabsorptive aspects of the diet-induced MFD phenotype. Furthermore, the response occurs in every cow and the magnitude of the response is very predictable ($R^2 = 0.86$[25]). *Trans*-9, *cis*-11 CLA and *cis*-10, *trans*-12 CLA have also been reported as potential inhibitors of milk fat synthesis,[26,27] although they are less potent than *trans*-10, *cis*-12 CLA. Additional unidentified bioactive isomers likely play a role in MFD, as the known CLA isomers do not account for the entire reduction in milk fat observed during diet-induced MFD.[28]

Cellular and Molecular Mechanisms of Conjugated Linoleic Acid Causing Milk Fat Depression

The fatty acids in milk come from approximately an equal contribution from de novo synthesis within the mammary cell and uptake of preformed fatty acids from circulation (for a review see Ref.[13]). The fatty acids are esterified in the endoplasmic reticulum (ER) and are assembled into lipid droplets that move to the apex of the cell. Several proteins are associated with the milk fat globular membrane that surrounds the lipid droplet, and they are essential for fat secretion.[29,30] The number of essential enzymes and processes required for milk fat synthesis provide the opportunity for regulation at multiple steps and levels. Of note, diet-induced MFD results in up to a 50% reduction in milk fat synthesis, but BH intermediates are not able to reduce milk fat beyond this

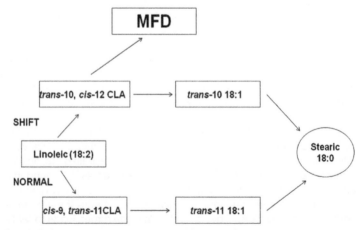

Fig. 4. The shift in intermediates produced from biohydrogenation of linoleic acid in ruminal contents as a result of a diet-induced microbial shift. MFD, milk fat depression.

point. One interpretation of this is that half of the milk fat is under dietary control of and responsive to dietary factors while a basal level of milk fat is constant or regulated by other factors. Milk fat provides a significant portion of the energy for a growing calf, so this may ensure adequate energy for the calf.

During both CLA-induced and diet-induced MFD, the decrease in milk fat includes both de novo and preformed fatty acids, although a larger decrease in the de novo synthesized portion is observed especially with larger reductions in milk fat. This finding suggests a coordinated regulation of the enzymes of lipid synthesis, and that the regulation could occur at the level of gene expression, enzyme abundance, or enzyme activity. Previous work clearly shows a coordinated decrease in mammary expression of many lipid synthesis enzymes during both CLA-induced and diet-induced MFD,[31–34] and regulation of gene expression is considered the predominant level of regulation during MFD. Coordinated suppression of mammary lipogenic genes suggests involvement of a central regulator of lipid synthesis, and a transcription factor called sterol response element binding protein 1 (SREBP1) has become a focus of investigation.[32,33] This transcription factor functions as a global regulator of lipid synthesis, and mammary expression of SREBP1 decreases during CLA-induced and diet-induced MFD. In addition, most lipid synthesis enzymes that are downregulated during CLA-induced and diet-induced MFD contain a SREBP1 response element in their promoter and are regulated by SREBP1c.[32] Other regulators have been investigated and a role for thyroid hormone responsive spot 14 has been proposed,[32] although functional roles of other transcription factors are not supported by current data (eg, LXRs and PPARs).

Investigation of MFD has provided key insights into the mechanisms regulating milk fat synthesis. This understanding of the molecular regulation of milk fat synthesis provides a foundation for the development of methods to increase milk fat. For example, single nucleotide polymorphisms (SNPs) that may explain genetic differences in milk fat yield and fatty acid composition have been identified in SREBP1, SREBP1 regulatory proteins, and S14.[35,36]

Recovery from Milk Fat Depression

The mammary gland is acutely sensitive to absorption of CLA, with reduced milk fat synthesis observed within 12 hours of abomasal infusion.[37] Recent time-course experiments have characterized the timing of induction and recovery of diet-induced MFD.[38] MFD was induced by feeding a diet lower in fiber and high in unsaturated fatty acids (29.5% neutral detergent fiber [NDF] plus 3.7% PUFA) and then recovered by feeding a higher-fiber and low-oil diet (36.9% NDF plus 1.1% PUFA) while sampling milk every other day. Milk fat concentration and yield decreased progressively when the low-fiber and high-oil diet was fed, reaching the maximal decrease by 9 days (**Fig. 5**). When switched to the recovery diet, milk fat yield progressively increased and was fully recovered by 18 days. A key insight from the experiment is the expected lag between making diet adjustments and changes occurring in milk fat synthesis. Addition of a risk factor may cause MFD in 7 to 10 days, and elimination of a risk factor is expected to take 10 to 14 days to observe a benefit. Knowing the time course is very important in identifying what may have caused MFD and knowing how long to wait to determine whether a diet correction has been effective in improving milk fat. In subsequent work focusing on diets that accelerate recovery, it was determined that correction of dietary unsaturated fat was more important than correction of diet fermentability,[39] and that removal of monensin did not change the rate of recovery of normal rumen BH and mammary de novo fatty acid synthesis.[40]

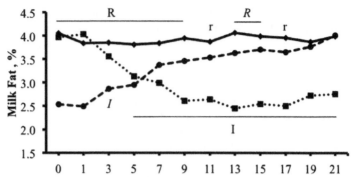

Fig. 5. Time course of induction of milk fat depression by feeding a low-fiber and high-oil diet, and recovery from milk fat depression by feeding a higher-fiber and low-fat diet. Cows were fed a high-fiber, low-oil diet (Control; *diamonds*), a low-fiber. high soy-oil diet to induce milk fat depression (*squares*), or a high-fiber, low-oil diet following high-fiber, low-oil diet that induced milk fat depression (Recovery; *circles*). Significant differences are shown between induction and control (R = $P<.01$, R = $P<.05$, and r = $P<.1$) and recovery and control (I = $P<.01$, I = $P<.05$, and i = $P<.1$). *From* Rico DE, Harvatine KJ. Induction of and recovery from milk fat depression occurs progressively in dairy cows switched between diets that differ in fiber and oil concentration. J Dairy Sci 2013;96(10):6621–30; with permission.

NUTRITIONAL FACTORS THAT CAUSE MILK FAT DEPRESSION
Key Nutritional Factors Targeted for Increased Risk of Milk Fat Depression

- Excessive unsaturated fat
- High rapidly degradable starch
- Amount and type of fiber
- Ionophores
- Feed management
- High yeasts and molds

These 6 independent nutritional factors are currently targeted for influencing rumen production of CLA_{MFI} and the development of MFD. More is known about the influence of forages, starch, and fat in the diet. These factors receive more detailed consideration in this article than yeast and management influences, which have been less tested and documented. Of importance is that MFD is commonly not due to a single factor but to an interaction of risk factors, allowing MFD to occur when more than 1 factor is only marginally high.

Fats

Too much fat in the diet of dairy cows is a classic cause of MFD. Nutritionists are keenly aware that fat must be limited to lower levels than protein or carbohydrate to avoid impaired rumen fermentation, reductions in feed intake, and MFD. It is tempting to push the limit on feeding fat when prices are favorable for high-fat by-products, when grain prices reach record levels making commercial fats more competitive, or when the farm has access to (perceptually inexpensive) high-fat waste products from a nearby food-processing plant. The key to preventing MFD from these high-fat ingredients is to fully understand the nutritional and chemical impact these ingredients have on both the rumen microorganisms and the cow, and to choose a feeding rate that will provide the most benefit with the least risk of detriment to the production of milk and components.

Fat supplements pose different degrees of MFD risk. Low-risk fats are those that cause little disruption of the microbial population in the rumen, and thus maintain normal fermentation and limited production of CLA_{MFI}. Low-risk fats are generally characterized by high saturated fatty acids or calcium salts of fatty acids. Most commercial bypass fats are based on one or both of these characteristics, so the risk of MFD is low. Calcium salts are most commonly made from palm fatty acids distillate, which is a lesser unsaturated plant oil. More recently calcium salts higher in PUFA have become available. Bypass fat feeding rate is usually limited by cost and availability. In addition, bypass fats are dry solid products rather than liquid fats, and therefore are easier to package, transport, and mix on the farm without specialized equipment. Bypass fats are also called rumen-inert fats to emphasize their lower risk for disrupting the rumen. However, MFD has been reported with inclusion of calcium salts, especially with products with more polyunsaturated fatty acids and when fed in higher-risk situations.[41]

High-risk fat supplements contain more unsaturated fatty acids that are typically found in forages, cereal grains, and oilseeds (cottonseed, soybeans, canola, sunflower, and so forth). A high concentration of unsaturated fatty acids in the rumen from 1 or more of these sources can inhibit some microbial species in the rumen. This change can favor species that produce CLA_{MFI}, the accumulation of which can lead to MFD. In addition, unsaturated fatty acids also increase the amount of substrate that must be biohydrogenated, resulting in increased CLA_{MFI} formation if the capacity of the pathway is limited. These high-risk, unsaturated fat supplements are referred to as rumen-active fats to emphasize their tendency to disrupt rumen conditions.

A convenient tool to monitor risky unsaturated fatty acid intake is called RUFAL or Rumen Unsaturated Fatty Acid Load. RUFAL reflects the total unsaturated fatty acid supply entering the rumen each day from feed. RUFAL accounts for unsaturated fatty acids from all feed ingredients rather than fatty acids only from fat supplements. RUFAL may better indicate potential rumen fermentation disruption than simply calculating the percentage of fat added to the diet. Studies show that increasing RUFAL causes fermentation disruption, which can hinder animal performance. Excessive RUFAL can lead to MFD. The interaction of risk factors makes it difficult to establish a RUFAL cutoff, but values below 3.5% DM are viewed as lower fat intakes, whereas those above 3.5% DM indicate fatty acid intakes that may be at risk of being too high. However, it should be noted that some herds with high milk fat (3.8% or more) have been fed RUFAL in excess of 3.5% DM, most likely because other risk factors were minimal. RUFAL suggests a guideline for identifying diets low or high in fat as a logical assessment of MFD risk.

Of the many strategies to feeding fat to dairy cows, perhaps the most important, yet most elusive, is the proper amount to feed. A proper feeding rate can usually prevent MFD associated with fat supplements. To effectively use the vast array of fat products available, practical guidelines must be developed that match sources of fat with proper supplementation. Many recommendations to limit rumen-active fats suggest a single feeding rate for added fat in dairy rations. These single numbers are easy to remember and calculate, but do not account for fatty acid contributions from the basal diet or adjust fat feeding rates in relation to fat supplement composition. An alternative approach includes the following 2 calculations:

1. Limit the total fat consumed from all sources (basal ingredients plus fat supplements) so that

   lbs total fatty acid intake = lbs milk fat produced

2. Limit rumen-active fats so that

$$\text{lbs rumen} - \text{active fatty acids} = \frac{4 \times \text{NDF} \times \text{DMI}}{\text{UFA} \times 100}$$

where NDF is % neutral detergent fiber (DM basis) of the dairy TMR; DMI is DM intake of cows in lb/d; UFA is % unsaturated fatty acids in the rumen-active fat supplement.

Starch

High-grain diets are also known to cause MFD. Rapid fermentation of starch can cause acid accumulation and lower pH in the rumen. Factors that can result in marked changes in rumen pH through any 24-hour period include: dietary carbohydrate profile and rates of degradation of the carbohydrate fractions as affected by source, processing, and moisture; physically effective NDF (peNDF) supply as affected by source and particle size; and production of salivary buffers as a function of peNDF supply and source. Despite our general understanding of these factors, the degree and duration of low rumen pH required for accumulation of CLA_{MFI} in the rumen is not known. Although data are limited, rumen pH changes are most likely associated with MFD because they alter bacterial populations by favoring those that use the alternative pathways of BH that form CLA_{MFI}.

Studies show that low pH alters the microbial population in the rumen and causes accumulation of CLA_{MFI}. In a study by Fuentes and colleagues,[22] the pH of rumen cultures was lowered from 6.5 to 5.5, causing a shift in CLA production that included increased CLA_{MFI}. Although milk fat percentages often decline as rumen pH values decrease, there is still a lot of variation seen as scatter around the line (**Fig. 6**). This finding indicates that rumen pH is not the only factor controlling CLA_{MFI} and milk fat percentage. Therefore, rumen acidosis should not be viewed as a prerequisite for MFD.

The rate of degradability of the starch fraction in grains also determines risk for MFD. Field observations and inferences from studies indicate that rapid rates of starch fermentability are linked to a greater risk of MFD. Fermented feeds with high grain content, such as corn silage and high-moisture corn, carry the highest risk. Differences in

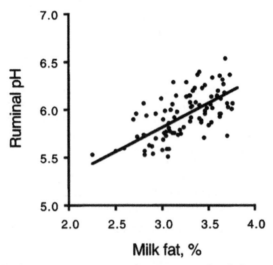

Fig. 6. Relationships between rumen pH and percentage of milk fat as reported by Allen (1997). (*Data from* Allen MS. Relationship between fermentation acid production in the rumen and the requirement for physically effective fiber. J Dairy Sci 1997;80:1447–62.)

corn varieties, silo storage time, and climate conditions for plant growth can all lead to rapid rates of starch degradation in silage and high-moisture corn. Longer storage can lead to higher rates of starch degradability. A study by Newbold and colleagues,[42] using an in vitro test in rumen fluid over 3 hours, found a 30% increase in degradability in corn silage stored for 2 months versus 10 months. If high rates of starch degradability in forages are suspected as a cause of MFD, usually there is little that can remedy the situation. One option is to dilute the forage with less degradable feed, but often this is not available. An alternative option is to focus on other risk factors (such as rumen pH and dietary fat) to minimize CLA_{MFI} production.

Forages/Fiber

Maintaining adequate forage levels in dairy diets decreases the risk of MFD. As explained previously, forage can help maintain rumen pH, slow rumen passage, and limit the synthesis of CLA_{MFI}. This approach emphasizes peNDF to sustain cud-chewing and production of salivary buffers. Nutritionists use specific forage guidelines tailored for specific dairies with individualized forage needs. Within those guidelines, however, maintaining a consistent forage program is the first line of defense against problems with MFD. Again, the rate of starch degradability in forage also affects CLA_{MFI} production. High rates of starch degradability in silage has been associated with an increased risk of MFD, which means that silage NDF alone, as a proxy of forage level and assumed peNDF, is not enough to explain all occurrences of MFD.

A lesser known and often ignored attribute of forages related to MFD is their contribution to the cow's total fat intake. For example, fatty acids in corn silage typically average around 1.5% to 2.0% of DM, but can reach 3.5% or higher. When requesting a forage analysis it is important to remember that fatty acid content is not the same as crude fat content. Fat content has traditionally been determined as the ether-extractable component of the feed. In addition to extracting fat, ether also extracts some carbohydrate, vitamins, and pigments. Therefore, crude fat in cereal grains, forages, and the TMR often contains less than 60% fatty acids. Forage containing 3.5% total fatty acids could contain 5% to 6% crude fat. Given the large quantities of corn silage fed to cows in some operations, this amounts to significant fat intakes just from silages alone.

Yeasts/Management

Yeasts/molds and management factors are both regarded as significant risk factors for MFD, but little is known about exactly how they affect rumen function and the accumulation of CLA_{MFI}. Speculative theories about molds and yeasts suggest they may produce antimicrobial substances as part of their metabolism, which in turn may negatively affect the rumen microbial population; however, much remains to be proved in this regard. High yeast and mold counts in fermented feeds is undesirable not only for the risk of MFD but also because it can reduce feed intake, negatively affect animal health, and decrease overall lactation performance, in addition to incurring additional feed losses through "shrink." In well-preserved silage, yeast counts less than 10,000 CFU/g are common. Counts that affect animal health and performance poorly are not well defined, and likely depend on the specific strain of yeast or mold infecting the plant. As a general rule, yeast counts at or higher than 1 million CFU/g should cause concern.

Several management factors also have been connected with the increased risk of MFD. Among these are bunk space, stocking density, and mixing of the TMR. These factors can all cause sorting and slug-feeding of grain, resulting in low rumen pH and subsequent production of CLA_{MFI} in the rumen. In general, all attempts to maintain cow comfort and maintain good overall herd management will minimize the risk of MFD.

Summary of Corn Silage Characteristics Often Associated with Increased Risk of Milk Fat Depression

- High fat content (such as fatty acids at 2.5% or more of plant DM)
- High free fatty acids (such as 50% or more of total fatty acids)
- High rates of starch degradability (such as 85% or more in a 7-hour in vitro test)
- High yeasts and molds (such as yeast counts exceeding 1 million CFU/g)

Feeding Strategies

Slug-feeding grain is commonly associated with subclinical rumen acidosis and MFD. Many assume that TMR feeding eliminates this issue because every bite has the same nutrient composition. However, the rate of intake of fermentable organic matter is variable over the day, owing to sorting and variable rates of intake. In general, cows sort for more fermentable feed particle early in the day but also consume feed at approximately a 3 times higher rate after delivery of fresh feed. Feed management may allow a more even distribution of intake across the day. The first consideration is continuous feed availability, as long periods without feed or away from feed is expected to promote high intake once feed becomes available. Increased feeding frequency may also distribute feed across the day, as offering fresh feed is a strong stimulus for feed intake.[43] For example, feeding 4 times per day in equal meals every 6 hours decreased the concentration of alternative BH fatty acids and increased milk fat yield and concentration compared with feeding once per day.[44]

Interactions Among Risk Factors

A single risk factor, such as starch source or feeding ionophores, might not contribute to MFD individually, but when combined interactions could suddenly trigger changes in BH that lead to MFD. As an example, continuous cultures of ruminal microorganisms were fed either a high-corn or high-barley diet along with 2 levels of soybean oil (0% and 5%) and 2 levels of monensin (0 and 25 ppm). Trans-10 18:1 was monitored as an indicator of a BH shift. The addition of soybean oil increased trans-10 18:1 concentrations in the cultures for both the corn and barley diets.[45] To a lesser extent, monensin also increased trans-10 18:1 for both corn and barley. However, an interaction occurred when monensin and soybean oil were combined. Adding monensin with soybean oil did not further elevate trans-10 18:1 when the diet was corn-based. When the diet was barley-based, adding monensin with soybean oil elevated trans-10 18:1 more than either risk factor alone.

A similar grain × monensin × fat interaction was examined in lactating dairy cows.[46] Eighty Holstein cows were assigned either a high (27.7%) or low (20.3%) starch diet for 21 days, followed by the addition of rumensin (13 ppm) or corn oil (1.25%) for an additional 21 days. Thereafter, cows were switched to diets with opposite corn-oil levels for a final 21-day period, giving 8 treatments in a 2 × 2 × 2 factorial design. Oil level was a higher risk factor for MFD in comparison with rumensin, with a decrease from 3.32% to 2.99% for corn oil versus 3.20% to 3.11% for rumensin. Feeding high-starch diets had borderline effects on MFD, causing milk fat to decline from 3.25% to 3.06% ($P = .10$). Starch degradability might also have been a contributing factor to MFD in this study. The diets used in this study contained steam-flaked corn, which has an inherently fast rate of ruminal starch degradation, therefore degradability, compounded by high DMI, may be a more potent MFD risk factor than starch intake alone.

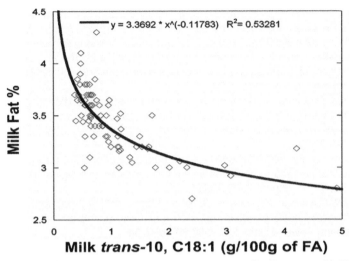

Fig. 7. Relationship between milk *trans*-10 C18:1 content and percentage of milk fat. (*Data from* Nydam DV, Overton TR, Mechor GD, et al. Risk factors for bulk tank milk fat depression in northeast and Midwest US dairy herds feeding monensin. Charlotte (NC): American Association of Bovine Practitioners; 2008.)

An on-farm epidemiologic study was done in 2008[47] to establish risk factors that contribute to MFD in commercial dairy herds feeding rumensin. This extensive study involved 79 commercial dairy herds across 10 states. Cow numbers ranged from 30 to 2800 across herds, with a mean herd size of 474 cows. Milk fat percentage ranged from 2.7% to 4.3% (mean 3.43%) and rumensin dose ranged from 150 to 410 mg/head/d (mean 258 mg/head/d). No significant associations with herd milk fat percentage were seen with stall types, cooling systems, or feeding design. Herds with higher formulated DMI, however, tended to have lower milk fat percentage. No relationships were seen between rumensin dose and herd milk fat percentage. Likewise, TMR concentrations of DM, acid detergent fiber, NDF, nonfiber carbohydrate, and crude fat did not relate to milk fat percentage.

Several significant relationships did surface from the study. Herd milk fat percentage was strongly associated with changes in *trans*-10 C18:1 isomers in milk fat (**Fig. 7**). An identical relationship was reported by Hinrichsen and colleagues[48] between milk fat yield and milk *trans*-10 C18:1 across published research studies. No single TMR characteristic or ration component measured in this study accounted for more than 10 percentage of the variation in herd milk fat percentage. When a multivariate regression was done on all measured TMR variables (such as DM, starch, NDF, and so forth) and herd management factors, followed by a stepwise regression that eliminated nonsignificant variables one at a time, the significant factors remaining in the model were TMR DM% and percentage of particles on the bottom pan of the Penn State particle separator. Together, TMR DM% and bottom-pan particles accounted for 21% of the variation in herd milk fat percentage in the study.

REFERENCES

1. Pond WG, Church DC, Pond KR, et al. Basic animal nutrition and feeding. 5th edition. Hoboken (NJ): John Wiley & Sons, Inc; 2005.

2. Hatfied R, Jung HG, Broderick G, et al. Nutritional chemistry of forages. In: Barnes RF, editor. Forages. The science of grassland agriculture, vol. 2, 6th edition. Ames (IA): Blackwell Publishing, Iowa State Press; 2007. p. 467–86.

3. Freeman-Pounders SJ, Hancock DW, Bertrand JA, et al. The fatty acid profile of rye and annual ryegrass pasture changes during their growth cycle. Forage and Grazinglands January 30, 2009.

4. Bauchart D, Verite R, Remond B. Long-chain fatty acid digestion in lactating cows fed fresh grass from spring to autumn. Can J Anim Sci 1984;64:330–1.

5. Thomas H. The role of polyunsaturated fatty acids in senescence. J Plant Physiol 1986;123:97–105.

6. Van Ranst G, Fievez V, De Riek J, et al. Influence of ensiling forages at different dry matters and silage additives on lipid metabolism and fatty acid composition. Anim Feed Sci Technol 2009;150:62–74.

7. Pires AV, Eastridge ML, Firkins JL, et al. Effects of heat treatment and physical processing of cottonseed on nutrient digestibility and production performance by lactating cows. J Dairy Sci 1997;80:1685 94.

8. Staples CR, Burke JM, Thatcher WW. Influence of supplemental fats on reproductive tissues and performance of lactating cows. J Dairy Sci 1998;81:856–87.

9. Bauman DE, Lock AL. Concepts in lipid digestion and metabolism in dairy cows. In Proc. Tri-State Dairy Nutr. Conf. 2006. p. 1–14. Available at: http://tristatedairy.osu.edu/. Accessed April 25 and 26, 2014.

10. Van Soest PJ. Ruminant fat metabolism with particular reference to factors affecting low milk fat and feed efficiency. A review. J Dairy Sci 1963;46:204–16.

11. Vyas D, Moallem U, Teter BB, et al. Milk fat responses to butterfat infusion during conjugated linoleic acid-induced milk fat depression in lactating dairy cows. J Dairy Sci 2013;96(4):2387–99.

12. Bauman DE, Griinari JM. Regulation and nutritional manipulation of milk fat: low-fat milk syndrome. Livest Prod Sci 2001;70(1–2):15–29.

13. Bauman DE, Griinari JM. Nutritional regulation of milk fat synthesis. Annu Rev Nutr 2003;23:203–27.

14. Davis CL, Brown RE. Low-fat milk syndrome. In: Phillipson AT, editor. Physiology of digestion and metabolism in the ruminant. Newcastle upon Tyne (United Kingdom): Oriel Press; 1970. p. 545–65.

15. McGuire MA, Griinari JM, Dwyer DA, et al. Role of insulin in the regulation of mammary synthesis of fat and protein. J Dairy Sci 1995;78(4):816–24.

16. Griinari JM, McGuire MA, Dwyer DA, et al. Role of insulin in the regulation of milk fat synthesis in dairy cows. J Dairy Sci 1997;80(6):1076–84.

17. Corl BA, Butler ST, Butler WR, et al. Short communication: regulation of milk fat yield and fatty acid composition by insulin. J Dairy Sci 2006;89(11):4172–5.

18. Bauman DE, Harvatine KJ, Lock AL. Nutrigenomics, rumen-derived bioactive fatty acids, and the regulation of milk fat synthesis. Annu Rev Nutr 2011;31:299–319.

19. Shingfield KJ, Griinari JM. Role of biohydrogenation intermediates in milk fat depression. Eur J Lipid Sci Technol 2007;109(8):799–816.

20. Lee YJ, Jenkins TC. Biohydrogenation of linolenic acid to stearic acid by the rumen microbial population yields multiple intermediate conjugated diene isomers. J Nutr 2011;141:1445–50.

21. Lee YJ, Jenkins TC. Identification of enriched conjugated linoleic acid isomers in cultures of ruminal microorganisms after dosing with 1-^{13}C-linoleic acid. J Microbiol 2011;49:622–7.

22. Fuentes MC, Calsamiglia S, Cardozo PW, et al. Effect of pH and level of concentrate in the diet on the production of biohydrogenation intermediates in a dual-flow continuous culture. J Dairy Sci 2009;92:4456–66.

23. Qiu X, Eastridge ML, Griswold KE, et al. Effects of substrate, passage rate, and pH in continuous culture on flows of conjugated linoleic acid and trans-C18:1. J Dairy Sci 2004;87:3473–9.

24. Baumgard LH, Corl BA, Dwyer DA, et al. Identification of the conjugated linoleic acid isomer that inhibits milk fat synthesis. Am J Physiol Regul Integr Comp Physiol 2000;278:R179–84.

25. de Veth MJ, Griinari JM, Pfeiffer AM, et al. Effect of CLA on milk fat synthesis in dairy cows: comparison of inhibition by methyl esters and free fatty acids, and relationships among studies. Lipids 2004;39(4):365–72.

26. Saebo AP, Saebo C, Griinari JM, et al. Effect of abomasal infusions of geometric isomers of 10,12 conjugated linoleic acid on milk fat synthesis in dairy cows. Lipids 2005;40:823–32.

27. Perfield JW II, Lock AL, Sæbø A, et al. Trans-9, cis-11 conjugated linoleic acid (CLA) reduces milk fat synthesis in lactating dairy cows. J Dairy Sci 2007;90: 2211–8.

28. Peterson DG, Matitashvili EA, Bauman DE. Diet-induced milk fat depression in dairy cows results in increased trans-10, cis-12 CLA in milk fat and coordinated suppression of mRNA abundance for mammary enzymes involved in milk fat synthesis. J Nutr 2003;133:3098–102.

29. Bauman DE, Mather IH, Wall RJ, et al. Major advances associated with the biosynthesis of milk. J Dairy Sci 2006;89(4):1235–43.

30. Cavaletto M, Giuffrida MG, Conti A. Milk fat globule membrane components–a proteomic approach. Adv Exp Med Biol 2008;606:129–41.

31. Ahnadi CE, Beswick N, Delbecchi L, et al. Addition of fish oil to diets for dairy cows. II. Effects on milk fat and gene expression of mammary lipogenic enzymes. J Dairy Res 2002;69(4):521–31.

32. Harvatine KJ, Bauman DE. SREBP1 and thyroid hormone responsive spot 14 (S14) are involved in the regulation of bovine mammary lipid synthesis during diet-induced milk fat depression and treatment with CLA. J Nutr 2006;136(10):2468–74.

33. Peterson DG, Matitashvili EA, Bauman DE. The inhibitory effect of trans-10, cis-12 CLA on lipid synthesis in bovine mammary epithelial cells involves reduced proteolytic activation of the transcription factor SREBP-1. J Nutr 2004;134(10):2523–7.

34. Piperova LS, Teter BB, Bruckental I, et al. Mammary lipogenic enzyme activity, trans fatty acids and conjugated linoleic acids are altered in lactating dairy cows fed a milk fat-depressing diet. J Nutr 2000;130(10):2568–74.

35. Medrano JF, Rincon G. SNP identification in genes involved in the SREBP1 pathway in dairy cattle. J Dairy Res 2012;79:66–75.

36. Hoashi S, Ashida N, Ohsaki H, et al. Genotype of bovine sterol regulatory element binding protein-1 (SREBP-1) is associated with fatty acid composition in Japanese Black cattle. Mamm Genome 2007;18(12):880–6.

37. Harvatine KJ, Bauman DE. Characterization of the acute lactational response to trans-10, cis-12 conjugated linoleic acid. J Dairy Sci 2011;94(12):6047–56.

38. Rico DE, Holloway AW, Harvatine KJ. Effect of dietary NDF and PUFA concentration on recovery from diet induced milk fat depression in monensin supplemented dairy cows. J Dairy Sci 2013;(96):659.

39. Rico DE, Harvatine KJ. Induction of and recovery from milk fat depression occurs progressively in dairy cows switched between diets that differ in fiber and oil concentration. J Dairy Sci 2013;96(10):6621–30.

40. Rico DE, Holloway AW, Harvatine KJ. Effect of monensin on recovery from diet-induced milk fat depression. J Dairy Sci 2014;97:2376–86.
41. Harvatine KJ, Allen MS. Effects of fatty acid supplements on milk yield and energy balance of lactating dairy cows. J Dairy Sci 2006;89(3):1081–91.
42. Newbold JR, Lewis EA, Lavrijssen L, et al. Effect of storage time on ruminal starch degradability in corn silage. J Dairy Sci 2006;89(Suppl 1):T94.
43. DeVries TJ, von Keyserlingk MA, Beauchemin KA. Frequency of feed delivery affects the behavior of lactating dairy cows. J Dairy Sci 2005;88(10):3553–62.
44. Rottman LW, Ying Y, Harvatine KJ. Effect of timing of feed intake on circadian pattern of milk synthesis. J Dairy Sci 2011;94(E-Suppl 1):830.
45. Jenkins TC, Fellner V, McGuffey RK. Monensin by fat interactions on trans fatty acids in cultures of ruminal microorganisms grown in continuous fermentors fed corn or barley. J Dairy Sci 2003;86:324–30.
46. Van Amburgh ME, Clapper JL, Mechor GD, et al. Rumensin and milk fat production. In: Proceedings of the 2008 Cornell Nutrition Conference. Syracuse (NY): 2008. p. 99–112.
47. Overton TR, Nydam DV, Bauman DE. Study to investigate the risk factors for milk fat depression (MFD) in dairy herds feeding rumensin. In: Proceedings of the 2008 Cornell Nutrition Conference. Syracuse (NY): 2008. p. 113–24.48.
48. Hinrichsen T, Lock AL, Bauman DE. The relationship between trans-10 18:1 and milk fat yield in cows fed high oleic acid or high linoleic acid plant oil supplements. Euro-Fed Lipid Congress. Madrid (Spain), September 11–14, 2006.

Calcium and Magnesium Physiology and Nutrition in Relation to the Prevention of Milk Fever and Tetany (Dietary Management of Macrominerals in Preventing Disease)

CrossMark

Javier Martín-Tereso, PhD[a],*, Holger Martens, VMD[b]

KEYWORDS

- Calcium • Magnesium • Hypocalcemia • Hypomagnesemia • Milk fever • Tetany
- Adaptation • Prevention

KEY POINTS

- Calcium and magnesium play similar and distinct roles in physiology as divalent cations in extracellular or intracellular compartments, respectively. As nutrients they are differently regulated, but still share enough common characteristics to be best understood together. Dairy cows may suffer events of hypocalcemia and hypomagnesemia, commonly known as milk fever and tetany.
- Milk fever is a nonnutritional, nondegenerative production disease, characterized by hypocalcemia at parturition as a consequence of a sudden increase in Ca demand and an unavoidable delay in Ca metabolism adaptation.
- Tetany is due to impaired Mg absorption from the rumen that cannot be compensated by absorptive or excretory adaptation, resulting in a net nutritional shortage of Mg, culminating in hypomagnesemia.
- Gastrointestinal and renal transepithelial transport mechanisms of Ca and Mg play key roles in the etiology of milk fever and tetany. Prevention strategies require triggering activation of Ca gastrointestinal absorption and avoiding factors limiting ruminal Mg absorption.

Continued

J. Martín-Tereso works for Nutreco, an animal nutrition company with commercial interests in dairy cattle nutrition. H. Martens has no conflicts of interest.
Disclosures: None.
[a] Nutreco Ruminant Research Centre, Nutreco Research & Development, Veerstraat 38, 5831JN Boxmeer, The Netherlands; [b] Department of Veterinary Physiology, School of Veterinary Medicine, Free University of Berlin, Oertzenweg 19b, Berlin 14163, Germany
* Corresponding author.
E-mail address: javier.martin-tereso@nutreco.com

Vet Clin Food Anim 30 (2014) 643–670
http://dx.doi.org/10.1016/j.cvfa.2014.07.007
0749-0720/14/$ – see front matter © 2014 Elsevier Inc. All rights reserved.

Continued

- Milk fever prevention strategies have focused on adaptation of Ca metabolism by challenging Ca balance weeks before parturition, either by reducing nutritional Ca availability or by inducing hypercalciuria with a lower dietary cation-anion difference. Oral Ca supply at calving can be complementary to adaptation strategies, whereas the standard use of intravenous Ca infusions may be detrimental. Assurance of high Mg supply is a prerequisite to preventing milk fever.
- Prevention of tetany should focus on supporting nutritional Mg supply by avoiding low Mg intakes, high K intakes, insufficient Na supply, and sudden dietary changes, especially those affecting rumen ammonia concentrations.

INTRODUCTION
Calcium and Magnesium Homeostasis, a Priority at Cellular and Animal Levels

Calcium (Ca) and Magnesium (Mg) are nutritionally essential minerals that present obvious elemental similarities given their proximity in the periodic table. This proximity confers sometimes analogous and at other times complementary roles in biology, the most evident being that Ca is the divalent extracellular cation while Mg is the intracellular one. Many cell functions need to be preserved by accurate regulation of these cations, and this is in both cases achieved by regulation of gastrointestinal absorption, renal reabsorption, and exchange with bone tissue.[1]

At both the animal and cellular levels, Ca is precisely controlled. Cells maintain very low ionic Ca by the expression of membrane Ca channels and complexation with proteins.[2] In the extracellular compartments, Ca is kept at constant levels to help cellular Ca regulation to sustain physiologic functions for which Ca is required, while managing Ca reserves and its skeletal function. An adult cow contains about 10 kg of Ca, of which 98% is in its bones, the rest being in the extracellular compartments.

Magnesium takes part in many functions such as activation of enzymes,[3] modulation of channels,[4] and bone formation.[5] A dairy cow with a body weight of 700 kg has a total amount of Mg of some 450 to 500 g. Most of the Mg is found in bones (60%–70%), the rest being located in intracellular spaces. Only about 1% is found in the extracellular space including the blood.

HYPOCALCEMIA AND HYPOMAGNESEMIA IN DAIRY COWS

Despite the importance of homeostatic control of these minerals, dairy cows often suffer from production diseases based on events of Ca and Mg dyshomeostasis. Causes and consequences of these negative fluctuations in blood Ca and Mg concentrations are different, but they share some fundamental characteristics and are better understood together.

Hypocalcemia

Breeding dairy cattle for production has generated milk yields severalfold greater than requirements of the offspring, which creates a unique physiologic condition, a discontinuity between Ca utilization for fetal growth and milk production.[6] Parturition requires redirection of Ca transfer from cow-to-calf to cow-to-mammary-gland, which nondairy cattle breeds and other mammals seem to cope with without problems. Dairy cows suffer from a very large and sudden increase of Ca clearance from their blood, and for this reason most of them develop some degree of hypocalcemia.

Serum Ca levels of 2.0 and 1.4 mM (8.0 and 7.6 mg/dL) have respectively been proposed as thresholds of subclinical or clinical hypocalcemia (**Table 1**),[7] although these do not unequivocally correlate with the appearance of external signs displayed by the animal at calving, commonly referred to as milk fever.

Serum Ca at calving can decrease to below 2.0 mM (8.0 mg/dL) in 25% of heifers, 41% of second-lactation cows, and up to 54% of fifth-lactation cows.[8] In practice, animals requiring Ca infusion treatments are considered clinical cases of milk fever. Farmers in the United States have declared an incidence of milk fever in 4.9% of the herds,[9] including first-lactation animals. Assuming a negligible fraction of cases being in heifers, this would suggest a 7.5% incidence of clinical milk fever in multiparous cows in the United States herd.

Milk Fever Is Neither a Nutritional Nor an Age-Related Degenerative Condition

Milk fever is not a nutritional deficiency of Ca. Hypocalcemia takes place in the days around calving, and does not persist later in lactation when Ca loss into milk is greatest in comparison with nutritional supply of Ca. Milk fever is caused by the insufficient speed of adaptation and not by the Ca deficit created between dietary supply and lactation Ca requirements.

Heifers are substantially less susceptible than multiparous cows to milk fever,[10] and as they age the latter increase in incidence by 9% in every additional lactation.[11] Milk fever is unlikely to be a degenerative condition because the cows are very young, considering that bovines can live up to 30 years.[12] Therefore, rather than by any degenerative process, the link between parity and milk fever incidence is more likely to be explained by a greater milk yield and precalving feed (and Ca) intake, which amplify the contrast in Ca metabolism before and after calving.

Hypomagnesemia

Blood Mg concentration reflects the difference between Mg influx and renal clearance. Renal Mg clearance is responsive to Mg intake[13] and also to parathormone (PTH) in concert with Ca regulation, with greater reabsorption under PTH influence. Under normal conditions Mg absorption is greater than Mg clearance, resulting in Mg serum concentration between 0.8 and 1.2 mM (1.95 and 2.92 mg/dL). Because magnesemia does not correlate very closely with externally observable clinical signs,[14] there are ranges of uncertain diagnosis (**Table 2**).

This state of Mg shortage resulting in hypomagnesemia causes a variety of clinical symptoms such as reduced feed intake, neurologic disorders such as ataxia, and tetanic muscle spasms, commonly referred to as tetany or grass staggers.

Table 1
Proposed criteria of hypocalcemia conditions in dairy cows

Hypocalcemic Status	Ca in Blood	
	mM	mg/dL
Normal Ca homeostasis	>2.0	>8.0
Subclinical hypocalcemia	1.4–2.0	7.6–8.0
Clinical hypocalcemia	<1.4	<7.6

Data from Roche J, Berry D. Periparturient climatic, animal, and management factors influencing the incidence of milk fever in grazing systems. J Dairy Sci 2006;89(7):2775–83.

Table 2
Concentration of Mg in blood and Mg status

Mg Status	Mg in Blood	
	mM	mg/dL
1. Normal Mg	0.9–1.2	2.19–2.92
2. Uncertainty	0.8–0.9	1.95–2.19
3. Suspicion of hypomagnesemia	0.7–0.8	1.70–1.95
4. Hypomagnesemia	<0.7	<1.70

Tetany

In cattle, the complex set of symptoms associated with hypomagnesemia has been well known for at least 80 years.[15] Low blood Mg concentrations are not always associated with convulsions and tetany.[14] Meyer and Scholz[16] and Allsop and Pauli[17] concluded from their studies that a decrease in Mg concentration in the cerebrospinal fluid is the major factor causing clinical symptoms by activation of noncontrolled contraction of muscle from the central nervous system. Treatment of hypomagnesemia by rectal infusion of Mg salts corrected Mg levels in blood within 5 minutes and in cerebrospinal fluid after 30 minutes, after which clinical signs were abolished.[18] Hence, the clinical symptoms of hypomagnesemia are very likely caused by Mg-related malfunctions of the central nervous system.

CALCIUM AND MAGNESIUM HOMEOSTASIS

Serum Ca is controlled by hormonal signals, the most important being PTH and 1,25-dihydroxyvitamin D (calcitriol), which mainly modulate renal tubular Ca reabsorption and gastrointestinal Ca transepithelial transport,[19] and bone Ca turnover.[20] Calcitonin primarily regulates opposing effects of PTH in response to hypercalcemic conditions. Serum Mg, on the contrary, has no known hormonal mechanisms of control, and its regulation relies on the renal regulation of excess Mg derived from dietary and osseous influxes.

Calcium Homeostasis

Main framework of the homeostatic system of calcium in dairy cows
Homeostatic regulation of Ca in mammals is mainly controlled by PTH and calcitriol; this is also the case in the bovine species,[11,21,22] but wide differences in the digestive system of ruminants result in minor specific differences, in particular in gastrointestinal absorption.[23]

Blood calcium monitoring and the action of parathormone
The parathyroid gland secretes PTH on detection of negative fluctuations of calcemia by the Ca^{2+} sensing receptor.[24] Evidence of this receptor in ruminants[25] demonstrates analogy with the generally accepted parathyroid role in serum Ca sensing.

PTH signals are responsible for the short-term fine tuning of Ca homeostasis by controlling renal Ca reabsorption. Urinary Ca excretion is small (<1 g/d[26]), but can be rapidly reduced further[27] or greatly increased[28] by positive or negative PTH signals. Therefore, renal regulation is useful to correct hypercalcemia, but not so much so for hypocalcemia.

Indirectly, PTH affects other Ca regulation mechanisms by inducing renal hydroxylation of 25-hydroxyvitamin D to calcitriol, which in turn will have its own effects on

Ca regulation, alone or in coordinated action with PTH. Calcitonin downregulates renal 1α-hydroxylase activity while increasing the activity of 24- or 26-hydroxylases to generate biologically inactive forms.

Calcitriol actions on the gastrointestinal tract and bone tissue

Calcitriol has a direct effect on gastrointestinal Ca absorption, which can provide substantial amounts of Ca to compensate Ca deficits; this is assumed to be the main means for Ca regulation in animals. However, there is direct evidence in rodents that this activation can take more than 24 hours to take effect,[29] and in dairy cows there is indirect evidence that inactivation of Ca absorption is delayed by about 2 days.[28,30] The significance of ruminal Ca absorption is still controversial. Rumen epithelium can absorb Ca in vitro,[31] but proof in vivo[32] and the evaluation of its relevance to Ca regulation[33] still need further study. Recent evidence in goats points toward absorption taking place in both rumen and intestine.[34] Nevertheless, independently from the relative importance of the different sites of absorption, it can be assumed that overall the role of the gastrointestinal tract of ruminants in Ca regulation is similar to that of the intestine in single-stomach animals.

Bone Ca can help compensate for the Ca deficit in early lactation when milk Ca output largely exceeds nutritionally available Ca,[35] but the readily available fraction of Ca in bone is very small.[36] Extensive bone mobilization is only induced by calcitriol when the PTH signal does not cease. Only if Ca absorption fails to sustain calcemia[20] will bone catabolism come into play.

Hormonal control of bone remodeling

PTH is the main hormone affecting bone remodeling which, together with calcitriol, triggers bone tissue to play its role in Ca homeostasis.[37] Nevertheless, bone anabolism and catabolism is also subject to local regulation,[38] which serves purposes other than Ca homeostasis. Responses to PTH and calcitriol are conditioned by the pattern of the hormonal signals received by the osseous tissue. A pulsatile PTH signal induces anabolism and a constant PTH stimulus induces osseous breakdown.[39] Instead, calcitriol cooperates with PTH in bone catabolism in acute applications to enhance bone resorption, but it is known to stop bone resorption in continuous applications.[20] As already described, calcitriol depends on PTH, and PTH rapidly reflects the effects observed in blood Ca, so the effects of these hormones cannot be understood separately and, more importantly, not independently from their reactions on blood Ca that are in turn highly conditioned by physiologic and nutritional conditions.

Magnesium Homeostasis

No hormonal regulation system exists to maintain body Mg or blood Mg concentration as in the case of Ca. Blood Mg concentration is achieved by a simple principle of Mg metabolism: Mg influx (gastrointestinal Mg absorption) must be matched by Mg efflux (Mg transport into cells, retention in bone, endogenous secretion, fetal growth, and milk production) as reflected in the following equation: Normal magnesemia = Influx (absorption) − (efflux + urinary Mg).

Magnesium absorption

Mg absorption is the main influx factor to sustain blood Mg, and the amount of Mg absorbed can be variable[40] in the ruminant. This variation is mostly explained by variable Mg intakes, the variation in the conditions of the site of absorption, which affects the mechanisms of absorption, and further by dietary components, such as potassium (K), which play an antagonistic role in the process of absorption.

It is now well established that Mg is absorbed from the rumen.[41,42] Net absorption from the small and large intestine is negligible[42] and is not able to compensate for impaired absorption from the forestomachs.[43] Therefore, ruminal Mg absorption is essential to maintain normomagnesemia[44] in adult ruminants. During calf development, Mg absorption switches from the intestine to the forestomachs.[45] The capability of the large intestine for Mg absorption is maintained and can be used for first-aid treatment of hypomagnesemia.[46,47]

Renal regulation of magnesium surplus

Because Mg influx rarely equals Mg efflux, additional mechanisms are necessary for adjustment of possible differences. This fine tuning is controlled by the kidneys. Any potential surplus (Mg influx > Mg efflux) is rapidly compensated by Mg excretion via kidneys. However, as with Ca, kidneys can handle only Mg surplus. If Mg influx is lower than Mg efflux, particularly via secretion into milk, urinary Mg excretion becomes very small (<1.0 mM) and finally hypomagnesemia occurs, because the missing mechanism of regulation hinders mobilization of Mg from bone and tissue or increase of absorption from the rumen.[48] This function of the kidney (excretion of Mg according the requirement) has led to recommendation of Mg concentrations in urine for diagnosis. Kemp[49] suggested a shortage of Mg uptake at urinary Mg of less than 0.87 mM. Hence, urinary Mg of less than 1 mM is likely a reliable indicator of insufficient intake/absorption and a better diagnostic tool of Mg status than blood Mg. According to the data of Kemp,[49] Mg uptake is sufficient at urinary Mg greater than 4.4 mM, and the range from 0.87 to 4.4 mM may indicate a risk for Mg shortage. This range of magnesemia means that Mg intake is either low but sufficient, marginal, or close to hypomagnesemia (**Fig. 1**).

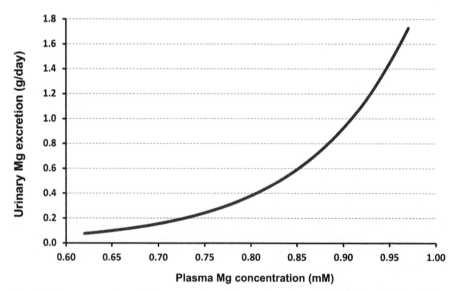

Fig. 1. Urinary excretion of Mg is nonlinearly correlated to plasma Mg. (*Adapted from* Schonewille JT, van't Klooster AT, Wouterse H, et al. Time courses of plasma magnesium concentrations and urinary magnesium excretion in cows subjected to acute changes in potassium intake. Vet Q 2000;22(3):136–40.)

TRANSEPITHELIAL TRANSPORT OF CALCIUM AND MAGNESIUM
Transepithelial Transport of Calcium

Calcium transport across epithelia can be active or passive. Transcellular active Ca transport is a saturable process subject to tight hormonal control.[50] Paracellular passive Ca diffusion is a nonsaturable process that depends on concentration gradients and presents limited regulation, although some degree of control is possible by modulation of epithelial permeability.[51,52]

Gastrointestinal calcium absorption

Transcellular gastrointestinal Ca transport often operates against a concentration gradient from lumen to blood, and for this reason requires energy expenditure. It consists of 3 basic steps (**Fig. 2**):

1. Ca entry to the cell. Calcium channels control the passive entry of Ca from gastrointestinal lumen into the cell cytosol. The expression of these proteins is controlled[53] by calcitriol, and could be the main regulatory step of the whole process. The main protein described to facilitate Ca entry is gastrointestinal TRPV6.[24]
2. Ca buffering in the cell. Very low intracellular free Ca does not permit quantitatively relevant transcellular Ca transport. Greater intracellular Ca buffering and diffusion is achieved by the gastrointestinal Ca-binding protein Calbindin-D9k,[50] which is also controlled by calcitriol.[54]
3. Ca export from the cell to the blood. Calcium ions are exported by the common mechanisms that extrude Ca from all cells. At a cost of energy, Ca–adenosine triphosphatase (ATPase) protein and the Na^+/Ca^{2+} exchanger[53] bring Ca ions into the bloodstream. This step plays little regulatory role in the process,[54] although it has been shown to be sensitive to calcitriol signal.[50]

Renal calcium reabsorption

Transcellular renal Ca transport is mostly analogous to that described for gastrointestinal absorption, with certain molecular differences (**Fig. 3**) and also differences in its hormonal control. In the kidney, Ca is also transported against the concentration gradient, and the process is therefore energy dependent. Calcium entry is facilitated by TRPV5,[55] a channel of the same family of TRPV6. Intracellular buffering is achieved also by a different Ca-binding protein, Calbindin-D28k.[50] The expression of these proteins determines the rate of active transport, which is regulated by PTH.[56] Export of Ca is the energy-dependent step of all cells mediated by Ca-ATPase protein and the Na^+/Ca^{2+} exchanger.[53]

Transepithelial Transport of Magnesium

Ruminal magnesium absorption

Early suggestions excluded passive absorption from the rumen.[57] In vitro studies revealed that passive permeability of the paracellular pathway of the rumen epithelium is very low and does not allow a sufficient passive flow of Mg, which indeed is a negligible pathway for Mg. Later in vivo and in vitro studies characterized active Mg transport[58] and, accordingly, 2 absorption and 1 common export mechanisms have been proposed: (**Fig. 4**)

1. Mg^{2+} uptake (as ion through a channel) is driven by the potential difference of the apical membrane, PD_a. This mechanism is called PD-dependent or K-sensitive Mg uptake, because PD_a is mainly modulated by the ruminal K concentration.[59] It is suggested that this transport is mediated by the epithelial apical membrane channel TRPM7[60] (TRPM6 in the intestine[61]).

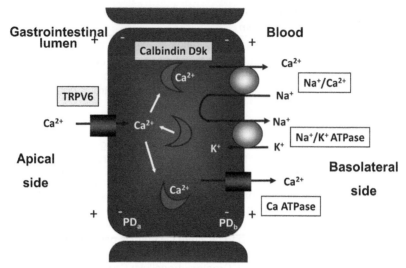

Fig. 2. Transepithelial gastrointestinal transport of Ca.

2. The second uptake mechanism is a cotransport together with an anion, which neutralizes the charge of Mg^{2+}. The driving force for this uptake is the gradient of the involved ions. Hence, it is called PD-independent or K-insensitive mechanism and is mainly driven by the ruminal Mg concentration. The molecular basis is still unknown.

3. Basolateral extrusion of Mg is mediated by Na^+/Mg^{2+} exchange using the electromotive force derived from Na influx into the cell down its electrochemical gradient, because Na concentration is much larger extracellularly than intracellularly, and the charge of voltage inside the cell is negative in comparison with the positive exterior. The best molecular candidate is the *SLC41A1* Na^+/Mg^{2+} exchanger.[62] Na is then pumped out of the cell across the basolateral membrane via Na,K-ATPase, which

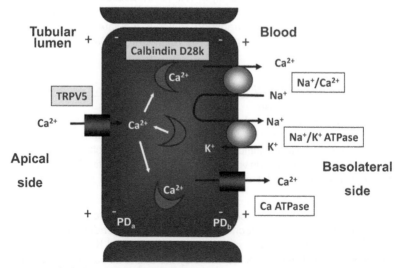

Fig. 3. Transepithelial renal transport of Ca.

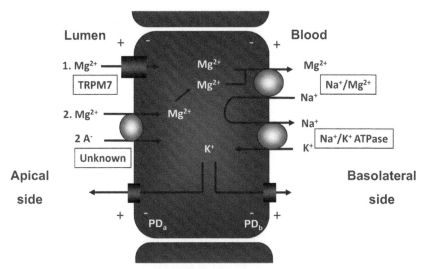

Fig. 4. Secondary active ruminal Mg transport. The two uptake mechanisms are working in parallel.

provides the Na electromotive force to move another Mg ion out of the cell and into the blood.

Two parallel working mechanisms in one epithelium are somewhat unusual, and the possible justification may be the need for ruminal Mg absorption at low and high Mg concentrations. Therefore, it is proposed that the two working uptake mechanisms exhibit complementary functions: The PD-dependent and K-sensitive mechanism has the capability of high affinity and low capacity for low Mg and, vice versa, the PD-independent one has a high capacity and low affinity for high Mg concentration (**Table 3**).

This conclusion is derived from early observations of Care and colleagues[58] in studies of Mg absorption from a rumen pouch of sheep. High ruminal K concentration depressed Mg absorption, particularly at low Mg concentration. The hypothesis of complementary function of the 2 ruminal Mg transport routes has been tested in a balance study with sheep.[63] Sheep were fed with increasing amounts of Mg and at 2 levels of K intake. Mg digestibility was depressed at all Mg intakes and that the amount of decrease was almost the same at all Mg levels, indicating that the K-sensitive Mg transport was likely to be saturated (**Fig. 5**).

The obvious agreement between the model of Mg transport derived from in vitro studies and the consequences of this model on balance data in vivo permits the conclusion that a higher risk of hypomagnesemia is given at low Mg and high K intake.

Table 3
Characteristics of Mg transport across the rumen epithelium

Apical Uptake Mechanism	Driving Force	Transport Functions	Attributes	Basolateral Extrusion
Mg^{2+} (electrogenic)	Apical potential difference (PD_a)	High affinity Low capacity	PD-dependent K-sensitive	Na/Mg Exchanger
Mg^{2+} + anion (electroneutral)	Chemical gradient	Low affinity High capacity	PD-independent K-insensitive	Na/Mg Exchanger

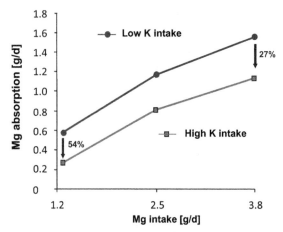

Fig. 5. Effect of 2 levels of K intake on Mg absorption. The decrease on Mg absorption is much more pronounced at low Mg and high K intake (54%; K-sensitive transport). Vice versa, Mg transport (%) is much less reduced at high Mg intake. This reduction is almost the same at all Mg intake and represents the K-sensitive Mg transport. The increase of Mg absorption with increasing Mg intake is very likely mediated by the K-insensitive Mg transport. (*Adapted from* Ram L, Schonewille JT, Martens H, et al. Magnesium absorption by wethers fed potassium bicarbonate in combination with different dietary magnesium concentrations. J Dairy Sci 1998;81(9):2485–92.)

Renal magnesium reabsorption

The filterable part of blood Mg is approximately 70%, and 3% to 5% is finally excreted. Three mechanisms have been described for reabsorption of Mg in the nephron:

1. In the proximal tubule 20% to 30% of the filtered Mg is reabsorbed, probably passively, together with water.
2. Most Mg (60%–70%) is reclaimed in the thick ascending limb of Henle. This paracellular transport is mainly driven by the transepithelial potential difference (lumen positive). This pathway is also used by Ca and mediated by paracellin-1. There is some evidence for competition between these 2 ions.[13] This interaction could explain the increase of magnesemia at low concentration of Ca[64] and the sensitivity to PTH.
3. Approximately 10% of the filtered Mg is reabsorbed in the distal convoluted tubule by an active transport mechanism.

Uptake is mediated by TRPM6, as in ruminal epithelium. Renal TRPM6 is regulated by epidermal growth factor (EGF) and dietary Mg.[13] Magnesium deficit increases mRNA and TRPM6 protein in kidneys of mice,[13] and it is believed that the Ca-sensing receptor detects the levels of Ca and Mg and regulates the absorption of these ions.[65] Hence, the TRPM6 is considered as a gatekeeper of Mg handling in the kidney.[66] It is likely that this transport mechanism limits Mg excretion and determines the low renal threshold of Mg. The efflux mechanism across the basolateral membrane is still uncertain.[66]

The regulation of TRPM6 could explain renal regulation of Mg surplus (Mg influx > Mg efflux). This activity of Mg transport is illustrated by Schonewille and colleagues[67] (see **Fig. 1**), who describe the correlation between urinary Mg and magnesemia. The exponential correlation clearly showed a turning point in blood Mg between 0.8 and 0.9 mM (1.95–2.19 mg/dL).

PHYSIOLOGIC BACKGROUND OF MILK FEVER AND TETANY
Mechanisms of Calcemia Control and Milk Fever

Calcium metabolism in the course of the lactation

In early lactation, there is a gap between supply and requirements despite efficient gastrointestinal absorption, and this is filled by bone mobilization. Later, when nutritional supply exceeds lactation needs, absorption remains active, driven by calcitriol stimulation, and the surplus replenishes bone reserves. At a certain point at the end of lactation, bone anabolism ceases along with active gastrointestinal absorption, resulting in a dormant Ca metabolism until the next calving.

In the weeks before calving, cows are in a physiologic state whereby Ca clearance is minimal, bone reserves lost in early lactation have already been replenished, and dietary Ca supply is severalfold greater than net nutritional requirements. Osseous tissue is in equilibrium, and calcemia is maintained by renal corrections of the small surplus created by unregulated passive gastrointestinal absorption.

The start of this dormancy depends on dietary Ca supply during lactation. The US National Research Council (NRC),[68] in common with other reference systems, base Ca supply recommendations on a factorial model aiming to satisfy net requirements by nutritional supply for any given milk yield or physiologic state. Traditionally Ca feeding recommendations have neglected this natural cycle whereby deficits and surplus are regulated with great flexibility. Calculated NRC recommendations for lactating cows range from 5 to 8 g/kg dry matter (DM) depending on yields, intakes, and days in milk. In practice, cows fed a diet as low in Ca as 5 g/kg DM during their lactation present a positive Ca balance as early as the fifth month of lactation.[69] Feeding high levels of Ca during lactation will reduce the extent and shorten the period of bone mobilization, but in turn will create a longer period of dormancy in Ca metabolism.

Limitations of bone mobilization Bone turnover controls calcemia by switching between anabolism and catabolism through processes of cell differentiation in osseous tissue. Regulation of the capture and release of bone Ca sets calcemia as a priority with respect to Ca replenishment after mobilization and bone anabolism connected with growth. Osseous tissue can support calcemia with Ca from its extracellular compartments. However, this resource is quantitatively negligible, being less than 10 g.[36] Bone matrix Ca is the main resource from which more than 1 kg of Ca is mobilized in the early months of lactation.[68]

Bone anabolism and catabolism depend on the action of osteoblasts and osteoclasts, respectively. The activity of these cell types is hormonally controlled, but the differentiation and maturation of these cell lineages is required for their action, and this is also regulated.[70]

Reaction of bone tissue to a hypocalcemic signal

PTH is secreted in response to hypocalcemia, acting directly on renal reabsorption and inducing bone catabolism. At the same time, PTH induces renal activation of calcitriol, which in turn activates Ca absorption. Two nutritional conditions are then possible:

1. Calcitriol activation of Ca absorption compensates hypocalcemia. PTH, having a short half-life of about 4 minutes,[71] will shortly cease interrupting the signal to bone tissue and reducing renal reabsorption, and eventually the calcitriol signal will fade until stimulated again by PTH. The result is the control of calcemia by iterative signals between calcitriol and its Ca absorption reaction and PTH reactions to blood Ca.
2. Calcitriol activation of Ca absorption is insufficient to compensate calcemia. Calcitriol signal will then persist and bone mobilization will sustain calcemia, releasing

bone Ca to maintain Ca homeostasis by iterative corrections between bone reactions to PTH and PTH reactions to blood Ca.

These mechanisms result in a prioritization for calcemia correction by dietary means, leaving bone mobilization as a backup system for situations in which dietary correction is insufficient.

Delayed adaptations in the mechanisms of control

Delayed adaptation of gastrointestinal calcium absorption Renal reabsorption quickly responds to PTH signals, whereas gastrointestinal absorption fails to respond to hypocalcemia in the days around calving. The reason for this may be found in differences in the life span of epithelial cells. Gastrointestinal cells live for a few days[72,73] and renal epithelial cells live for several months.[72,74] Enterocytes acquire Ca transport configuration in early stages of development in the crypts, but only use this competence during maturity,[75] days after calcitriol signal has taken place.[76] Configuration seems to be fixed for the entire life span of these cells. This unavoidable delay in adaptation of the gastrointestinal tract has been pointed out as the intrinsic cause of transient hypocalcemia in dairy cows at calving.[26] By contrast, long-lived renal cells cannot have a fixed Ca transport configuration and react to hormonal signals within their life span.

Delay of bone remodeling reaction Bone also shows a delayed reaction to hypocalcemia. Osteoclast activity can be induced within hours, but recruitment of new osteoclasts takes place by differentiation of osteoblasts[77] that receive PTH and calcitriol signals and become active osteoblasts only after 2 days. Hence, pregnant cows take 48 hours of PTH stimulation for their osseous tissue to start mobilizing Ca,[78] and the reason for this delay is associated with the time it takes to induce the cell-differentiation process.

Metabolic acidification activates calcium metabolism

pH sensitivity of renal calcium transport Acid-base balance has been extensively studied in its relationship with the incidence of milk fever. Urinary pH is a predictor of milk fever incidence,[79] and is highly correlated with urinary Ca.[26,80] The rate-limiting protein for renal Ca reabsorption is strongly affected by pH,[81] reducing its activity to half at low physiologic pH,[24] which results in excessive urinary Ca. This pH sensitivity is mediated by retrieval of this protein from the cellular membrane on acidification of the extracellular compartment.[82] TRPV5 knock-out mice combine excessive urinary Ca losses with permanent activation of TRPV6 in the intestine, resulting from a constant calcitriol signal.[83] This molecular evidence connects milk fever prevention and hypercalciuric effects of diets rich in anions for dairy cows.

Activation of calcium metabolism before calving

Link between active gastrointestinal absorption before calving and milk fever incidence Anticipation of the hypocalcemic challenge seems to be the mode of action for the most common approaches to dietary prevention of milk fever, and also explanatory of the main risk factors.[26] Quantitative analysis of nutritional and physiologic factors creating this state of dormancy and how to stimulate Ca metabolism before calving can help to reduce the incidence and severity of peripartum hypocalcemia. **Fig. 6** describes the nutritional and physiologic partitioning of Ca in a dairy cow at the onset of lactation. **Table 4** breaks down blood Ca clearance into its different fractions and the factors defining the gastrointestinally available Ca pool.

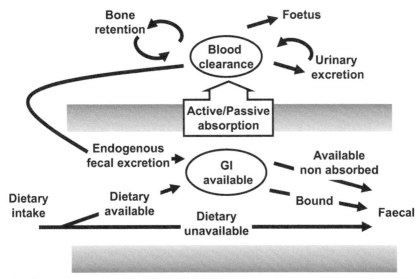

Fig. 6. Digestive and physiologic fate of Ca in precalving dairy cows. GI, gastrointestinally. (*Adapted from* Martín-Tereso J, Verstegen MW. A novel model to explain dietary factors affecting hypocalcaemia in dairy cattle. Nutr Res Rev 2011(24):228–43.)

To maintain normocalcemia in the precalving cow, Ca clearance will be compensated by gastrointestinal Ca absorption from the available enteric pool. Should this be insufficient, bone mobilization will come into play. In general, the gastrointestinally available pool will be greater than Ca clearance, resulting in an available but not absorbed fraction going into feces (see **Fig. 6**). The fraction of the gastrointestinally available pool needing to be absorbed is predictive of upregulation of gastrointestinal absorption efficiency. If this fraction is high, passive absorption alone will be insufficient to maintain normocalcemia, thus requiring active absorption.[26] This activation prepares the cow for the upcoming hypocalcemic challenge.

Summary of adaptive mechanisms and milk fever etiology

Of the 3 control mechanisms that act on hypocalcemia, renal reabsorption cannot correct large Ca deficits, and gastrointestinal absorption and bone resorption are unable to proceed in less time than 1 or 2 days. These facts explain the transient hypocalcemia observed in dairy cows between gestation and lactation, from which animals normally fully recover in the first week of lactation, coping from then on, without problems, with the high Ca demand of peaking lactation by efficient Ca absorption and bone mobilization.

Inducing adaptation of Ca metabolism earlier than the onset of lactation seems to mitigate the magnitude of this transient hypocalcemia. This goal can be achieved by

Table 4	
Factors defining Ca clearance and gastrointestinal available pool before calving	
Factors Defining Ca Clearance	**Fractions of Gastrointestinally Available Ca Pool**
Endogenous gastrointestinal secretions	Endogenous gastrointestinal secretions
Urinary losses (relevant to low DCAD diets)	Dietary available supply
Bone Ca retention (relevant to heifers)	Gross supply
Fetal growth	Ca availability (intrinsic or precipitate)

challenging Ca supply or demand to trigger adaptation and receive the metabolic challenge of calving with the appropriate configuration of Ca metabolism.

Magnesium Absorption and Tetany

Modeling magnesium absorption as effected by potassium content in the diet

In vivo[43,84] and in vitro studies[85] have shown the importance of ruminal K concentration on reduced Mg absorption, which is not compensated for by the small and large intestine.[43] This negative effect has been confirmed by a meta-analysis of Mg absorption in dairy cows by Weiss,[86] which generated Equation 1 (**Table 5**). Schonewille and colleagues[40] extended this meta-analysis and obtained Equation 2 (see **Table 5**). True Mg absorption is corrected in apparent Mg absorption by subtracting endogenous Mg, which for a body weight of 700 kg would be 2.8 g (700 kg × 4 mg) resulting in Equation 3, which confirms the previous findings of Weiss.[86]

Three conclusions can be drawn from Equations 1 and 2:

1. The effect of K is canceled out by 1% K in the DM.
2. The depressive effect of K on digestible Mg is more pronounced at high K content and low Mg intake which has been predicted by in vitro models and confirmed in vivo in sheep.
3. The digestibility of Mg is within the same range at 1% K in DM (24% and 20%).

Apparent Mg absorption must cover the Mg requirement for milk, endogenous secretion, and tissue uptake (soft tissue, bone, pregnancy). In an adult, nonpregnant cow Mg is used for milk production and endogenous secretion. It is assumed that Mg uptake in tissue is zero in the absence of growth rate and that no fetal Mg is required.

Equation 3 can be rearranged with Equation 4 to determine Equation 5, which by solving for Mg intake permits with Equation 6 an approach for the assessment of Mg intake according to milk production and K content.

This last equation has been used to calculate Mg intake at increasing milk production and K content (**Table 6**). At low Mg requirement (milk 0 L/d), the necessary increase of Mg intake was 57% from 1% to 4% dietary K. This additional amount of Mg was only 24% at high Mg intake for 60 L/d. Again, the effect of K is pronounced at low Mg and high K intake. Mg absorption is calculated according Equation 3 and covers the Mg requirement (see **Table 6**).

It must be emphasized that this calculation used the mean values of Equation 3 and the mean of requirement for milk and endogenous secretion. The variation of these values is high, and a safety margin should be included. Schonewille and Beynen[88] have proposed a factor of 1.6.

Effect of ruminal ammonium and sodium on magnesium absorption

Ruminal ammonium The available data support the conclusion that a rapid increase of NH_4^+ disturbs ruminal Mg absorption,[89] which is vanishing after 2 to 3 days of adaptation of the rumen epithelium to high ruminal NH_4^+.[90] Hence, a rapid change from low-nitrogen to a high-nitrogen diet and rapid increase of ruminal NH_4^+ impairs ruminal Mg absorption, which has not been observed in normal balance studies[91] and meta-analysis,[86] but may explain field observations.[49] Hence, the negative effect of NH_4^+ on Mg absorption appears to be transient for few days.

Dietary sodium Butler[92] found a negative correlation between Na content of the grass and the incidence of tetany. Lower Na supply results in a decrease of Na and an increase in K concentration in saliva, and subsequently in the ruminal fluid. These alterations are identical with consequences of a high K intake and cause a decrease of

Table 5
Set of equations used to determine Mg requirements

Equation		Reference
Intake of digestible Mg (apparent Mg absorption) = 4.5 + 0.24 × Mg intake (g/d) − 4.4 × K (%DM)	(1)	Weiss,[86] 2004
True Mg absorption = 3.6 + 0.2 × Mg intake (g/d) − 0.08 × dietary K (%DM)	(2)	Schonewille et al,[40] 2008
Apparent Mg absorption = 0.8 + 0.2 × Mg intake (g/d) − 0.08 × dietary K (%DM)	(3)	Schonewille et al,[40] 2008 corrected by endogenous secretion (3.6−2.8 = 0.8)
Mg Requirement[a] = Milk (0.12 g/L) + endogenous secretion (2.8 g/d)	(4)	Martens and Stumpff,[87] 2011
Milk (0.12 g/L) + endogenous secretion (2.8 g/d) = 0.8 + 0.2 × Mg intake − 0.08 × dietary K	(5)	Martens and Stumpff,[87] 2011
Mg intake for requirement (g/d) = 10 g/d + Milk (L/d) × 0.6 (g/L) + 0.4 × dietary K (g/kg DM)	(6)	Martens and Stumpff,[87] 2011

[a] Nonpregnant and adult cow.
Data from Refs.[40,86,87]

Table 6
Mg intake at increasing milk yield and dietary K using Equation 6

| Milk Yield (L/d) | Mg Milk (g/d) | Mg (g/d) | | Mg Intake (g/d) | | | Mg Absorption (g/d) |
		Maintenance	Requirement	1% K	2% K	4% K	
0	0	2.8	2.8	14.0	18.0	22.0	2.8
20	2.4	2.8	5.2	26.0	30.0	38.0	5.2
40	4.8	2.8	7.6	38.0	42.0	50.0	7.6
60	7.2	2.8	10.0	50.0	54.0	62.0	10

Absorption was calculated with Equation 3. 12 mg/L milk and endogenous secretion 700 kg BW × 4 mg/kg (2.8 g/d). The absorption of Mg covers at all K-intake Mg requirement.

Mg absorption. Insufficient Na intake impairs Mg absorption and is a very often overlooked risk factor for cattle at pasture, particularly for beef cattle.

PRACTICAL APPROACHES TO MILK FEVER PREVENTION

The most common preventive actions for milk fever are nutritional and are implemented in the close-up diet, although milk fever is not a nutrient imbalance but a failure of physiologic adaptation. First proposals included vitamin D supplementation and modified Ca-to-phosphorus ratios.[93] Later, low Ca diets received some attention, and for decades anionic salts became the standard preventive strategy. In addition, Ca drenches and intravenous infusions are used as treatments in clinical cases or are applied during the calving routine to prevent the effects of clinical and subclinical hypocalcemia.

Nowadays, prevention of milk fever is mostly multifactorial and is integrated in a general close-up nutrition strategy aiming to prevent this and other production diseases. Dietary strategies and nutritional risk factors have been sufficiently described by comprehensive reviews.[11,94] This section discusses the practical utility of these practices and the metabolic implications from the perspective of their physiologic mode of action.

Supranutritional Supply of Forms of Vitamin D

Vitamin D in its different forms has been studied as a way to prevent milk fever.[95] These applications have not been nutritional but acute treatments, often using doses that are nearly toxic,[96] which act as an exogenous calcitriol signal and can result in responses in serum Ca.[97]

The main pitfall of these practices is that when an exogenous vitamin D signal is introduced in the system, this will induce reactions but it will also activate counterreactions. Exogenous vitamin D will raise calcemia by activation of absorption, but this in turn will depress PTH, resulting in renal Ca excretion.[98] At the same time, exogenous vitamin D, being independent from PTH regulation, sustains its signal, ultimately being able to induce soft-tissue calcification.[96] Therefore, cows only benefit from exogenous vitamin D signals if they are induced at the correct time in relation to calving.[99] Too early or too late introduction of supranutritional vitamin D will not result in decreased hypocalcemic risk, but it might in fact reduce the ability of the animal to maintain calcemia.

Calcium Infusions and Oral Acute Calcium Applications

A straightforward approach to correct calcemia is to supply Ca during the hypocalcemic event, although this is an intervention more than a preventive measure, and it is often necessary to avoid the risk of death associated with clinical hypocalcemia. However, these practices have metabolic implications.

Intravenous infusions of Calcium

Treating with intravenous Ca is the most direct intervention to correct hypocalcemia, and this is sometimes understood as an easy and inexpensive solution to milk fever by incorporating this practice in the calving protocol on the farm. However, there are negative consequences to consider. Calcemia is in itself a signal in the system, and when applied to animals that do not definitively require this treatment will induce the counterreaction of PTH depression, renal correction of hypercalcemia, and reduced rate of activation of calcitriol, which will cause a delay in adaptation of Ca metabolism, even inducing hypocalcemia in initially healthy animals (**Fig. 7**).[100] Artificially correcting calcemia should be a tool to save cows from acute hypocalcemia, but never a standard calving procedure, because it interferes in the natural homeorhetic adaptation of Ca metabolism.

Oral acute Calcium applications

Supplying cows with high oral doses of Ca in solution or suspension is a fairly common management practice on dairy farms. This approach can be more or less labor demanding and invasive, depending on whether the product is supplied as a drench or as a palatable drink. Increasing the amount of Ca in the gastrointestinal tract of a precalving cow will result in 2 main effects. First, the total amount of absorbable Ca is increased. This effect is especially positive in combination with precalving diets that activate Ca absorption. Second, this greater Ca availability will allow for some passive influx, which directly contributes to sustained calcemia.

In contrast to intravenous infusions, oral Ca is unlikely to result in delayed regulation consequent to a positive calcemia signal. Passive absorption should be moderate and expanded in time. Ruminal pH results in low Ca solubility limiting passive Ca

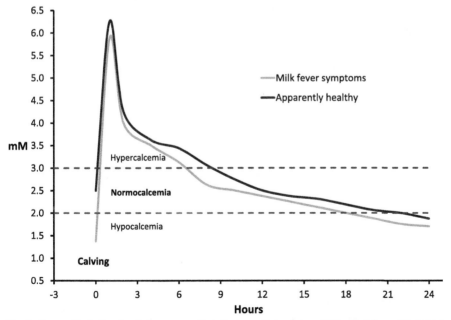

Fig. 7. Serum Ca following intravenous Ca infusion after calving. (*Adapted from* Albright J, Blosser T. Blood levels and urinary excretion of calcium in normal cows and cows with parturient paresis after intravenous injections with calcium borogluconate. J Dairy Sci 1957;40(5):477–86.)

absorption in the forestomachs. Furthermore, the rate of passage to lower gastrointestinal compartments buffers the release of ruminal contents into the abomasum and duodenum to a small percentage per hour.

Aqueous solutions of Ca chloride can result in epithelial damage during application.[94] At the same time one should not expect a large difference in Ca availability, as the rumen environment will precipitate Ca ions at high pH and high carbonate concentrations. Suspensions of other forms of Ca seem to be a safer and more palatable approach to acute oral supplementation at calving.

Decreased Dietary Calcium Supply Weeks Before Calving

Low calcium diets

Lowering dietary Ca in the close-up diet can prevent milk fever,[101–106] especially if Ca intake is as low as 20 g per day.[94] Meta-analyses[79,107] of disease risk confirm this very low risk observed when Ca intakes are very low. Furthermore, mechanistic analysis explains empirical evidence as a result of metabolic adaptation.[26]

Reducing Ca intake is difficult in practice because it seems incompatible with limiting energy intake before calving. Concentrates are poor in Ca whereas forages are rich in Ca, and traditionally high forage diets have been fed to close-up dairy cows. However, there are exceptions to this general rule. Corn silage and cereal straws are relatively low in Ca. Furthermore, straw limits total DM intake (DMI). In practice, it is feasible and beneficial to reduce Ca intake by avoiding green forages such as grasses and alfalfa in close-up rations, but reaching extremely low levels of Ca remains difficult to combine with the general nutritional objectives of precalving rations.

Reduction of calcium availability using nutritional antagonists of calcium availability

Zeolites To reduce Ca supply, the use of Ca antagonists has been proposed. The first approach studied was zeolite clays, which improved calcemia around calving.[108–116] The apparent drawback of zeolite feeding is the effect on feed intakes.[114,115] Nevertheless, at moderate doses (23 g/kg DM) intake suppression is controlled without compromising effectiveness.[115] Zeolite feeding prevents milk fever by reducing Ca availability before calving, but also has shown negative effects on magnesemia and phosphatemia. This latter finding may also be related to zeolites' mode of action, as dietary compensation by phosphorus supplementation seems to reduce the preventive value of the application regarding milk fever.[116]

Bypass phytic acid Rumen bypass phytic acid from treated rice bran also has been proposed to reduce the dietary availability of Ca. This cereal by-product is the feed with the highest phytic acid content and is ranked first as a Ca antagonist.[117] However, this is not necessarily true for a ruminant because phytic acid is rumen degradable,[118] but its ruminal breakdown can be prevented by technological treatments.[119] This by-product of rice milling can induce adaptation of Ca metabolism by its naturally low Ca content, which lowers Ca intake, and also by lowering Ca availability.[30] Feeding 2 kg of treated rice bran in the close-up diet has been shown to improve the rate of recovery of calcemia around calving and to have a positive impact on feed intake in the days after calving.[120]

Reduction of Dietary Cation-Anion Difference

The most commonly used approach for the prevention of milk fever in nutritional practice is the induction to moderate metabolic acidosis by the modification of dietary cation-anion difference (DCAD). This goal is achieved by feeding mineral supplements that contain sulfur (S) or chlorine (Cl) without Na or K, commonly known as anionic salts. DCAD balance is calculated by adding Na and K intakes and subtracting Cl and S intakes in milliequivalents.[121] The effectiveness is monitored by measuring urine pH. This approach has been extensively studied,[10,80,121–123] and found to be consistently successful.

Extent of decrease of dietary cation-anion difference and effectiveness of milk fever prevention

High DCAD in close-up diets is mostly caused by K content in forages, which in itself is an indirect negative factor for milk fever through its effect on Mg availability. Meanwhile, formulation to low DCAD is a dietary intervention to prevent milk fever. It is important to separate these 2 effects even if they point in the same direction, because the application of anionic salts in close-up diets mostly seems to be effective when DCAD reaches low values and metabolic acidosis is achieved.[11,79,123] This effect seems to be linked with the effect on urine pH[79,80,123] and urinary Ca,[80] which substantially changes at DCAD values around −50 to −150 mEq/kg DM (**Fig. 8**).

A negative effect on feed intake has been described for low DCAD diets,[123] and palatability of anionic salts has been studied for this reason.[122] This effect does not seem a problem if the minerals are mixed in the total diet, and if the total supply required is moderate in association with moderate K content in the basal diet. Nevertheless, on farms where animal numbers limit the use of total mixed rations in close-up diets, concentrations of anionic salts in supplemental compound feeds can lead to refusals, limiting the practical applicability of this strategy in certain production environments.[120]

Mode of action of dietary cation-anion difference

Traditionally, metabolic alkalosis associated with high K forage in close-up diets has been explained as a burden for Ca metabolism.[124–127] This situation should arise

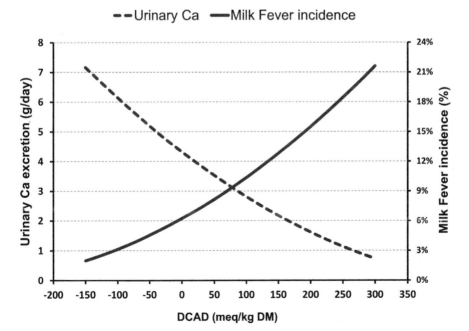

Fig. 8. Equations describing the relation between DCAD and daily urinary Ca excretion (equation from Roche and colleagues[80] adapted by Martín-Tereso and Verstegen[26]) and milk fever incidence (equation from Charbonneau and colleagues[123]). (*Data from* Refs.[26,80,123])

through reduced PTH[128] responsiveness during metabolic alkalosis or improved calcitriol responsiveness at lower DCAD.[125] Nevertheless, these potential negative effects are not evident in conditions of high Na supplementation in high fermentable diets[129] or in high K intakes in late lactation forage-rich diets, which in particular puts pressure on tetany, but calcemia is adequately sustained. A more recent explanation proposes that lower pH would release bone Ca, which would result in higher urinary Ca, which in turn would activate intestinal absorption by an increased calcitriol signal.[11]

The already discussed inhibition of TRPV5 during metabolic acidosis and the counterreaction of gastrointestinal TRPV6 represent a more plausible explanation for milk fever prevention by low DCAD diets. A PTH-independent increase of renal Ca excretion would create the signal chain leading to activated gastrointestinal absorption: negative calcemia deviation, release of PTH, and activation of calcitriol, just as observed in TRPV5 knock-out mice.[83] Greater apparent Ca absorption has been described for low-DCAD fed cows,[82] as a response to increased urinary Ca excretion. Hypercalciuria induced by ionic salts has been estimated to create a Ca deficit sufficient to activate Ca absorption.[26] Furthermore, if dietary Ca would be unable to compensate this deficit, sustained and combined PTH and calcitriol signals would induce bone mobilization.

However, the effect of dietary Ca intake on low DCAD has been controversial. Although higher dietary Ca has traditionally been recommended to compensate hypercalciuria,[130] benefits from this recommendation have remained elusive to validation.[124] Although meta-analysis[79] and mechanistic study of Ca balance[26] suggest a benefit from lower Ca, empirical validation of this recommendation remains pending.

Low DCAD strategy can be an effective approach to the prevention of milk fever. Nevertheless, it is important to monitor urinary pH. Moderate doses of anionic salts will not result in milk fever prevention if they do not result in an acidic urinary pH.[120]

Magnesium as a Risk Factor for Milk Fever

Hypomagnesemia impairs the release of PTH[131] and the effects of PTH at the target organ.[126] Hence, hypomagnesemia reduces the capacity for Ca mobilization from the bone and increases the risk for milk fever. Indeed, Sansom and colleagues[132] demonstrated in cows that hypomagnesemia significantly reduced Ca mobilization. The important role of sufficient Mg intake at parturition is underlined by the results of meta-analysis of possible causal reasons of milk fever. A change in dietary Mg from 0.3% to 0.4% DM was estimated to reduce the risk for milk fever by 62%.[79] This high Mg concentration is far higher than the German recommendation of 0.2%, but can easily be explained by a calculation of Mg intake and necessary requirement, which includes Mg for maintenance (2.8 g/d) and in colostrum: (3.6 g/d) (5 L × 0.733 mg/L) = 6.4 g/d.

The amount of Mg in colostrum is an approximation. Kehoe and colleagues[133] reported Mg concentration in the colostrum of 0.733 mg/kg (range 230–1399 mg/kg) of fully milked out cows (55 cows from 55 herds) within 4 hours of calving. The amount of colostrum was not published. The assumed 5 L (5 × 0.733 mg/kg = 3.6 g) is probably an underestimation, particularly for the whole day, and underlines the risk of Mg shortage.

It is well known that DMI is severely reduced at parturition, varying between 6 and 10 kg/d. This DMI is accompanied by an Mg intake of 18 to 30 g/d (Mg 0.3%) or 24 to 40 g/d (Mg 0.4%) (**Table 7**).

Because Mg digestibility is generally low,[40] the calculated Mg digestibility for covering the requirement of 6.4 g/d shows (see **Table 7**) that the assumed Mg intake with 6 or 8 kg/d DMI is low, even at these high Mg concentrations of 0.3% or 0.4% Mg.

Table 7
Dry matter intake, Mg intake, and necessary Mg digestibility for Mg requirement at parturition

Dry Matter Intake (kg/d)	Mg (%DMI)	Mg Intake (g/d)	Mg Requirement (g/d)	Necessary Mg Digestibility (%)
6	0.3	18	6.4	36[a]
8	0.3	24	6.4	27[a]
10	0.3	30	6.4	21
6	0.4	24	6.4	27[a]
8	0.4	32	6.4	20
10	0.4	40	6.4	16

[a] Unlikely high Mg digestibility for the necessary requirement.

Summary of Milk Fever Prevention Strategies

Preventing milk fever requires multifactorial approaches that should be made compatible with general nutritional objectives of close-up diets. A strategy to induce the adaptation of Ca metabolism should be combined with assuring the Mg supply by supplementation and control of K intakes. Limiting Ca availability or inducing renal hypercalciuria are the 2 most effective strategies to prevent milk fever by inducing the activation of Ca absorption weeks before calving. Furthermore, intravenous infusions should be limited to extreme clinical cases, and acute oral supply, preferably in the form of a palatable Ca suspension, should be complementary and should not replace a close-up diet aiming to induce metabolic adaptation.

PRACTICAL RECOMMENDATIONS FOR THE PREVENTION OF TETANY

The impact of classic grass tetany is generally low in dairy cattle fed with concentrate diet for milk production. Concentrates are supplemented with minerals (Mg and Na) and dilute the K content of the total ration. Rapid changes of diet (N and NH_4^+) are rare. A significant risk is given for dairy cows in countries with traditional grassland feeding, as in Ireland and New Zealand. If concentrates are offered to increase milk production, Mg and Na must be included to cover the requirement. Furthermore, use of molasses-based licks/buckets is a method of choice to supplement cows with Mg and Na.

The classic risk of grass tetany still arises in beef cattle if they are suddenly moved from the barn to young grassland in spring. The sudden change (nitrogen and NH_4^+), the low Na and Mg content, and the high K content of the new grass are the known risk factors, which can be avoided by a stepwise change of diet and availability of licks/buckets with enough Na and Mg.

REFERENCES

1. Thébault S, Hoenderop JG, Bindels RJ. Epithelial Ca^{+2} and Mg^{+2} channels in kidney disease. Adv Chronic Kidney Dis 2006;13(2):110–7.
2. Case RM, Eisner D, Gurney A, et al. Evolution of calcium homeostasis: from birth of the first cell to an omnipresent signalling system. Cell Calcium 2007;42(4–5): 345–50.
3. Günther T. Stoffwechsel und Wirkungen des intrazellulären Magnesium. J Clin Chem Clin Biochem 1977;15:433–8.

4. Stumpff F, Martens H. The rumen and potassium homeostasis: a model. Anim Feed Sci Technol 2007;16(Suppl 2):436–41.
5. Zhou H, Clapham DE. Mammalian MagT1 and TUSC3 are required for cellular magnesium uptake and vertebrate embryonic development. Proc Natl Acad Sci U S A 2009;106(37):15750–5.
6. Ramberg C, Johnson E, Fargo R, et al. Calcium homeostasis in cows, with special reference to parturient hypocalcemia. Am J Physiol Regul Integr Comp Physiol 1984;246(5):698–704.
7. Roche J, Berry D. Periparturient climatic, animal, and management factors influencing the incidence of milk fever in grazing systems. J Dairy Sci 2006;89(7): 2775–83.
8. Reinhardt TA, Lippolis JD, McCluskey BJ, et al. Prevalence of subclinical hypocalcemia in dairy herds. Vet J 2011;188(1):122–4.
9. USDA. Dairy 2007, Part II: changes in the U.S. dairy cattle industry, 1991-2007. Fort Collins (CO): USDA-APHIS-VS; 2008.
10. Moore S, VandeHaar M, Sharma B, et al. Effects of altering dietary cation-anion difference on calcium and energy metabolism in peripartum cows. J Dairy Sci 2000;83(9):2095–104.
11. DeGaris P, Lean I. Milk fever in dairy cows: a review of pathophysiology and control principles. Vet J 2008;176(1):58–69.
12. Barja G. Rate of generation of oxidative stress-related damage and animal longevity. Free Radic Biol Med 2002;33(9):1167–72.
13. Groenestege WM, Hoenderop JG, van den Heuvel L, et al. The epithelial Mg^{2+} channel transient receptor potential melastatin 6 is regulated by dietary Mg^{2+} content and estrogens. J Am Soc Nephrol 2006;17(4):1035–43.
14. Todd J, Horvath D. Magnesium and neuromuscular irritability in calves, with particular reference to hypomagnesaemic tetany. Br Vet J 1970;126:333–46.
15. Sjollema B. On the nature and therapy of grass staggers. Vet Rec 1930; 10(425–430):450–3.
16. Meyer H, Scholz H. Studies on the pathogenesis of hypomagnesemic tetany. I. Relationships between the magnesium contents in blood and cerebrospinal fluid. Dtsch Tierarztl Wochenschr 1972;79(3):55 [in German].
17. Allsop T, Pauli J. Responses to the lowering of magnesium and calcium concentrations in the cerebrospinal fluid of unanesthetized sheep. Aust J Biol Sci 1975; 28(5–6):475–81.
18. Reynolds CK, Bell MC, Sims MH. Changes in plasma, red blood cell and cerebrospinal fluid mineral concentrations in calves during magnesium depletion followed by repletion with rectally infused magnesium chloride. J Nutr 1984;114(7): 1334–41.
19. Breves G, Schröder B, Muscher A. Luminal and endocrine factors for regulation of intestinal monosaccharide and Ca^{2+} transport. Livest Prod Sci 2010;134: 4–10.
20. Erben R. Vitamin D analogs and bone. J Musculoskelet Neuronal Interact 2001; 2(1):59–69.
21. Goff J. Macromineral physiology and application to the feeding of the dairy cow for prevention of milk fever and other periparturient mineral disorders. Anim Feed Sci Technol 2006;126(3–4):237–57.
22. Horst R. Regulation of calcium and phosphorus homeostasis in the dairy cow. J Dairy Sci 1986;69(2):604–16.
23. Schröder B, Breves G. Mechanisms and regulation of calcium absorption from the gastrointestinal tract in pigs and ruminants: comparative aspects with

special emphasis on hypocalcemia in dairy cows. Anim Health Res Rev 2007; 7(1–2):31–41.

24. Suzuki Y, Landowski C, Hediger M. Mechanisms and regulation of epithelial Ca^{2+} absorption in health and disease. Annu Rev Physiol 2008;70:257–71.

25. Brown EM, Gamba G, Riccardi D, et al. Cloning and characterization of an extracellular Ca^{2+}-sensing receptor from bovine parathyroid. Nature 1993; 366(6455):575–80.

26. Martín-Tereso J, Verstegen MW. A novel model to explain dietary factors affecting hypocalcaemia in dairy cattle. Nutr Res Rev 2011;24:228–43.

27. Schonewille J, van't Klooster A, Wouterse H, et al. Hypocalcemia induced by intravenous administration of disodium ethylenediaminotetraacetate and its effects on excretion of calcium in urine of cows fed a high chloride diet. J Dairy Sci 1999;82(6):1317–24.

28. Martín-Tereso J, Derks M, van Laar H, et al. Urinary calcium excretion in nonlactating dairy cows in relation to intake of fat-coated rice bran. J Anim Physiol Anim Nutr (Berl) 2010;94:129–36.

29. Armbrecht HJ, Boltz MA, Christakos S, et al. Capacity of 1,25-dihydroxyvitamin D to stimulate expression of calbindin D changes with age in the rat. Arch Biochem Biophys 1998;352(2):159–64.

30. Martín-Tereso J, van Puijenbroek R, van Laar H, et al. Effect of feeding rumen protected rice bran on calcium homeostasis of non-lactating multiparous cows. J Anim Physiol Anim Nutr (Berl) 2011;95:236–44.

31. Schröder B, Rittmann I, Pfeffer E, et al. In vitro studies on calcium absorption from the gastrointestinal tract in small ruminants. J Comp Physiol B 1997; 167(1):43–51.

32. Wilkens MR, Kunert-Keil C, Brinkmeier H, et al. Expression of calcium channel TRPV6 in ovine epithelial tissue. Vet J 2009;182(2):294–300.

33. Wilkens MR, Mrochen N, Breves G, et al. Gastrointestinal calcium absorption in sheep is mostly insensitive to an alimentary induced challenge of calcium homeostasis. Comp Biochem Physiol B Biochem Mol Biol 2011;158:199–207.

34. Sidler-Lauff K, Boos A, Kraenzlin M, et al. Influence of different calcium supplies and a single vitamin D injection on vitamin D receptor and calbindin D9k immunoreactivities in the gastrointestinal tract of goat kids. J Anim Sci 2010;88(11):3598–610.

35. Taylor M, Knowlton K, McGilliard M, et al. Blood mineral, hormone, and osteocalcin responses of multiparous Jersey cows to an oral dose of 25-hydroxyvitamin D_3 or vitamin D_3 before parturition. J Dairy Sci 2008;91(6):2408–16.

36. Liesegang A, Eicher R, Sassi ML, et al. The course of selected bone resorption marker concentrations in response to short-term hypocalcemia experimentally induced with disodium EDTA infusions in dairy cows. J Vet Med A Physiol Pathol Clin Med 2000;47(8):477–87.

37. Parfitt A. The actions of parathyroid hormone on bone. Relation to bone remodelling and turnover, calcium homeostasis, and metabolic bone disease. Part II. Metabolism 1976;25:909–55.

38. Hadjidakis D, Androullakis I. Bone remodeling. Ann N Y Acad Sci 2006;1092(1 women's health and disease: gynecologic, endocrine, and reproductive issues): 385–96.

39. Lemaire V, Tobin F, Greller L, et al. Modeling the interactions between osteoblast and osteoclast activities in bone remodeling. J Theor Biol 2004;229(3): 293–309.

40. Schonewille J, Everts H, Jittakhot S, et al. Quantitative prediction of magnesium absorption in dairy cows. J Dairy Sci 2008;91(1):271–8.

41. Ruckebusch Y, Thivend P. Magnesium metabolism and hypomagnesaemia. Digestive physiology and metabolism in ruminants. Clermont-Ferrand: MTP Press; 1980. p. 447–66.
42. Martens H, Schweigel M. Pathophysiology of grass tetany and other hypomagnesemias. Implications for clinical management. Vet Clin North Am Food Anim Pract 2000;16(2):339.
43. Tomas F, Potter B. The effect and site of action of potassium upon magnesium absorption in sheep. Aust J Agric Res 1976;27(6):873–80.
44. Pfeffer E, Rahman K. Untersuchungen zur Lokalisierung der Magnesium-Absorption beim Wiederkäuer. Z Tierphysiol Tierernahr Futtermittelkd 1974;33: 209–10.
45. Smith R. Absorption of major minerals in the small and large intestines of the ruminant. Proc Nutr Soc 1969;28(1):151–60.
46. Meyer H, Busse F. Zur rektalen absorption von magnesium beim wiederkaeuer. Dtsch Tierarztl Wochenschr 1975;82:140–1.
47. Bell M, Oluokun J, Ramsey N, et al. Magnesium treatment of cows for grass tetany [Hypomagnesemia]. Feedstuffs; 1978. p. 24–32, 50.
48. Martens H, Stössel EM. Magnesium absorption from the temporarily isolated rumen of sheep: no effect of hyper- or hypomagnesaemia. Exp Physiol 1988; 73(2):217–23.
49. Kemp A. The effect of fertilizer treatment of grassland on the biological availability of magnesium to ruminants. In: Fontenot JP, editor. Role of magnesium in animal nutrition. Blacksburg (VA): Polytechnic Institute State University Blacksburg; 1983. p. 143–57.
50. Hoenderop JG, Nilius B, Bindels RJ. Calcium absorption across epithelia. Physiol Rev 2005;85(1):373–422.
51. Pérez A, Picotto G, Carpentieri A, et al. Minireview on regulation of intestinal calcium absorption. Emphasis on molecular mechanisms of transcellular pathway. Digestion 2008;77(1):22–34.
52. Wasserman R. Vitamin D and the dual processes of intestinal calcium absorption. J Nutr 2004;134(11):3137–9.
53. Bouillon R, Van Cromphaut S, Carmeliet G. Intestinal calcium absorption: molecular vitamin D mediated mechanisms. J Cell Biochem 2003;88(2):332–9.
54. Bronner F. Mechanisms of intestinal calcium absorption. J Cell Biochem 2003; 88(2):387–93.
55. Khanal R, Nemere I. Regulation of intestinal calcium transport. Annu Rev Nutr 2008;28:179–96.
56. van Abel M, Hoenderop JG, van der Kemp AW, et al. Coordinated control of renal Ca^{2+} transport proteins by parathyroid hormone. Kidney Int 2005;68(4):1708–21.
57. Scott D. Factors influencing the secretion and absorption of calcium and magnesium in the small intestine of the sheep. Exp Physiol 1965;50(3):312–29.
58. Care A, Brown R, Farrar A, et al. Magnesium absorption from the digestive tract of sheep. Exp Physiol 1984;69(3):577–87.
59. Leonhard-Marek S, Martens H. Effects of potassium on magnesium transport across rumen epithelium. Am J Physiol Gastrointest Liver Physiol 1996;271(6): G1034–8.
60. Schweigel M, Kolisek M, Nikolic Z, et al. Expression and functional activity of the Na/Mg exchanger, TRPM7 and MagT1 are changed to regulate Mg homeostasis and transport in rumen epithelial cells. Magnesium Res. 2008;21:1–6.
61. Van Der Wijst J, Hoenderop JG, Bindels RJ. Epithelial Mg^{2+} channel TRPM6: insight into the molecular regulation. Magnes Res 2009;22(3):127–32.

62. Kolisek M, Nestler A, Vormann J, et al. Human gene SLC41A1 encodes for the Na$^+$/Mg^{2+} exchanger. Am J Physiol Cell Physiol 2012;302(1):C318–26.

63. Ram L, Schonewille JT, Martens H, et al. Magnesium absorption by wethers fed potassium bicarbonate in combination with different dietary magnesium concentrations. J Dairy Sci 1998;81(9):2485–92.

64. Martinez N, Sinedino L, Bisinotto R, et al. Effect of induced subclinical hypocalcemia on physiological responses and neutrophil function in dairy cows. J Dairy Sci 2014;97(2):874–87.

65. Chattopadhyay N, Vassilev P, Brown E. Calcium-sensing receptor: roles in and beyond systemic calcium homeostasis. Biol Chem 1997;378(8):759–68.

66. San-Cristobal P, Dimke H, Hoenderop JG, et al. Novel molecular pathways in renal Mg^{2+} transport: a guided tour along the nephron. Curr Opin Nephrol Hypertens 2010;19(5):456–62.

67. Schonewille JT, van't Klooster AT, Wouterse H, et al. Time courses of plasma magnesium concentrations and urinary magnesium excretion in cows subjected to acute changes in potassium intake. Vet Q 2000;22(3):136–40.

68. NRC. Nutrient requirements of dairy cattle. 7th revised edition. Washington, DC: National Academy Press; 2001.

69. Taylor M, Knowlton K, McGilliard M, et al. Dietary calcium has little effect on mineral balance and bone mineral metabolism through twenty weeks of lactation in Holstein cows. J Dairy Sci 2009;92(1):223–37.

70. Pivonka P, Zimak J, Smith D, et al. Model structure and control of bone remodeling: a theoretical study. Bone 2008;43(2):249–63.

71. Bieglmayer C, Prager G, Niederle B. Kinetic analyses of parathyroid hormone clearance as measured by three rapid immunoassays during parathyroidectomy. Clin Chem 2002;48(10):1731–8.

72. Norman A, Friedlander E, Henry H. Determination of the rates of synthesis and degradation of vitamin D-dependent chick intestinal and renal calcium-binding proteins. Arch Biochem Biophys 1981;206(2):305–17.

73. Creamer B, Shorter R, Bamforth J. The turnover and shedding of epithelial cells. Gut 1961;2(2):110–8.

74. Vogetseder A, Karadeniz A, Kaissling B, et al. Tubular cell proliferation in the healthy rat kidney. Histochem Cell Biol 2005;124(2):97–104.

75. Walters J, Weiser M. Calcium transport by rat duodenal villus and crypt basolateral membranes. Am J Physiol Gastrointest Liver Physiol 1987;252(2):170–7.

76. Halloran BP, De Luca HF. Intestinal calcium transport: Evidence for two distinct mechanisms of action of 1, 25-dihydroxyvitamin D3. Arch Biochem Biophys 1981;208(2):477–86.

77. Greenfield E, Bi Y, Miyauchi A. Regulation of osteoclast activity. Life Sci 1999; 65(11):1087–102.

78. Goff J, Littledike E, Horst R. Effect of synthetic bovine parathyroid hormone in dairy cows: prevention of hypocalcemic parturient paresis. J Dairy Sci 1986; 69(9):2278–89.

79. Lean I, DeGaris P, McNeil D, et al. Hypocalcemia in dairy cows: meta-analysis and dietary cation anion difference theory revisited. J Dairy Sci 2006;89(2): 669–84.

80. Roche J, Dalley D, Moate P, et al. Dietary cation-anion difference and the health and production of pasture-fed dairy cows 2. Nonlactating periparturient cows. J Dairy Sci 2003;86(3):979–87.

81. de Groot T, Bindels RJ, Hoenderop JG. TRPV5: an ingeniously controlled calcium channel. Kidney Int 2008;74(10):1241–6.

82. Lambers TT, Oancea E, de Groot T, et al. Extracellular pH dynamically controls cell surface delivery of functional TRPV5 channels. Mol Cell Biol 2007;27(4): 1486–94.
83. Hoenderop J, van Leeuwen J, van der Eerden B, et al. Renal Ca^{2+} wasting, hyperabsorption, and reduced bone thickness in mice lacking TRPV5. J Clin Invest 2003;112(12):1906–14.
84. Martens H, Blume I. Effect of intraruminal sodium and potassium concentrations and of the transmural potential difference on magnesium absorption from the temporarily isolated rumen of sheep. Exp Physiol 1986;71(3):409–15.
85. Martens H, Gäbel G, Strozyk H. The effect of potassium and the transmural potential difference on magnesium transport across an isolated preparation of sheep rumen epithelium. Exp Physiol 1987;72(2):181–8.
86. Weiss W. Macromineral digestion by lactating dairy cows: factors affecting digestibility of magnesium. J Dairy Sci 2004;87(7):2167–71.
87. Martens H, Stumpff F. Ruminal Mg transport and assessment of Mg intake in dairy cows. Two sides of one coin [abstract]. J Dairy Sci 2011;94(Suppl 1):510.
88. Schonewille J, Beynen A. Reviews on the mineral provision in ruminants (III): magnesium metabolism and requirement in ruminants. CVB Documentation Report Nr. 35. Lelystad (The Netherlands): Central Veevoederbureau; 2005. p. 14.
89. Martens H, Heggemann G, Regier K. Studies on the effect of K, Na, NH$_4^+$, VFA and CO$_2$ on the net absorption of magnesium from the temporarily isolated rumen of heifers. Zentralbl Veterinarmed A 1988;35(1):73–80.
90. Gäbel G, Martens H. The effect of ammonia on magnesium metabolism in sheep. J Anim Physiol Anim Nutr (Berl) 1986;55(1–5):278–87.
91. Fontenot J, Wise M, Webb K Jr. Interrelationships of potassium, nitrogen, and magnesium in ruminants. Fed Proc 1973;32:1925–8.
92. Butler E. The mineral element content of spring pasture in relation to the occurrence of grass tetany and hypomagnesaemia in dairy cows. J Agric Sci 1963; 60:329–40.
93. Boda J, Cole H. Calcium metabolism with special reference to parturient paresis (milk fever) in dairy cattle: a review. J Dairy Sci 1956;39(7):1027–54.
94. Thilsing-Hansen T, Jørgensen R, Østergaard S. Milk fever control principles: a review. Acta Vet Scand 2002;43(1):1–19.
95. Horst R, Goff J, Reinhardt T. Role of vitamin D in calcium homeostasis and its use in prevention of bovine periparturient paresis. Acta Vet Scand Suppl 2003;97:35–50.
96. Littledike E, Horst R. Vitamin D$_3$ toxicity in dairy cows. J Dairy Sci 1982;65(5): 749–59.
97. Gast D, Horst R, Jorgensen N, et al. Potential use of 1, 25-dihydroxycholecalciferol for prevention of parturient paresis1. J Dairy Sci 1979;62(6):1009–13.
98. Hove K, Horst R, Littledike E. Effects of 1 [alpha]-hydroxyvitamin D$_3$, 1, 25-dihydroxyvitamin D$_3$, 1, 24, 25-trihydroxyvitamin D$_3$, and 1, 25, 26-trihydroxyvitamin D$_3$ on mineral metabolism and 1, 25-dihydroxyvitamin D concentrations in dairy cows. J Dairy Sci 1983;66(1):59–66.
99. Hibbs J, Conrad H. Studies of milk fever in dairy cows. VI. Effect of three prepartal dosage levels of vitamin D on milk fever incidence. J Dairy Sci 1960;43(8): 1124–9.
100. Albright J, Blosser T. Blood levels and urinary excretion of calcium in normal cows and cows with parturient paresis after intravenous injections with calcium borogluconate. J Dairy Sci 1957;40(5):477–86.

101. Goings R, Jacobson N, Beitz D, et al. Prevention of parturient paresis by a prepartum, calcium-deficient diet. J Dairy Sci 1974;57(10):1184–8.
102. Wiggers K, Nelson D, Jacobson N. Prevention of parturient paresis by a low-calcium diet prepartum: a field study. J Dairy Sci 1975;58(3):430–1.
103. Yarrington J, Capen C, Black H, et al. Effects of a low calcium prepartal diet on calcium homeostatic mechanisms in the cow: morphologic and biochemical studies. J Nutr 1977;107(12):2244–56.
104. Green H, Horst R, Beitz D, et al. Vitamin D metabolites in plasma of cows fed a prepartum low-calcium diet for prevention of parturient hypocalcemia. J Dairy Sci 1981;64(2):217–26.
105. Kichura T, Horst R, Beitz D, et al. Relationships between prepartal dietary calcium and phosphorus, vitamin D metabolism, and parturient paresis in dairy cows. J Nutr 1982;112(3):480–7.
106. Shappell N, Herbein J, Deftos L, et al. Effects of dietary calcium and age on parathyroid hormone, calcitonin and serum and milk minerals in the periparturient dairy cow. J Nutr 1987;117(1):201–7.
107. Oetzel G. Meta-analysis of nutritional risk factors for milk fever in dairy cattle. J Dairy Sci 1991;74(11):3900–12.
108. Thilsing-Hansen T, Jorgensen R, Enemark J, et al. The effect of zeolite A supplementation in the dry period on periparturient calcium, phosphorus, and magnesium homeostasis. J Dairy Sci 2002;85(7):1855–62.
109. Enemark J, Frandsen A, Thilsing-Hansen T, et al. Aspects of physiological effects of sodium zeolite A supplementation in dry, non-pregnant dairy cows fed grass silage. Acta Vet Scand Suppl 2003;97:97–117.
110. Enemark J, Kirketerp-Møller C, Jørgensen R. Effect of prepartum zeolite A supplementation on renal calcium excretion in dairy cows around calving and evaluation of a field test kit for monitoring it. Acta Vet Scand Suppl 2003;97:119–36.
111. Thilsing-Hansen T, Jørgensen R, Enemark J, et al. The effect of zeolite A supplementation in the dry period on blood mineral status around calving. Acta Vet Scand Suppl 2003;97:87–95.
112. Katsoulos P, Roubies N, Panousis N, et al. Effects of long-term dietary supplementation with clinoptilolite on incidence of parturient paresis and serum concentrations of total calcium, phosphate, magnesium, potassium, and sodium in dairy cows. Am J Vet Res 2005;66(12):2081–5.
113. Thilsing T, Larsen T, Jorgensen R, et al. The effect of dietary calcium and phosphorus supplementation in zeolite A treated dry cows on periparturient calcium and phosphorus homeostasis. J Vet Med A Physiol Pathol Clin Med 2007;54(2): 82–91.
114. Grabherr H, Spolders M, Flachowsky G, et al. Influence of zeolite A supplementation during the dry period of dairy cows on feed intake, on the macro and trace element metabolism around calving and milk yield in the following lactation. Berl Munch Tierarztl Wochenschr 2008;121(1–2):41–52.
115. Grabherr H, Spolders M, Furll M, et al. Effect of several doses of zeolite A on feed intake, energy metabolism and on mineral metabolism in dairy cows around calving. J Anim Physiol Anim Nutr (Berl) 2009;93(2):221–36.
116. Pallesen A, Pallesen F, Jørgensen R, et al. Effect of pre-calving zeolite, magnesium and phosphorus supplementation on periparturient serum mineral concentrations. Vet J 2008;175(2):234–9.
117. Siener R, Heynck H, Hesse A. Calcium-binding capacities of different brans under simulated gastrointestinal pH conditions. In vitro study with ^{45}Ca. J Agric Food Chem 2001;49(9):4397–401.

118. Clark W Jr, Wohlt J, Gilbreath R, et al. Phytate phosphorus intake and disappearance in the gastrointestinal tract of high producing dairy cows. J Dairy Sci 1986; 69(12):3151–5.

119. Martín-Tereso J, Gonzalez A, Van Laar H, et al. In situ ruminal degradation of phytic acid in formaldehyde-treated rice bran. Anim Feed Sci Tech 2009; 152(3–4):286–97.

120. Martín-Tereso J, Wijlen H, Laar H, et al. Peripartal calcium homoeostasis of multiparous dairy cows fed rumen-protected rice bran or a lowered dietary cation/anion balance diet before calving. J Anim Physiol Anim Nutr (Berl) 2014;98(4):775–84.

121. Block E. Manipulating dietary anions and cations for prepartum dairy cows to reduce incidence of milk fever. J Dairy Sci 1984;67(12):2939–48.

122. Oetzel G, Fettman M, Hamar D, et al. Screening of anionic salts for palatability, effects on acid-base status, and urinary calcium excretion in dairy cows. J Dairy Sci 1991;74(3):965–71.

123. Charbonneau E, Pellerin D, Oetzel G. Impact of lowering dietary cation-anion difference in nonlactating dairy cows: a meta-analysis. J Dairy Sci 2006;89(2): 537–48.

124. Goff J, Horst R. Effects of the addition of potassium or sodium, but not calcium, to prepartum rations on milk fever in dairy cows. J Dairy Sci 1997;80(1):176–86.

125. Goff J, Horst R, Mueller F, et al. Addition of chloride to a prepartal diet high in cations increases 1, 25-dihydroxyvitamin d response to hypocalcemia preventing milk fever. J Dairy Sci 1991;74(11):3863–71.

126. Goff J. The monitoring, prevention, and treatment of milk fever and subclinical hypocalcemia in dairy cows. Vet J 2008;176(1):50–7.

127. Goff J, Liesegang A, Horst R. Diet-induced pseudohypoparathyroidism: a hypocalcemia and milk fever risk factor. J Dairy Sci 2014;97(3):1520–8.

128. Horst R, Goff J, Reinhardt T. Calcium and vitamin D metabolism in the dairy cow. J Dairy Sci 1994;77(7):1936–51.

129. Hu W, Murphy M. Dietary cation-anion difference effects on performance and acid-base status of lactating dairy cows: a meta-analysis. J Dairy Sci 2004; 87(7):2222–9.

130. Oetzel G. Management of dry cows for the prevention of milk fever and other mineral disorders. Vet Clin North Am Food Anim Pract 2000;16(2):369–86.

131. Anast CS, Mohs JM, Kaplan SL, et al. Evidence for parathyroid failure in magnesium deficiency. Science 1972;177(4049):606–8.

132. Sansom B, Manston R, Vagg M. Magnesium and milk fever. Vet Rec 1983; 112(19):447–9.

133. Kehoe S, Jayarao B, Heinrichs A. A survey of bovine colostrum composition and colostrum management practices on Pennsylvania dairy farms. J Dairy Sci 2007;90(9):4108–16.

Trace Mineral Feeding and Assessment

William S. Swecker Jr, DVM, PhD

KEYWORDS

- Trace minerals or elements • Dairy nutrition • Liver biopsy • Nutrient requirements

KEY POINTS

- Trace minerals are an essential component of a feeding program for dairy herds. Deficiencies are unlikely when the cows are fed amounts to meet National Research Council (NRC) requirements.
- The need for additional trace elements to support high milk production is supported by the increased dry matter intake associated with lactation.
- Dietary analysis is needed to identify the relative concentrations of the antagonists and potentially the antagonists may be removed rather than increasing supplementation.
- Organic and alternate forms of trace elements have received wide acceptance throughout across multiple food animal production systems.
- Blood and liver analysis can be effectively used to confirm diagnoses or monitor the efficacy of the feeding program.

INTRODUCTION

Practitioners may be asked to evaluate the trace mineral status of dairy herds or offer opinions on the mineral supplementation program. Many times this request comes based on reduced reproductive success, udder health problems, or nonspecific increases in morbidity or mortality. As McClure[1] noted, deficiencies of almost all nutrients have been thought to cause infertility, yet few have been proven to do so cattle. Trace minerals fit in a somewhat unique position because either deficient or excessive amounts can lead to disorders.

Before an investigation on trace mineral inadequacy or excess, the author recommends an approach suggested by Clark and Ellison in the article aptly titled "Mineral testing–the approach depends on what you want to find out."[2] The strategy of who and what to test depends on the question at hand.

Disclosure: W.S. Swecker has received funding from Zinpro Corporation (<$10k) in 2004 for evaluation of trace mineral content of ovaries. Results presented at 2006 ADSA meeting.
Department of Large Animal Clinical Sciences, Virginia-Maryland Regional College of Veterinary Medicine, Virginia Tech, 205 Duckpond Drive, Blacksburg, VA 24061-0442, USA
E-mail address: cvmwss@vt.edu

Vet Clin Food Anim 30 (2014) 671–688
http://dx.doi.org/10.1016/j.cvfa.2014.07.008   vetfood.theclinics.com
0749-0720/14/$ – see front matter © 2014 Elsevier Inc. All rights reserved.

1. Is the poor performance owing to a mineral deficiency?
2. Are animals on this farm ever likely to suffer from a mineral deficiency?
3. Are animals going into a period where demand is increasing or availability is decreasing? If so, do they have adequate reserves to prevent a deficiency?
4. Is the supplementation program on this farm adequate?

The author suggests the addition of a potential fifth category based on herds that recycle manure on farm.

5. Does the supplementation program pose an environmental risk?

The goal is to provide trace minerals at a concentration that provides for the needs of the cattle without incurring an economic or toxicologic expense.

The objectives of this article are to:

1. Provide a brief overview of the essential trace elements for dairy cows;
2. Provide a description of the determination of the requirements of essential trace elements for dairy cows;
3. Describe the relative contribution of common feeds to meeting the trace element needs of dairy cows;
4. Describe common classes of trace element supplements; and
5. Describe sampling both feeds and animals to determine trace mineral adequacy.

WHICH TRACE ELEMENTS ARE REQUIRED BY DAIRY COWS?

Dairy cattle, like other animals, have a requirement for essential trace minerals. Currently, cobalt (Co), copper (Cu), iodine (I), iron (Fe), manganese (Mn), selenium (Se), and zinc (Zn) are deemed essential and thus must be supplied in the diet.[3] A critical aspect of essentiality is that a biologic function has been established for that mineral and that dysfunction or disease can be identified when the element is not present at adequate amounts in the ration. To that end, both chromium and molybdenum (Mo) may have biologic functions within cattle, but the deficiency state has not been established thus they are currently not considered essential trace elements **Table 1**.

Requirements for the Trace Elements for Dairy Cows

The maintenance requirement of these minerals is the amount needed to prevent the deficient state or development of classic lesions associated with deficiency. Many of these elements are involved in immune and reproductive function and the amount needed for optimal immune or reproductive function may be at a higher level that the amount required to prevent deficiency; however, data are limited to affirm those amounts. Although trace mineral supplementation is a relatively low-cost portion of a cow's ration, a sensible approach is needed to provide adequate amounts in the ration.

Likewise, some elements like Cu, Se, and I, when fed at higher levels, may be associated with toxicoses. The potential for trace mineral accumulation should be considered when manure and urine are recycled on crop fields. Manure and urine represented 90% or more of the output of Cu, Mn, and Zn on Swedish dairy farms.[7] Sheppard and Sanipelli[8] proposed that Cu and Zn could accumulate in soils that are managed to prevent accumulation of phosphorus, because most harvested crops would take up less Cu and Zn, relative to phosphorus. Currently, there are proposals to add trace mineral balance to nutrient management plans.[9] Therefore, the goal of a dairy ration is provide essential amounts to support productivity without leading to toxicoses or soil accumulation.

Table 1
Function and classic signs of deficiencies of essential trace elements

Mineral	Function (s)	Signs of Deficiency	Comments/Interactions
Cobalt (Co)	Utilized by rumen microbes to make cyanocobalamin or vitamin B_{12}	Anemia	Deficiency not commonly seen in United States
Copper (Cu)	Multiple enzymes or proteins *Ceruloplasmin:* prepares Fe for mobilization or incorporation into hemoglobin *Lysyl oxidase:* allows cross-linking of collagen *Tyrosinase:* converts tyrosine to melanin *Cytochrome oxidase:* last enzyme in electron transport chain of bacteria and eukaryotes *Dopamine β-hydroxylase:* conversion of dopamine to norepinephrine Cu-Zn SOD: antioxidant	Achromotrichia – or graying of black hair on cattle Lameness associated with physitis in weaned dairy calves[4]	Jersey cows tend to have higher liver Cu than Holsteins when fed similar diets[5]
Iodine (I)	Thyroid hormone	Enlarged thyroid glands, weak or dead hairless calves[4]	
Iron (Fe)	Carry O_2 in blood	Anemia	
Manganese (Mn)	Cofactor for multiple enzymes; Mn SOD	Classic deficiencies poorly described	Deficiencies rare
Selenium (Se)	Multiple forms of GSH-Px Iodothyronine deiodinases	White muscle disease	
Zinc (Zn)	300 enzymes, eg, alkaline phosphatase, carbonic anhydrase, LDH, Cu-Zn SOD Conversion of β-carotene to vitamin A at the intestine	Deficiency has been related to Foot problems and increased mastitis	Highest concentration of trace elements in milk; higher milk Zn in Jerseys than Holsteins when fed similar diets[6]

Abbreviations: GSH-Px, glutathione peroxidase; LDH, lactate dehydrogenase; SOD, superoxide dismutase.

Determination of Requirements

The authors of Nutrient Requirements of Dairy Cows utilized factorial estimates to determine trace mineral requirements for Cu, Mn, and Zn. The factorial approach is based on adding gestational, lactational requirements, or both to the maintenance requirement. Requirements for Co, Fe, I, and Se were based on dietary concentrations that prevent deficiency in maintenance and imply that the increased intake associated with lactation should meet requirements (**Table 2**).

Holsteins, Jerseys, and Cu

Several workers over the years have proposed that Jerseys may need less Cu in the diet or are more susceptible to Cu toxicosis than Holsteins. Du and colleagues[5] fed high or low Cu diets as either $CuSO_4$ or Cu proteinate to Holsteins and Jerseys. Jerseys had higher liver Cu and Fe, and lower liver Zn than Holsteins. Of interest, the Jerseys fed the low supplementation level of Cu (11 ppm in the diet) attained adequate Cu status. Jersey cows consumed 7% more feed than the Holsteins on a metabolic body weight basis; thus, the difference in liver Cu may be owing to increased intake or a difference in Cu metabolism between the breeds. Bidewell and colleagues[12] reported a case of chronic Cu toxicosis in a UK herd with both Jersey and Holstein–Friesian cows fed a high Cu ration (30–50 ppm Cu). Herd incidence of chronic Cu poisoning was 5% in the Jersey cows and 0.4% in the Holstein–Friesians. Likewise, plasma Cu and liver leakage enzymes were higher in the Jerseys compared with the Holsteins–Friesians. Although the data are limited, the author suggests that Jersey cows should be fed Cu at the required concentration and over-supplementation should be avoided.

TRACE MINERAL CONCENTRATION IN COMMON DAIRY FEEDS

Most of the research published on trace minerals and cattle comes from beef and dairy cattle in grazing environments where the basal ration is forage from the farm. Trace mineral content of feeds is highly variable and reflects trace mineral content of soils, which is highly variable between regions. In addition, soil contamination can contribute to the trace element content of a feedstuff. Within feeds, forages tend to have a higher content of soil compared with grains owing to harvesting methods. The total mineral content of feed is represented by the ash content, which can be up to 10% of the dry weight of the forage, especially with soil contamination. A simple tool that veterinarians can use to benchmark trace mineral and ash content of forages is the DairyOne feed composition library (available at: http://www.dairyone.com/Forage/FeedComp/mainlibrary.asp).

Another method to determine soil contamination of feeds is measuring the aluminum or titanium concentrations of the feed sample. Most forages contain less than 400 ppm aluminum, and concentrations of aluminum above 1000 ppm indicate soil contamination.[13] The practical application of minimizing soil contamination is to reduce the presence of antagonists like Fe and Mo.

Historically, trace mineral deficiencies were associated with regions in the country owing to variation in mineral content between regions. For example, Dargatz and Corah[14] reported regional variation in trace mineral content of forages across the United States. The US Geological Survey provides an online database from the National Geochemical Survey that provides maps of soil mineral concentration (available at: http://mrdata.usgs.gov/geochem/doc/home.htm). The practitioner can use this online tool to quickly identify soil concentrations of key minerals in their region. An example from US Geological Survey is given in **Fig. 1**.

A key point is alfalfa sourced from a different regions of the country may have similar protein and fiber concentrations however, the Cu, Se, and Zn concentrations may be very different.

Table 2
Current nutrient requirements for trace elements in a 650-kg, mature Holstein making 45 kg milk

Mineral	Digestibility Coefficient	Dietary Requirement in mg/kg DM (ppm)	Comments
Cobalt (Co)		0.11 mg/kg DM	Amount needed for rumen microbial production to maintain vitamin B_{12} concentrations in tissue from rumen microbial production. Higher dietary concentrations (0.15–0.20 ppm) have been suggested for beef bulls based on other markers of B_{12} status (folate, methylmalonic acid and homocysteine).[10]
Copper (Cu)	Absorption coefficient ranges from 2%–5% in dairy NRC depending on S and Mo content	11 mg/kg DM; used factorial model	Increases in S above 0.2% decreases Cu absorption; increases in Mo above 0.5 ppm decreases Cu absorption
Iodine (I)	80%–90% absorbed	0.45 mg/kg DM; thyroid activity increases during lactation	Most incorporated into thyroid hormones; toxic dietary concentration 5 mg/kg
Iron (Fe)	Absorption coefficient of 10% in dairy NRC	20 mg/kg DM	Fe is recycled efficiently in body; >250 mg/kg Fe in diet depletes Cu; 1000 ppm Fe is toxic; preferred dietary sources are $FeSO_4$, FeCl vs Fe oxide and Fe carbonate
Manganese (Mn)	Absorption coefficient of 0.75% in dairy NRC	Used factorial model; 15 mg/kg DM	Excreted in bile; High Ca, K, and phosphorus increases Mn in feces; high Fe decreases retention
Selenium (Se)	Absorption coefficient of 30%–60%	Regulated by FDA; 0.3 mg/kg DM	Increased S may decrease digestibility; can increase Se in milk with higher dietary concentrations
Zinc (Zn)	Absorption coefficient of 15% in dairy NRC	Factorial approach; 55 mg/kg DM; nonlactating 25–30 mg/kg DM	Zn is the most abundant trace mineral in milk (associated with the Casein fraction) and thus higher concentrations may be needed for high milk production[11]

Abbreviations: DM, dry matter; FDA, US Food and Drug Administration; Mo, molybdenum; NRC, National Research Council.

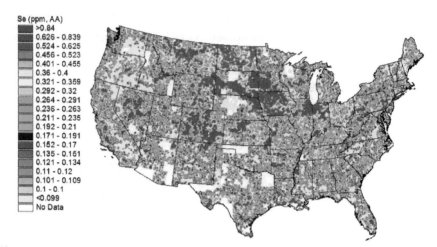

Fig. 1. Analysis of soil selenium by hydride-generation atomic absorption spectrometry. (*From* U.S. Geological Survey. Mineral Resources On-Line Spatial Data. Available at: http://mrdata.usgs.gov/geochem/doc/lower48maps/se_aa.jpg. Accessed July 24, 2014.)

Sampling Feeds

Determination of mineral content is based on taking a representative sample. Sampling strategy for forages should be the same as taking samples for other nutrients: Coring of multiple hay bales or taking silage samples from multiple sites on the face of the bunker or silo. Mineral sources are occasionally sampled to ensure content. Care must be taken to get a representative sample, which can mean actually coring a mineral bag like a bale of hay. As the sources of the differing minerals may differ in particle size, settling of particles can occur during transport. Thus, grab samples from the top of the bag or mineral pile are not representative.

Analysis of Feeds

Trace elements are present in feeds at concentrations 1000-fold lower than macrominerals; thus, analytical variation between laboratories and methodologies is important. Within the trace elements, concentrations of Co, I, and Se are approximately 100-fold less than the concentrations of Cu, Fe, Mn, and Zn. The advent of technologies like inductively coupled plasma mass spectrometry has allowed for identification of multiple minerals at very low concentrations on a single sample. Near-infrared reflectance spectroscopy is utilized for rapid analysis of feed samples for feed components such and protein. Although near-infrared reflectance spectroscopy may be reasonably accurate for some of the macrominerals in alfalfa (Ca, K, phosphorus), the accuracy of near-infrared reflectance spectroscopy for accurately predicting trace mineral concentrations, compared with other nutrients, is limited.[15,16] The author recommends traditional wet chemistry methods for accurate determination of trace minerals in feeds.

Within feeds, feed processing has limited effect on trace mineral availability, with 1 exception. Hansen and Spears[17] reported in a series of in vitro assays, that the ensiling process of corn silage may increase the bioavailability of Fe, especially when the silage is contaminated with dirt.

FORMS OF TRACE MINERALS IN RATIONS: ORGANIC TRACE MINERALS VERSUS INORGANICS
Production and Reproduction

Minerals have been commonly supplemented to cattle in the form of inorganic salts. Among different forms of salts, the sulfate form (Cu sulfate, Zn sulfate, Fe sulfate) is preferred, because sulfates are generally more available than the respective oxide forms of the salts. The development of organic forms of trace minerals provides an additional option for supplementation. Organic forms, such as chelates of mineral with amino acids, minimize the risk of mineral antagonism and thus chelated forms tend to be absorbed more efficiently. A consistent and predictable increase in production or reproduction after supplementation with organic or inorganic trace minerals is not evident or, as Overton and Yasui[18] noted, "there is heterogeneity of responses for outcome variables for all minerals listed." Many studies, however, lack power to detect relevant differences.[19] Likewise, the variation in trace mineral concentrations among feeds from varied regions may lead to the variation in responses. Rabiee and colleagues[20] reported in a metaanalysis that supplementation with organic trace minerals (Zn, Cu, Mn, and Co) increased milk production by 0.93 kg/d and reduced days open by 13.5 d. Conversely, supplementation of organic Fe from of 60 days before calving to 63 days in milk (DIM) did not increase production or change blood measures of Fe status. The authors noted that the control diets exceeded 280 ppm Fe on a dry matter (DM) basis, which vastly exceeds the requirement of 15 to 25 ppm.[21]

Organic Trace Minerals and Immune Function

Nemec and colleagues[22] fed either inorganic or organic trace minerals to 2 cohorts of Holstein cows starting at 32 or 77 DIM, respectively. Cows supplemented with organic trace minerals had higher rabies antibody titers 4 weeks after inoculation than cows fed inorganic trace minerals; however, a difference in neutrophil function was not detected. Scaletti and Harmon infused *Escherichia coli* into one quarter of first-calf Holstein heifers fed no supplemental Cu, Cu sulfate, or Cu proteinate from 60 days precalving to 49 DIM. Clinical score was higher (worse) in unsupplemented cows at several but not all time periods postinfection. Likewise, cows supplemented with Cu proteinate tended to have higher milk production compared with unsupplemented and Cu sulfate–supplemented cows at some but not all time periods postinfection.[23] Cu, Se, and Zn, have a defined role in the immune system of cattle and deficiencies of these minerals have been associated with impaired immune function. Consistent evidence to provide these minerals above concentrations suggested by the NRC to improve immune function in all cows is lacking, in the author's opinion.

ASSESSING TRACE MINERAL STATUS OF CATTLE
Se in Blood or Plasma/Serum

Whole blood or plasma/serum can be utilized to evaluate Se status. The majority of Se in a blood sample is in the form of glutathione peroxidase deposited into erythrocyte during formation.[24] Thus, whole blood Se tends to increase or decrease over a periods of weeks to months because turnover is related to red blood cell lifespan, which is about 5 months in cattle. Serum or plasma also contains glutathione peroxidase; however, this isoform is secreted by the liver.[25] Serum or plasma Se concentrations are approximately 50% the concentration of whole blood Se[26] and are more sensitive to recent changes in dietary intake; thus, serum or plasma Se will change in days to weeks. Maas and colleagues[27] concluded that serum Se was only useful to detect the deficient state (<0.05 ppm) when serum Se concentrations were compared with blood Se concentrations.

Cu and Zn in Serum/Plasma

Most classical texts report that serum or plasma Cu and Zn can be utilized to diagnose severe deficiencies; however, the utility of those samples to determine marginal status or response to supplementation is not recommended. Macrae and colleagues[28] reported on variation in serum Cu in more than 17,000 UK dairy cows sampled as part of metabolic profiling project. They did note that more dry cows groups (26%) had mean serum Cu levels below 9.4 μmol/L than lactating groups (7.5%). Balemi and colleagues[29] measured liver and serum Cu concentrations in nonpregnant, non-lactating Friesians fed baled ryegrass silage in New Zealand. Liver Cu concentrations increased in cows supplemented with organic or inorganic Cu compared with unsupplemented controls. A difference in serum Cu concentrations was not detected between Cu-supplemented and unsupplemented cows during the original 116-day study or a follow-up 56-day study.[30] Grace and colleagues[31] compared liver and serum Cu in lactating and cull Friesian crossbred and Jersey cows in New Zealand. Serum and liver concentrations were not correlated in individual cows or herds.

Conversely, Guyot and colleagues,[32] compared serum concentrations of Zn, Cu, inorganic I, and glutathione peroxidase between "sick" (n = 65) and "healthy" dairy herds (n = 20) in Belgium. The classification of sick and healthy was based on threshold percentages of common calf and adult disorders. Within herds, they sampled 8 adult cows and avoided sick animals and cows within 2 weeks of calving. Mean serum Zn, Cu, inorganic I, and glutathione peroxidase was lower in the sick herds. Only 69% of the sick herds reported mineral supplementation of the cows versus 100% for the healthy herds. Hussein and Staufenbiel[33] measured serum Cu, plasma Cu, serum ceruloplasmin (a Cu-containing acute phase protein), and plasma ceruloplasmin in 240 Holstein cows across a lactation. The goal was to determine if a ratio of Cu/ceruloplasmin would enhance the determination of Cu status. The number of cows classified as marginal or deficient were substantially different between the ratios used and the authors concluded that the "values should be interpreted with caution during assessment of Cu status." Spolders and colleagues[34] reported an increase in serum Zn in lactating Holstein cows fed approximately twice the recommended amount of Zn compared with cows fed the recommended amount.

The author concludes that serum or plasma concentrations of Cu and Zn have minimal diagnostic validity for dairy herds fed rations balanced for trace mineral. If the practitioner chooses assess serum concentrations of Zn, specialized trace mineral tubes (Royal Blue) should be used for collection of the sample.

Trace Elements in the Liver

The liver is the recommended sample of choice to evaluate status of Cu, Zn, Fe, and Mn. The advent of multimineral assays like inductively coupled plasma mass spectrometry now allows the diagnostic laboratory the ability to measure a panel of trace elements on one small sample that can be obtained with a 14- or 16-gauge biopsy needle. Trace mineral content from a small biopsy of 1 lobe of the liver seems to be highly correlated to the trace mineral content of liver homogenate.[35]

Procedure for liver biopsy in cows

Location The liver can be approached from the right side of the cow, at the 10th or 11th intercostal space. The biopsy needle crosses the pleural space in this site, but the lungs are usually cranial to the site. Two site guidelines should be remembered:

(1) Enter the cow on the right side on a line from the tuber coxae to point of the shoulder and (2) aim the biopsy needle cranially and ventrally toward the point of the left shoulder. An ultrasound probe can also be used to identify the location of the liver (**Fig. 2**).

Site preparation Clip hair from an approximate 15 × 15-cm square site centered over the 10th or 11th intercostal space. The first goal is to remove hair and dirt located on the skin, which can be accomplished a brush followed by a surgical scrub. The author's preference is to use isopropyl alcohol on a white sponge as the intermediate and final cleansing solution. The sponge can be visually evaluated for residual dirt or surgical scrub, and if present, continue to wipe until the skin is clean.

Local nerve block The author uses approximately 10 mL of 2% lidocaine injected with an 18-gauge, 1.5-inch needle. The needle is fully inserted to the hub and approximately 5 mL is injected along the needle track while the needle is slowly being withdrawn to the subcutaneous region. The remaining 5 mL is placed in the subcutaneous space in a fanlike pattern craniodorsal to the needle site. On dark-hided cattle, the author scratches the skin at biopsy site so it can be identified later. Apply 1 more scrub and then check the sensitivity of the biopsy site by gently poking the skin with a needle (**Fig. 3**).

Skin incision Perform a stab incision through the skin with a #10 blade. The incision does not need to be long, but must penetrate the skin. Penetrating the skin with the biopsy needle dulls the tip and results in a less than adequate biopsy specimen (**Fig. 4**).

Biopsy procedure The biopsy needle is now advanced through the intercostal muscles and diaphragm (approximately 4 cm). You may actually feel the needle "pop" through the liver capsule. Advance the needle another 1 or 2 cm into the liver, but leave enough of the needle exposed to manually take the biopsy (**Fig. 5**).

Most needles must be manually operated to obtain the biopsy. The author uses a Tru-Cut 14-guage X6″ needle. The cost is $30 to $35 per needle. You first hold the sleeve associated with the outer portion of the needle and slowly advance the stylet portion of the needle to full depth. You then hold the stylet still and advance the sleeve over the stylet. Once completed, withdraw the closed biopsy needle and check the

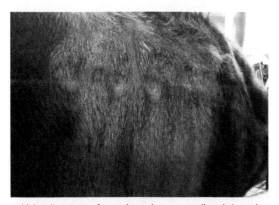

Fig. 2. The horizontal blue line goes from the tuber coxae (hooks) to the point of the shoulder. The blue dots represent the 12th, 11th, and 10th intercostal spaces from left to right, respectively. The vertical blue line represents the 11th rib.

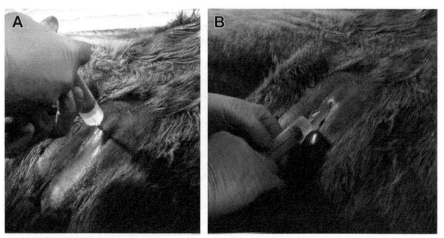

Fig. 3. Demonstration of local nerve block with 5 mL deposited along the needle tract (*A*) and 5 mL deposited under the skin cranial to the biopsy site (*B*).

chamber of the needle for a liver specimen. The author commonly takes a second sample from the same skin site if the first biopsy specimen did not completely fill the chamber. Automated biopsy needles that have a trigger mechanism to obtain the sample are available. These needles are usually smaller bore and more expensive.

Handling the biopsy The small biopsy sample can now be placed in an appropriate receptacle. The author prefers a 6-mL trace element tube (BD Vacutainer Trace Element Serum plus Blood Collection Tube) because it is big enough to write appropriate identifying information on the label. Use a clean needle to tease the biopsy

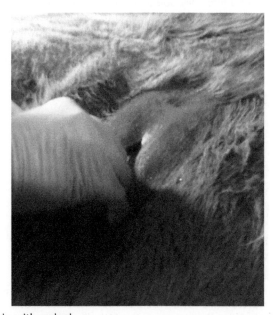

Fig. 4. Incising skin with scalpel.

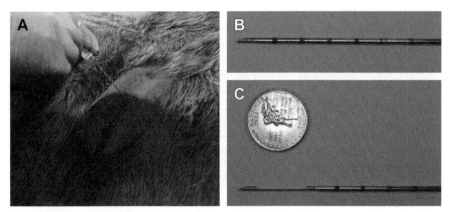

Fig. 5. Advancing the 14-gauge biopsy needle into the liver (*A*). Biopsy needle in closed position (*B*) and open position (*C*). US Quarter for reference.

sample out of the chamber into the tube. Like collection of milk for mastitis samples, holding the tube in a horizontal plane minimizes the risk of contamination with dirt and debris. Other plastic receptacles may be used, but check with your reference laboratory on the appropriateness of the receptacle for the sample (**Fig. 6**).

The skin can be closed with nonabsorbable suture or surgical staples. If reusing the biopsy needle on multiple cattle, thoroughly rinse with distilled water and sanitize with alcohol. Once the needle becomes dull, you will have difficulty getting an adequate sample. The use of antimicrobials is left to clinician preference. Based on personal communication, you may consider antibiotics in regions where *Clostridium novyii* or *C hemolyticum* are prevalent. Consider the class of animal and appropriate withdrawal periods if antimicrobials are used. You will note in all pictures that gloves are worn when performing biopsies. The author finds it easier to keep hands clean and minimize contamination of the sample when gloves are worn. An excellent review and guidelines for the procedure are available from the Nutrition Section of Diagnostic Center for Population and Animal Health at Michigan State (available at: http://www.animalhealth.msu.edu/Sections/Nutrition/WEBCD. NUTR.REF.002.pdf).

Rogers and colleagues[36] reported a decrease in gain and intake on day 7 after liver biopsy procedure in yearling beef steers; however, they also performed ruminocentesis and orogastric intubation on the steers. In a second trial with stocker heifers, a difference in gain after 7 days was not detected.

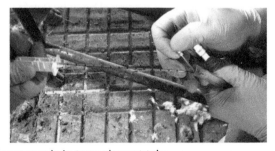

Fig. 6. Placing biopsy sample in trace element tube.

Effect of exsanguination on liver Fe

On occasion, slaughtered cattle may be used as a source of liver for trace mineral analyses. Exsanguination either at the slaughter house or via bleeding before death (eg, rupture of an aortic aneurysm) is associated with reduced Fe concentrations in the liver; thus, the Fe concentrations may be interpreted as falsely low on those cattle.[37]

Hair

Across species, hair has been a tantalizing sample to evaluate trace mineral status. Minerals enter through the hair follicle during formation; thus, long hairs, like those of the tail switch, could provide a longitudinal reference for intake over time. This strategy also applies to long-term toxicoses with heavy metals such as mercury or lead.[38] Unfortunately, routine hair analysis of cattle is problematic for 2 reasons.

- Tail hair is contaminated with feces, urine, and dirt. A reliable cleaning method that removes mineral contaminants from the surface of the hair, yet maintains the minerals within the hair, has not been identified.
- Hair color in cattle Influences mineral content.[38]

Milk

Milk is considered a poor source of trace minerals for neonates, yet this comment should be balanced by the increased absorption of minerals in neonates relative to adults. Zn is at a $10\times$ higher concentration in milk compared with other trace minerals, but does not seem to be responsive to dietary concentrations. Van Hulzen and colleagues[39] estimated the heritability of milk Zn as moderate ($h^2 = 0.41$) and the inter-farm phenotypic variation was low. Thus, diet would have a low impact on milk Zn concentration. Conversely, concentrations of Se and I have been associated with dietary intake and increased concentrations of these minerals in milk may be considered beneficial (Se) or detrimental (I) to human health.[40,41] Cows supplemented with an organic form of Se (selenized yeast) have higher milk Se concentrations than cows fed inorganic sources of Se like sodium selenite.[42] Herd variation on milk Se among herds was relatively high compared with intraherd heritability, which also implies a response to dietary supplementation.[39] Milk I concentrations increase when dietary concentrations exceed the requirement. A second contribution of I to milk is the use of iodophor teat dips. Use of iodophor teat dips without complete cleaning premilking or spraying postmilking is associated with higher I content in milk.[43] The increased concentration may be owing to direct contamination of iodophors from teat dips or absorption of I through the teat skin into the cow.

INTERPRETATION OF TRACE MINERAL CONCENTRATIONS IN ANIMALS AND FEEDS

Many diagnostic laboratories have used a seminal book by Puls[44] for reference concentrations of both deficient and toxic concentrations of trace elements in blood and liver. Most laboratory directors would acknowledge that the Pul's references are based on potentially outdated analytical methods and were established on cattle that were less productive than today's cattle. Many laboratories actively update their methodology and reference intervals so the author recommends that practitioners talk to the laboratory before taking the samples and about interpretation of results. Reference intervals and methodology can differ between laboratories and your best results will be obtained when you talk to the laboratory. Laboratories may report liver trace mineral results on a wet basis or DM basis. Ludwick and associates[45] noted that samples may dry out between collection and analyses and suggested that potassium concentrations could be used to standardize trace mineral concentrations reported on a wet basis.

The formation of a reference interval for most blood analytes is based on sampling a normal population and setting a confidence interval around the average.[46] For trace elements, most diagnostic laboratories use the terms deficient, marginal, adequate, and high/toxic. There are no international definitions of these terms, but consider the following guideline.

1. *Deficient*: Concentrations are associated with classic clinical signs of disease associated with this mineral. Additional supplementation is recommended.
2. *Marginal*: Classic clinical signs are usually not evident, but the performance may be impaired. Additional supplementation may help.
3. *Adequate*: Concentrations are similar to animals that have been fed adequate concentrations of the mineral in question. Additional supplementation is not needed.
4. *High/Toxic*: Concentrations are associated with signs of toxicosis and supplementation of this mineral should be limited or removed.

Who to Sample

The general recommendation is to sample 5 to 10 animals from the group to make a reasonable estimate of the group's status. Chronically diseased animals should not be sampled because feed intake is usually diminished for a period of time and stress or disease can cause alterations in serum and liver mineral concentrations. The practitioner may be led to the investigation by the mineral results from a single necropsy of a diseased animal, yet be very cautious in applying the results of 1 animal to the entire herd.

Neonates or fetuses can be a potential source of liver for diagnostic sampling. Liver samples can be obtained from dead calves, for example, stillbirths, dystocias, and neonatal deaths. Again, the author would advise against using chronically ill calves. Different reference intervals have been reported in neonates.[47–49] Neonates may give an assessment of late lactation and dry cow feeding. A suggested guideline for herd sampling is given in **Table 3**.

Sample Herd

The following is an example of liver biopsies from a dairy herd.

The client was interested in evaluation of the trace mineral status of first calf heifers owing to an increased rate of infectious problems (metritis and mastitis). Heifers were selected to avoid those within 10 days of calving or a minimum of 10 DIM with a total of 5 fresh heifers and 6 close-up heifers. Results are presented in **Table 4**.

Observations of liver trace mineral concentrations

1. Co is marginal in both the close-up and fresh heifers. Evaluate Co in the pregnant heifer rations and consider additional supplementation.
2. Cu is marginal in 1 fresh heifer; however, mean Cu for both groups is adequate. No change is needed.
3. Mo is above normal range in both groups. There is an increased risk of Cu antagonism. It may be advisable to try to find feed ingredient that is contributing Mo and remove it, if cost effective.
4. Zn is marginal in the fresh group, yet adequate in the close-up group. Decline may be associated with the stress of calving and deposition in milk. Consider additional Zn in close-up ration and sample cohorts at peak lactation to see if marginal status persists.

Table 3
Expansion of Clark and Ellison's guidelines on sampling herds

Reason	Who to Sample	Interpretation
Is the poor performance owing to a mineral deficiency?	5–10 representative cohorts for blood Se and 10–12 representative cohorts for liver Cu[50]	Mean concentrations in marginal or deficient range
Are animals on this farm ever likely to suffer from a mineral deficiency?	5–10 high-producing animals	Mean concentrations in adequate range
Do the cows have adequate reserves to prevent a deficiency?	5–10 animals before increased demands, eg, late lactation or dry cows	Mean concentration in adequate range
Is the supplementation program on this farm adequate?	5–10 animals before and 30–90 d after supplementation	Compare mean concentration before and after
Does the supplementation program pose an environmental risk based on the nutrient management plan?	Ration or feces	Compare with environmental standards

Data from Clark RG, Ellison RS. Mineral testing–the approach depends on what you want to find out. N Z Vet J 1993;41(2):98–100; and Laven RA, Nortje R. Diagnosis of the Cu and Se status of dairy cattle in New Zealand: how many samples are needed? N Z Vet J 2013;61(5):269–73.

Table 4
Liver mineral concentrations from a dairy herd (µg/g dry weight basis)

Specimen	Co	Cu	Fe	Mn	Mo	Se	Zn	Status
Liver	0.29	183	300	11.5	3.3	2.5	94	Fresh
Liver	0.29	111	432	12.1	4	2.1	93	Fresh
Liver	0.21	111	275	8.8	3.2	1.4	66	Fresh
Liver	0.26	86	333	9.4	3.1	1.8	78	Fresh
Liver	0.34	230	315	9.1	3.5	2	105	Fresh
Liver	0.28	74	344	9.2	3.8	1.6	133	Close up
Liver	0.28	142	563	7.9	4	2	100	Close up
Liver	0.3	106	391	9.6	4.2	1.5	132	Close up
Liver	0.25	119	451	9.2	4	1.7	107	Close up
Liver	0.23	177	368	6.9	3.7	1.4	328	Close up
Liver	0.18	43	451	8.4	3.3	1.6	124	Close up
Mean fresh	0.28	144.2	331	10.2	3.4	2.0	87	
Mean close up	0.25	117.4	445	8.4	3.8	1.6	128	
Normal range	0.3–0.6	50–300	200–450	5–9	1.5–3.0	0.7–2.5	100–300	
Deficient	0.1	10	150	4.5		0.4	80	

Abbreviations: CO, cobalt; Cu, copper; Fe, iron; Mn, manganese; Mo, molybdenum; Se, selenium; Zn, zinc.

5. Will increased Co and Zn in the ration for the heifers decrease metritis and mastitis? The author would suggest increasing concentrations in the rations for at least 60 days before calving and to monitor metritis and mastitis outcomes for the next 3 months. If no response is noted, look for other risk factors for metritis and mastitis.

SUMMARY

Trace minerals are an essential component of a feeding program for dairy herds. Deficiencies are unlikely when the cows are fed amounts to meet NRC requirements. The need for additional trace elements to support high milk production is supported by the increased DM intake associated with lactation. Zn is the only trace element that is secreted in concentrations in milk that would suggest an increase in dietary concentration. Mineral antagonisms do influence trace mineral absorption, especially Cu antagonism by S, Fe, and Mo. Dietary analysis is needed to identify the relative concentrations of the antagonists and potentially the antagonists may be removed rather than increasing Cu supplementation. Organic and alternate forms of trace elements have received wide acceptance throughout across multiple food animal production systems. The author recommends cost analysis of all sources of trace minerals relative to potential benefits in feeding above requirements. Blood and liver analyses can be effectively used to confirm diagnoses or monitor the efficacy of the feeding program.

REFERENCES

1. McClure TJ. Nutritional and metabolic infertility in the cow. Wallingford (England): CAB International; 1994.
2. Clark RG, Ellison RS. Mineral testing–the approach depends on what you want to find out. N Z Vet J 1993;41(2):98–100.
3. Nutrient requirements of dairy cattle, 7th revised edition. Washington, DC: National Academy Press; 2001.
4. Mulligan FJ, O'Grady L, Rice DA, et al. A herd health approach to dairy cow nutrition and production diseases of the transition cow. Anim Reprod Sci 2006;96(3–4):331–53.
5. Du Z, Hemken RW, Harmon RJ. Copper metabolism of Holstein and jersey cows and heifers fed diets high in cupric sulfate or copper proteinate. J Dairy Sci 1996;79(10):1873–80.
6. Sol Morales M, Palmquist DL, Weiss WP. Milk fat composition of Holstein and Jersey cows with control or depleted copper status and fed whole soybeans or tallow. J Dairy Sci 2000;83(9):2112–9.
7. Gustafson GA, Salomon E, Jonsson S. Barn balance calculations of Ca, Cu, K, Mg, Mn, N, P, S and Zn in a conventional and organic dairy farm in Sweden. Agr Ecosyst Environ 2007;119(1–2):160–70.
8. Sheppard SC, Sanipelli B. Trace elements in feed, manure, and manured soils. J Environ Qual 2012;41(6):1846–56.
9. Castillo AR, St-Pierre NR, del Rio NS, et al. Mineral concentrations in diets, water, and milk and their value in estimating on-farm excretion of manure minerals in lactating dairy cows. J Dairy Sci 2013;96(5):3388–98.
10. Stangl GI, Schwarz FJ, Muller H, et al. Evaluation of the cobalt requirement of beef cattle based on vitamin B-12, folate, homocysteine and methylmalonic acid. Br J Nutr 2000;84(5):645–53.

11. Fransson GB, Lonnerdal B. Distribution of trace elements and minerals in human and cow's milk. Pediatr Res 1983;17(11):912–5.

12. Bidewell CA, Drew JR, Payne JH, et al. Case study of copper poisoning in a British dairy herd. Vet Rec 2012;170(18):464.

13. Robinson DL, Hemkes OJ, Kemp A. Relationships among forage aluminum levels, soil contamination on forages, and availability of elements to dairycows. Neth J Agr Sci 1984;32(2):73–80.

14. Dargatz DA, Corah LR. Forage analyses from cow/calf herds in 18 states. Fort Collins (CO): Centers for Epidemiology and Animal Health, NAHMS, USDA: APHIS:VS; 1996.

15. Cozzolino D, Moron A. Exploring the use of near infrared reflectance spectroscopy (NIRS) to predict trace minerals in legumes. Anim Feed Sci Tech 2004; 111(1–4):161–73.

16. Halgerson JL, Sheaffer CC, Martin NP, et al. Near-infrared reflectance spectroscopy prediction of leaf and mineral concentrations in alfalfa joint contribution of the Minnesota agric. Exp. Stn. and USDA-ARS. Agron J 2004;96(2): 344–51.

17. Hansen SL, Spears JW. Bioaccessibility of iron from soil is increased by silage fermentation. J Dairy Sci 2009;92(6):2896–905.

18. Overton TR, Yasui T. Practical applications of trace minerals for dairy cattle. J Anim Sci 2014;92(2):416–26.

19. Karkoodi K, Chamani M, Beheshti M, et al. Effect of organic zinc, manganese, copper, and selenium chelates on colostrum production and reproductive and lameness indices in adequately supplemented Holstein cows. Biol Trace Elem Res 2012;146(1):42–6.

20. Rabiee AR, Lean IJ, Stevenson MA, et al. Effects of feeding organic trace minerals on milk production and reproductive performance in lactating dairy cows: a meta-analysis. J Dairy Sci 2010;93(9):4239–51.

21. Weiss WP, Pinos-Rodriguez JM, Socha MT. Effects of feeding supplemental organic iron to late gestation and early lactation dairy cows. J Dairy Sci 2010; 93(5):2153–60.

22. Nemec LM, Richards JD, Atwell CA, et al. Immune responses in lactating Holstein cows supplemented with Cu, Mn, and Zn as sulfates or methionine hydroxy analogue chelates. J Dairy Sci 2012;95(8):4568–77.

23. Scaletti RW, Harmon RJ. Effect of dietary copper source on response to coliform mastitis in dairy cows. J Dairy Sci 2012;95(2):654–62.

24. Scholz RW, Hutchinson LJ. Distribution of glutathione peroxidase activity and selenium in the blood of dairy cows. Am J Vet Res 1979;40(2):245–9.

25. Takahashi K, Avissar N, Whitin J, et al. Purification and characterization of human plasma glutathione peroxidase: a selenoglycoprotein distinct from the known cellular enzyme. Arch Biochem Biophys 1987;256(2):677–86.

26. Walker GP, Dunshea FR, Heard JW, et al. Output of selenium in milk, urine, and feces is proportional to selenium intake in dairy cows fed a total mixed ration supplemented with selenium yeast. J Dairy Sci 2010;93(10):4644–50.

27. Maas J, Galey FD, Peauroi JR, et al. The correlation between serum selenium and blood selenium in cattle. J Vet Diagn Invest 1992;4(1):48–52.

28. Macrae AI, Whitaker DA, Burrough E, et al. Use of metabolic profiles for the assessment of dietary adequacy in UK dairy herds. Vet Rec 2006;159(20):655.

29. Balemi SC, Grace ND, West DM, et al. Accumulation and depletion of liver copper stores in dairy cows challenged with a Cu-deficient diet and oral and injectable forms of Cu supplementation. N Z Vet J 2010;58(3):137–41.

30. Smith SL, Grace ND, West DM, et al. The impact of high zinc intake on the copper status of dairy cows in New Zealand. N Z Vet J 2010;58(3):142–5.
31. Grace ND, Knowles SO, Hittmann AR. High and variable copper status identified among dairy herds in the Waikato region by concentrations of Cu in liver sourced from biopsies and cull cows. N Z Vet J 2010;58(3):130–6.
32. Guyot H, Saegerman C, Lebreton P, et al. Epidemiology of trace elements deficiencies in Belgian beef and dairy cattle herds. J Trace Elem Med Biol 2009; 23(2):116–23.
33. Hussein HA, Staufenbiel R. variations in copper concentration and ceruloplasmin activity of dairy cows in relation to lactation stages with regard to ceruloplasmin to copper ratios. Biol Trace Elem Res 2012;146(1):47–52.
34. Spolders M, Höltershinken M, Meyer U, et al. Assessment of reference values for copper and zinc in blood serum of first and second lactating dairy cows. Vet Med Int 2010;2010:1–8.
35. Ouweltjes W, de Zeeuw AC, Moen A, et al. Measurement of trace elements in liver biopsy samples from cattle. Tijdschr Diergeneeskd 2007;132(3):76–83.
36. Rogers GM, Capucille DJ, Poore MH, et al. Growth performance of cattle following percutaneous liver biopsy utilizing a Schackelford-courtney biopsy instrument. The Bovine Practioner 2001;35(2):177–84.
37. Lamm CG, Bischoff KL, Erb HN, et al. Trace mineral concentrations in dairy cattle with rupture of abdominal artery aneurysms. The Bovine Practioner 2010; 44(1):38–40.
38. Combs DK, Goodrich RD, Meiske JC. Mineral concentrations in hair as indicators of mineral status: a review. J Anim Sci 1982;54(2):391–8.
39. van Hulzen KJ, Sprong RC, van der Meer R, et al. Genetic and nongenetic variation in concentration of selenium, calcium, potassium, zinc, magnesium, and phosphorus in milk of Dutch Holstein-Friesian cows. J Dairy Sci 2009;92(11):5754–9.
40. Stockdale CR, Gill HS. Effect of duration and level of supplementation of diets of lactating dairy cows with selenized yeast on selenium concentrations in milk and blood after the withdrawal of supplementation. J Dairy Sci 2011;94(5):2351–9.
41. Norouzian MA. Iodine in raw and pasteurized milk of dairy cows fed different amounts of potassium iodide. Biol Trace Elem Res 2011;139(2):160–7.
42. Ceballos A, Sanchez J, Stryhn H, et al. Meta-analysis of the effect of oral selenium supplementation on milk selenium concentration in cattle. J Dairy Sci 2009; 92(1):324–42.
43. Castro SI, Berthiaume R, Robichaud A, et al. Effects of iodine intake and teat-dipping practices on milk iodine concentrations in dairy cows. J Dairy Sci 2012;95(1):213–20.
44. Puls R. Mineral levels in animal health diagnostic data. 3rd edition. Clearbrook (BC): Sherpa International; 1988.
45. Ludwick TP, Poppenga RH, Green PG, et al. The correlation of potassium content and moisture in bovine liver samples analyzed for trace mineral concentrations. J Vet Diagn Invest 2008;20(3):314–20.
46. Geffré A, Friedrichs K, Harr K, et al. Reference values: a review. Vet Clin Pathol 2009;38(3):288–98.
47. Graham T, Thurmond M, Mohr F, et al. Relationships between maternal and fetal liver copper, iron, manganese, and zinc concentrations and fetal development in California Holstein dairy cows. J Vet Diagn Invest 1994;6(1):77–87.
48. Van Saun RJ, Poppenga RH. Breed effects on bovine fetal and maternal hepatic mineral concentrations. 13th International Conference on Production Diseases in Farm Animals. Leipzig, Germany, August 2007.

49. Van Saun RJ, Poppenga RH. Factors influencing bovine maternal and fetal hepatic mineral concentrations. Paper presented at 13th International Conference on Production Diseases in Farm Animals, Leipzig, Germany, August 2007.
50. Laven RA, Nortje R. Diagnosis of the Cu and Se status of dairy cattle in New Zealand: how many samples are needed? N Z Vet J 2013;61(5):269–73.

Transition Cow Nutrition and Feeding Management for Disease Prevention

Robert J. Van Saun, DVM, MS, PhD[a],*, Charles J. Sniffen, PhD[b]

KEYWORDS

- Transition period • Metabolic disease • Dry cow • Periparturient disease
- Ration formulation • Metabolizable protein

KEY POINTS

- No single nutritional program or management scheme provides consistent outcome performance for transition cows.
- Management of late lactation cows should focus on controlling variation in body condition score.
- Feeding higher amounts of metabolizable protein in the dry diets may help to ensure adequate intake in the face of variable dry matter intake within a group.
- Metabolic adaptations of maternal metabolism are essential to maintain nutrient availability in support of fetal development and lactation.
- Use of 1-group or 2-group dry cow feeding system depends on dry period length, with a 1-group system for shorter dry periods.
- Separate grouping of springing heifers throughout the transition period is desirable.

INTRODUCTION

The last issue of *Veterinary Clinics* dedicated to dairy nutrition was published more than 22 years ago.[1] In that issue, the dry cow was identified as the key to fresh cow performance, and current dry cow management approaches were described as "management by neglect."[2] By the end of the decade, Drackley[3] published a seminal article describing "the final frontier" as the need to understand transition cow biology in improving dairy cow productivity. Over the last 2 decades, much intensive research

Funding sources: Pennsylvania Department of Agriculture Grant #44123907, Zoetis unrestricted funds (Dr R.J. Van Saun); none (Dr C.J. Sniffen).
Conflict of interest: none.
[a] Department of Veterinary and Biomedical Sciences, College of Agricultural Sciences, Pennsylvania State University, 115 W.L. Henning Building, University Park, PA 16802-3500, USA;
[b] Fencrest, LLC, PO Box 563, Holderness, NH 03245, USA
* Corresponding author.
E-mail address: rjv10@psu.edu

has been completed in addressing transition cows relative to nutrient requirements, physiologic adaptations, and metabolic associations with periparturient disease; yet, dairy farms continue to be plagued by high prevalence of costly fresh cow disorders adversely affecting productivity and reproductive performance (**Table 1**). This may be a pessimistic view of the state of affairs, because over this same period, milk production continued to rapidly increase, and diagnostic method sensitivity increased as well as recognition of subclinical disease syndromes; all resulting in postpartum disease events maintaining stable or slightly increasing prevalence rates. Most in the dairy industry believe that there are tremendous opportunities to improve transition cow health and reproductive performance without compromising milk production, yet the solution is not clearly evident.

In this article, a historical perspective is provided on transition cow nutrition and management research and its impact on current practices. Underpinning principles of metabolic adaptations necessary to successfully navigate the transition from pregnancy to lactation are described, with particular emphasis on the role of amino acids. Our objectives are to provide practical guidance, based on available research and field experience, in defining nutritional requirements for the pregnant cow relative to proper feeding management strategies and second, integrate other factors that may deter herd transition performance to ensure that a greater percentage of cows successfully complete this critical adaptation period. The transition period has typically been defined as the 3-week to 4-week period surrounding calving. For the purposes of this article, the entirety of the dry period and the last few weeks of lactation are included as part of the discussion of feeding and managing the transition cow for disease prevention.

PERSPECTIVES ON DRY COW FEEDING AND MANAGEMENT

In the current transition cow system, a range of feeding programs and grouping strategies are observed, with no one approach consistently resulting in the desired outcome (ie, cows are successful in metabolically adapting to lactation with minimal to no disease events, reduced involuntary culls, and having efficient productive and reproductive performance). To direct future management and feeding practices in an effort to minimize adverse health events, a historical perspective is needed to

Table 1
Compiled periparturient disease incidence rates and estimated costs from various published studies

Disease	Median Incidence Risk (%)	Range of Incidence Risk (%)	Estimated Cost ($/case)
Hypocalcemia	6.5	0.3–22	335
Subclinical hypocalcemia	22	8–54	125
Retained fetal membranes	8.6	1.3–39.2	285
Metritis	10.1	2–37	359
Subclinical metritis	53	37–74	???
Ketosis	4.8	1.3–18.3	145
Subclinical ketosis	43	26–55	67
Lameness	7.0	1.8–30	302–400
Clinical mastitis	14.2	1.7–54.6	185–205
Subclinical mastitis	30	15–60	???

Data from Refs.[4–11]

appreciate rationale for past management practices and reasons for success or failure.

Defining Nutritional Requirements

Fetal growth from time of conception to birth can be described by an exponential growth curve, with more than 70% of growth occurring in the last 60 to 70 days of pregnancy (**Fig. 1**).[12] This factor places the greatest nutritional burden of pregnancy on the cow just before parturition. More recent research has indicated a more critical role for early gestation to midgestation nutrition relative to fetal and placental development as well as neonatal metabolic, reproductive, and growth performance. This subject is epigenetics or what is termed fetal programming, and findings suggest maternal undernutrition (<70%) or overnutrition (>140%) in early to mid gestation can have long-lasting impacts on fetal development, health, and performance.[13,14] A more detailed discussion of this aspect of gestational nutrition is beyond the scope of this article, but the expanding influence of gestational nutrition, which was previously considered inconsequential, is emphasized.

The National Research Council (NRC) dairy[15–17] and beef[18,19] cattle publications have defined and improved on models to predict energy (**Fig. 2**) and protein (**Fig. 3**) requirements in support of pregnancy. All models depicted in **Figs. 2** and **3** are based on a 45-kg fetal birth weight for comparison. Before the work of Bell and colleagues,[20] the only publication describing growth characteristics of the Holstein fetus were from a 1950s Vermont extension circular.[21] The dairy NRC requirement models before 2001 were based on work describing fetal growth in Danish Red cattle, showing the limited scope of data on which our prediction models were based.[22]

Gestational energy

The dairy NRC models all initiate an energy need after 190 days or more of gestation, because this was the lower limit of collected data from the studies on which the data were based.[15–17] It is assumed that energy needs before this period are insignificant.

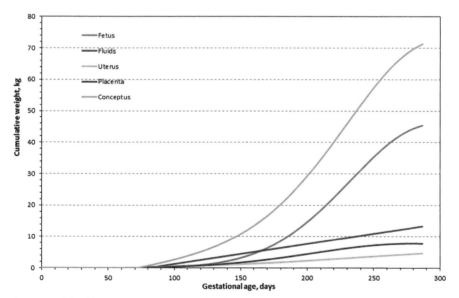

Fig. 1. Model of bovine conceptus growth where the conceptus includes fetus, uterine, and placental growth based on CNCPS model for a 45-kg birth weight.

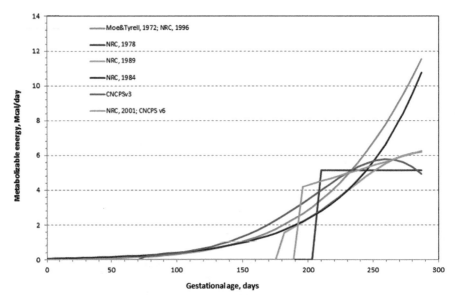

Fig. 2. Different models describing metabolizable energy (ME) requirement in support of pregnancy (45-kg birth weight).

The original metabolizable energy (ME) determinations of Moe and Tyrell[23] show a more continuous energy curve consistent with the fetal growth curve. The beef NRC models[18,19] used pregnancy energy models mimicking these data, although attempting to model full gestational energy needs results in some bias, given the range in fetal size from conception to birth.[20] Certainly, there are breed and compositional

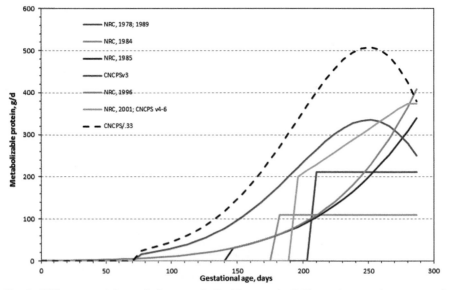

Fig. 3. Different models predicting metabolizable protein (MP) requirement in support of pregnancy (45-kg birth weight).

differences that may account for energy differences between dairy and beef cattle as well as modeling methods. Bell and colleagues'[20] energy data were consistent with previous NRC data,[16] and thus were considered to confirm the recommendation, yet did not provide insight as to fetal energy demands before 190 days' gestation. The question remains as to whether or not early gestation energy needs are significant and whether current models truly capture energy needs in final fetal growth.

Gestational protein

Modeling gestational protein requirements is more complicated, as shown by model variation in **Fig. 3**. A proportion of the differences among these models is caused by assumed efficiency of converting metabolizable protein (MP) (ie, absorbed amino acids) to net protein (ie, retained within the fetus). Models before 1995 used an efficiency of 50%,[24] whereas Bell[25] summarized data suggesting that this efficiency was lower, at 33%. This difference in efficiency increases pregnancy MP requirement 150%. Other challenges in predicting gestational protein requirements result from the dynamic metabolic functions of amino acids in supporting placental and uterine growth as well as the significant role that amino acids play in fetal energy metabolism; none of which contributes to fetal protein retention, which is the measured end point.[25,26] Another consideration is whether or not experimental diets were properly formulated to meet or exceed cow requirements to maintain a stable labile reserve protein pool in the cow. This is an underlying assumption of NRC models; maternal skeletal muscle is not used in support of pregnancy. McNeil and colleagues[27] showed that lamb birth weights are not different from ewes fed energy adequate diets with either 12% or 15% crude protein (CP) diets. However, body compositional analysis showed that ewes fed the 12% CP diet had significant skeletal muscle protein loss, accounting for the lack of difference in birth weights. Ewes fed the 15% CP diet had significant skeletal muscle accretion, suggesting that these ewes may be better positioned metabolically to adapt to negative energy balance and mobilize amino acids to support lactation. Cows in Bell and colleagues'[20] study consumed 10 to 12 kg dry matter (DM) of a total mixed ration containing 13% and 14% (after 250 days' gestation) CP diets. No measure of maternal protein status was determined in this study.

For demonstration purposes, we used the original Cornell Net Carbohydrate and Protein System (CNCPS, version 3.0) mechanistic model to predict gestational protein requirement, which accounted for an amino acid energy contribution, to predict MP requirement, using an efficiency factor of 0.33 rather than the original 0.5 factor.[28] From **Fig. 3**, it can be seen that this model greatly increases MP needs throughout gestation compared with other models. In addition, MP to support mammary development (120–200 g MP/d) would need to be added to this model.[25,29,30] How predicted MP and CP requirements are affected by these different models is compared in **Table 2**. This model shows MP needs before the 190-day cutoff used by NRC based on data extrapolation limitations. This exercise is hypothetical, but intriguing relative to potential implications for gestational MP requirements as well as explaining possible roles for amino acid nutritive status relative to health (ie, immunologic and metabolic), productive, and reproductive outcomes during transition.

Grouping Management

Grouping strategies for dry cows have also undergone considerable changes over the period of intensification of production of dairy cattle. Dry cows were initially considered second-class citizens or nonworking cows and thus received little attention and often received poor-quality forage (dry cow hay). Separation of dry cows into

Table 2
Comparison of CP and MP protein requirement models for a 650-kg mature cow at 270 days pregnant with a 45-kg birth weight calf

	NRC 1989	NRC 2001	NRC 2001 Modified	CNCPS[a]/.33
Maintenance				
Urinary	105	105	105	105
Scurf	15	15	15	15
MFN[b]	410	338	338	338
Conceptus	212	355	355	480
Mammary	0	0	120–200	120–200
Total MP	742 g/d	813 g/d	933–1013 g/d	1058–1138
CP[c]	1060 g/d	1160 g/d	1332–1447 g/d	1511–1625
	8.2%–9.6%	8.9%–10.5%	11.1%–13.1%	12.5–13.7

[a] CNCPS, version 3.0 with modification changing MP efficiency from 0.5 to 0.33.
[b] Metabolic fecal nitrogen.
[c] Assumed DM intake between 11 and 13 kg/d.

an independent group was not readily practiced, with dry cows often housed in the low-production group. Separation of dry cows for differential feeding was advocated, with the recognition of nutrient content of the lactating diets predisposing cows to milk fever and excessive body condition gain.

Dry cow grouping strategies evolved from 1 to multiple groups (ie, far-off, close-up) based on research addressing changes in nutritional requirements with rapid fetal growth and recognizing differences in intake capacity by time relative to calving and parity.[31] Feeding higher-concentrate diets in close-up groups to meet increasing energy needs, decreased intake, or some combination is not a new concept[32,33]; however, negative effects relative to reduced postpartum intake and health events were recognized.[34,35] Higher-energy diets with increased nonfiber carbohydrate (NFC) content were again recommended more recently as part of the close-up group to compensate for expected lower DM intake (DMI) and to promote maximal intake.[29,36,37] Negative effects of excess energy[38] or propionate precursors[39] have directed further consideration to grouping and nutrient content approaches. Issues related to excess energy intake and insulin insensitivity have supported a high-fiber single-group feeding system,[40] whereas regulation of energy metabolism (hepatic oxidation theory) supports a different feeding system for cow groups depending on predominate oxidative fuel.[39] Dietary fiber content also regulates intake, with lower capacity closer to parturition and for first-parity heifers. Neutral detergent fiber (NDF) intake as percent of live body weight (LBW) for far-off (0.9%–1.1% LBW, cows; 0.85%–1.0% LBW, heifers) and close-up (0.75%–0.95% LBW, cows; 0.65%–0.85% LBW, heifers) dry cow groups are suggested.[2]

With the continued disease prevalence challenges to cows navigating the transition period, some researchers have considered altering the traditional 50-day to 60-day dry period to minimize dramatic metabolic changes.[41–43] These approaches have ranged from complete elimination of the dry period with sustained somatotropin usage to shortening between 45 and 30 days.[42] Suggested benefits of the shorter dry period include capturing more milk in late lactation, better energy balance, and improved health and fertility post partum. A recent meta-analysis of 24 studies manipulating dry period length showed lower milk production, improved energy balance, and decreased risk of ketosis, but no difference in other diseases or fertility.[44] Adoption of shorter dry periods has been limited because of the milk loss concerns, although many farms have been successful using a 45-day minimum dry period.

Outcome Expectations and Assessment

Surveys of fresh cow health suggest that more than 50% of all cows experience 1 or more periparturient health events, although this is highly variable between farms.[45,46] Overall, it is desired to have cows and heifers transition from pregnancy into lactation with minimal disease problems, rapidly increase in milk yield and DMI, and be capable of becoming pregnant again within a defined period. The following parameters can be used to assess transition success.

- Disease prevalence goal and action levels for various postpartum disease conditions are provided in the article by Oetzel on dairy herd diagnostic investigation elsewhere in this issue.
- Herd turnover within the first 60 days of lactation, defined as the number of culled and dead cows as a percent of the total herd, is an acute metric for evaluating transition cow performance.[47] A turnover rate less than 6% is a desired goal.
- Number of cows having increased nonesterified fatty acids (NEFA) and β-hydroxybutyric acid (BHB) concentrations should be less than 15% to 20% of tested cows.[48] Criteria for NEFA and BHB suggesting adverse effects on reproduction, health, and milk production are:
  - NEFA pre partum: greater than 0.3 mEq/L (>0.3 mmol/L)
  - NEFA post partum: greater than 0.7 mEq/L (>0.7 mmol/L)
  - Postpartum BHB concentrations greater than 10 mg/dL (>0.96 mmol/L)
- Milk composition evaluation relative to fat % and fat/protein ratio (FPR) can be used to assess potential disease risk.[49]
  - Investigate when greater than 10% of cows have first test milk fat greater than 5% (Holsteins), greater than 6% (Jersey)
  - Investigate when greater than 40% of cows have FPR greater than 1.4 at first or second test dates. More often, high FPR on second test date is a result of low milk true protein (<2.7%), suggesting a protein deficiency component.
- Transition cow index is a metric available through some dairy herd improvement record systems providing a comprehensive assessment of herd transition success.[50] Within-herd benchmarking is based on assessing this average index level to 10th and 90th percentile values. More positive values indicate minimal transition cow problems.

PREPARTUM NUTRITION AND POSTPARTUM DISEASE

For a cow to transition from late pregnancy into lactation successfully, she needs to exquisitely coordinate metabolism in multiple tissues to provide sufficient glucose to support productive needs.[51] Daily requirements for glucose, amino acids, fatty acids, and calcium for an early lactation cow (4 days post partum; 30 kg milk, 4.7% fat, and 4.2% protein) are 2.7, 2.0, 4.5, and 6.8 times greater, respectively, than those needed for pregnancy.[25] These differences represent changes in nutrient requirements over a period of only 1 to 2 weeks and occur during a period of lowest DMI, highlighting the tremendous metabolic alterations necessary to adequately support lactation. The inability of the cow to metabolically adapt to this transition is the underpinning of most postpartum diseases. The late gestation diet has been shown to play a critical role in modulating a cow's predisposition to periparturient health disorders. Other nonnutritional factors affecting the cow's ability to consume sufficient nutrients also contribute, and may contribute more significantly, to postpartum disease susceptibility. Understanding the underlying metabolic processes during pregnancy allows for a better appreciation of prepartum nutritional role in transition success. Nuances of how management and environment alter stability of these metabolic changes remains to be elucidated.

Fetal and Maternal Metabolic Adaptations and Association with Disease Risks

A summary of the key metabolic nutrients relative to their supply and metabolic roles in the fetus and dam is shown in **Table 3** (see reviews).[5,25,52–54] Potential disease risks for either fetus or dam in the face of a given nutrient deficiency are provided. The coordination of metabolic processes occurring during transition in the dam to facilitate glucose availability to support either fetal development or milk production is shown in **Fig. 4**.

Protein Metabolism in Transition

Much emphasis has been placed on energy metabolism and markers of energy balance as underpinning metabolic disturbances of transition and risk for disease. Although increased concentrations of either NEFA or BHB are highly associated with disease risk, their presence is not a direct determinant. A population of cows can perform without evidence of disease with increased concentrations of NEFA, suggesting some other factor or protective element. As our understanding of transition metabolism sheds more light on its complicated nature, a more integrated perspective on transition metabolism is needed, and central to this is the supply and prioritization of amino acid metabolism (**Fig. 5**) as it relates to cow response to diet and management. Although the body of published literature does not strongly suggest improved cow performance with higher prepartum dietary protein, there is much interest and anecdotal observations suggesting benefits from feeding diets delivering greater MP (>1100 g/d) than models suggest is necessary to meet the cow's amino acid requirements. This observed response may be caused by an underestimation of the MP requirement, providing an essential amino acid or acids, accounting for intake variability within a group allowing for adequate MP intake for cows with lower intake, or some combination of these factors.

Most studies evaluating prepartum protein nutrition essentially looked at milk yield or composition as metrics for a measured response.[30] Most observations and research suggest that the primary benefit of prepartum protein feeding comes from disease prevention and improved reproductive performance.[55,56] Curtis and colleagues[57] first reported that higher prepartum protein diets decreased incidence of ketosis. Cows fed a higher protein prepartum diet, independent of energy content, had lower serum NEFA concentration, NEFA/cholesterol ratio, and fatty liver score.[58] Van Saun[59] also reported lower clinical ketosis prevalence for mature Holstein cows fed 1300 g MP/d compared with cows fed 1100 g/d. In this study, all cows maintained a higher body condition score (BCS; mean 3.9 BCS at calving), and thus, were more predisposed to ketosis problems. Using 3-methylhistidine (3-MH) as a marker of skeletal muscle degradation, van der Drift and colleagues[60] showed muscle mobilization occurring pre partum to 4 weeks post partum for dry cows fed a diet composed of grass silage and corn silage containing approximately 12.6% CP. Cows having higher 3-MH concentrations generally had lower BHB concentrations, suggesting a protective effect. Cows with extreme hyperketonemia had excessive muscle and fat mobilization. Amount of muscle mobilization was highly variable among cows in this study, although supplementing methionine may mitigate body protein mobilization.[61]

Feeding additional rumen undegradable protein pre partum showed improved insulin status in mature dairy cows relative to BCS and BCS score change.[62] In addition, cows fed a balanced protein diet post partum compared with a high rumen degradable protein (RDP) diet had higher insulin sensitivity across BCS.[63] Insulin not only is an important regulator of glucose homeostasis but also influences reproductive performance. Cows consuming more MP pre partum (>1300 g/d) had improved reproductive performance,[59] and ovulation time was not influenced by negative energy balance nadir.[64] In contrast, cows consuming lower prepartum MP intake (1100 g/d) followed by a postpartum diet high in RDP had their first ovulation time highly correlated with negative energy balance nadir.[59]

Using production data from 55,000 lactations, it was found that milk protein and milk FPR in early lactation were associated with reproductive performance.[65,66] Cows with low milk protein on first or second test day had lower first service and overall conception risks. Mobilized protein from skeletal muscle and involuting uterine tissue provide a primary source of amino acids to the mammary gland to support milk protein synthesis.[67] Lower milk protein content may reflect inadequate dietary MP supply and repartitioning of amino acids to support the immune response or gluconeogenesis.

Blood albumin concentration reflects dietary amino acid supply and metabolic responses repartitioning available amino acids. Increasing dietary protein in early lactation increased albumin concentration.[68] Albumin is synthesized in the liver and is considered a negative acute phase protein, meaning its rate of synthesis is decreased during an acute phase response to inflammatory cytokines.[69] Albumin concentration pre and post partum was associated with greater risk for postpartum disease.[70] Blood albumin concentration of 3.5 g/dL or greater was found in primarily healthy cows compared with lower concentrations being predominately associated with cows having 1 or more disease events.[70] Cows experiencing endometritis post partum had lower prepartum albumin concentration.[71] Lower prepartum albumin concentrations were observed in pasture-fed cows consuming a high-NFC (31.8%) compared with low-NFC (13.2%) diet.[72] Lower albumin concentration may reflect inadequate dietary MP supply, liver dysfunction, an active inflammatory response, or some combination and may provide a marker of transition cow health status.[73]

Amino acids play a critical role in stabilizing metabolism of carbohydrates and lipids during transition as well as supplying substrate for tissue protein synthesis, gluconeogenesis, and other metabolic mediators. All cows experience a period of negative protein balance in early lactation, which seems independent of prepartum protein feeding. However, if dietary protein is sufficiently deficient pre partum, tissue protein mobilization may occur, and the reservoir of labile protein to be used in early lactation may be compromised, resulting in greater risk for impaired health, productive efficiency, and reproductive performance.[74]

Role of Inflammation in Metabolic Regulation

A growing body of research is recognizing an association between the activated inflammatory response mediated by proinflammatory cytokines interleukin 1 (IL-1), IL-6, and tumor necrosis factor α (TNF-α) and altered metabolism leading to greater disease risk, poor production, and impaired reproduction.[69,75–80] Proinflammatory cytokines can be released from adipose tissue during mobilization as well as from any stress response.[76] Hepatic activation by these cytokines initiates the acute phase protein (APP) response, resulting in upregulated synthesis of positive APPs (+APP; ie, ceruloplasmin, haptoglobin, serum amyloid-A, C-reactive protein, complement components) as well as enzymes and other physiologic mediators. Both IL-1 and TNF-α have profound metabolic effects promoting an increased basal metabolic rate (BMR) to produce fever in concert with reducing appetite. Reduced appetite in the transition cow is a recognized lynchpin to metabolic disease susceptibility. Mobilized skeletal muscle provides amino acids to support gluconeogenesis in maintaining the

Table 3
Comparison of fetal and maternal nutrient sources and metabolic adaptations during transition and association with nutrient-specific deficiency disease risks

Key Nutrient	Fetal	Maternal
Energy		
Sources (% contribution)	Glucose and lactate (50–60), amino acids (30–40), acetate (10–15), fatty acids (<5)	Glucose, short and long chain fatty acids, ketone bodies, glycerol, amino acids
Metabolism	Metabolic rate is nearly twice that of the dam. Glucose utilization is dependent on maternal glucose status. When energy deprived, amino acids are oxidized at higher rates (>60%)	General shift from predominate glucose utilization to fat oxidation by maternal tissues, reduced insulin secretion and tissue sensitivity with advancing pregnancy status facilitating fat oxidation
Disease risks	Reduced birth weight, weak calf syndrome, altered placental development	Pregnancy toxemia; subclinical or clinical ketosis; hepatic lipidosis; impaired immune response leading to mastitis, metritis, RFM, secondary LDA
Protein		
Supply	Placental active transport of amino acids from maternal blood supply (70%–80% of maternal circulating amino acids)	Microbial and dietary bypass proteins provide the metabolic source of amino acids to support body functions; mobilization of labile proteins (blood proteins, skeletal muscle) can make up for dietary deficiencies
Metabolism	Amino acids deposited into fetal tissues and placenta to support growth, oxidized for energy in fetus, amino acid exchange between fetus and placenta	Amino acids used to support body protein turnover and new protein synthesis; upregulation of many metabolic regulatory enzymes in support of gluconeogenesis, lipid metabolism, milk protein synthesis; amino acids serve as intermediates in TCA cycle facilitating CHO and lipid metabolism; amino acids may be redirected toward acute phase protein synthesis in face of inflammatory response
Disease risks	Reduced birth weight, inability to thermoregulate, weak calf syndrome, FPT?	Subclinical and clinical ketosis; varying degrees of hepatic lipidosis; reduced blood transport proteins for minerals and vitamins; impaired immune response with increased infectious disease susceptibility, RFM, udder edema?

	Calf/fetus	Cow/dam
Minerals		
Supply	Provided from placental transfer from maternal blood; delivery dependent on maternal status	Dietary supply of macrominerals and microminerals; rumen microbes may alter availability of some microminerals (Cu, Se, Zn)
Metabolism	Maintain metabolic functions similar to adults; all minerals stored at high concentrations in liver for reserve to be used in postnatal life because milk is low in many trace minerals	Interactions between minerals affect bioavailability especially excessive K relative to Mg and Ca homeostasis; besides supporting metabolic functions, minerals are transferred to fetus and into colostrum
Deficiency disease	Inadequate trace minerals may result in abortion, stillbirth, or weak calves with compromised immune response	Inadequate calcium homeostasis leading to subclinical or clinical milk fever, hypomagnesemia, hypophosphatemia, immune dysfunction, RFM, mastitis, metritis, LDA
Vitamins		
Supply	B-vitamins transferred via placenta; fat-soluble vitamins not efficiently transported by placenta	Dietary supplementation, low amounts in silage and stored forage; vitamin A can be significantly degraded in rumen; vitamin E may also be reduced;
Metabolism	Metabolic functions similar to adult; lower status compared with dam in serum; receive primary source from colostrum consumption	vitamins perform many metabolic and immune support functions; vitamin D needed for calcium homeostasis; vitamins A and D transported on specific proteins, vitamin E on lipoproteins
Deficiency disease	Abortion or stillbirth (vitamin A, E?); weak calf, blindness (vitamin A); altered immune response	Low colostrum vitamin status; increased risk for RFM, mastitis, metritis, hypocalcemia (D only)

Abbreviations: FPT, failure of passive transfer; LDA, left displaced abomasum; RFM, retained fetal membranes; TCA, Tricarboxylic acid cycle.
Data from Refs. [5,25,52–54]

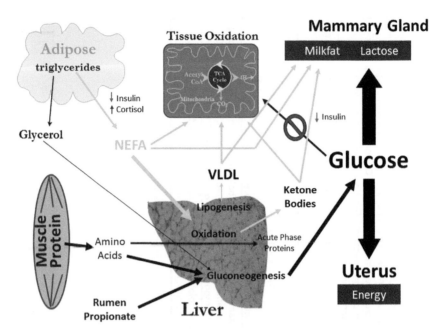

Fig. 4. Summarized metabolic adaptations occurring via homeorhetic regulation in the transition from pregnancy to lactation. VLDL, very low density lipoprotein.

higher BMR. This response is in an effort to promote the immune response in responding to some pathogen or stressor, but is costly nutritionally to the animal.[81]

Mobilization of skeletal muscle further exacerbates negative protein balance in early lactation and may account for the predilection for more than 1 disease process once one has been established.[74] In addition to mobilization of skeletal muscle, constitutive proteins synthesized by the liver such as albumin, retinol binding protein, apoproteins, and transferrin (eg, negative APPs) are not synthesized, most likely to further provide

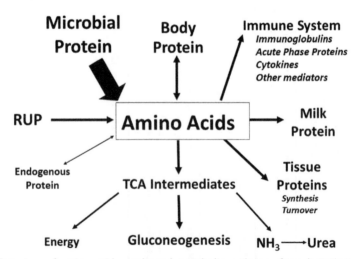

Fig. 5. Overview of amino acid supply and metabolic pathways for a lactating cow. RUP, rumen undegradable protein.

amino acids to support the APP response. Reduction of these constitutive proteins may adversely affect mineral and vitamin metabolism through the loss of transport proteins. In addition, loss of apoproteins reduces the ability of the liver to synthesize very low density lipoproteins and potentially increase fatty infiltration in the face of increased NEFA concentrations. An activated immune response is necessary during transition to deal with uterine clearance and protection from potential mastitis pathogens, but excessive stimulation of this response through environmental, social, or dietary factors predisposes to poor transition cow performance.

FORMULATING TRANSITION DIETS
Nutritional Modeling

Nutrition models have become more complex in the last 20+ years. The increased complexity started with the recognition that use of book values for feed analyses, especially forages, was no longer acceptable. There was a need for a more complex system in forage analyses to address nutrient availability and effect on rumen dynamics. There was also a need to recognize complexities of the rumen, contributions of the rumen microbial ecosystem, and predict rumen digestive extent as a function of microbial digestion rate (k_d) versus rate at which that nutrient escaped digestion and flowed out of the rumen (rate of passage, k_p). This recognition resulted in the development of a dynamic system modeling rumen function. This effort was started in the mid-1980s with the CNCPS and has continued with many versions.[82] The central concept of this effort is that the model had to be usable in the field, and nutrient inputs for feeds had to largely be amenable to analysis in a commercial laboratory. The NRC dairy model was released in 2001 with dynamic components in the protein area and with the introduction of a preweaned calf model as well as the introduction of an improved mineral submodel.[17] The NRC effort was a significant step forward.

Defining the Animal

The definition of dry cow requirements is based on carefully defining first the dry cow group that is to be fed. We often get into the mode of using 1 set of numbers. This strategy is inappropriate. **Fig. 6** is an example of an input for the early dry cow group

Animal type	u.m.		
Number of animals	n		30
Days in cycle	days		365
Breed type		Dairy	
Primary breed		Holstein	
Secondary Breed			
Lactation number	n		3.00
Calving interval	months		13.00
Age at first calving (AOFC)	months		24.00
Age (actual average)	months		50.00
Mean FBW	lbs		1,443.0
Mature FBW	lbs		1,503.6
Days pregnant	days		259
BCS (1–5)			3.25
Target BCS			3.25
Days to reach target BCS	days		100
Calf birth weight	lbs		100.0
ADG	lbs/day		0.153

Fig. 6. Descriptions used for formulating a far-off dry cow diet.

into the CNCPS system. The impetus of defining the animal correctly is to ensure that the diet provides sufficient nutrients to all individuals within the group. Obviously, some animals are overfed, but the desire is to minimize the underfeeding variation.

Frame size

We need to carefully start by identifying the mature frame size in the herd and then to carefully assess distribution of cows within the group; the mean frame body weight and average of the group. The days pregnant for this group is set at 259 days. This number should not be the average days pregnant but is the days pregnant when they leave the group. This number increases MP and ME requirements when formulating the ration. This number should be increased to 280 days pregnant when the cows move into the close-up group. The same concept holds; we need to be certain that we have adequate MP. We think in terms of projected calving, but there are deviations between projected and actual calving. This information can now be easily recorded at a dairy. The other information that changes in the figure for the close-up is the age and frame size weight to reflect the percentage of the group that are heifers calving for the first time (ie, springers).

Calf birth weight

Frame size is important because it defines a significant part of the nutrient requirements. Added to this factor is the conceptus requirement. This is a moving target with each day of pregnancy (see **Fig. 1**). The conceptus mass is predicted from the calf birth weight. It might be argued that calf birth weight should be lower (see **Fig. 6**); however, a certain percent of the births are more than 45 kg (100 lb). Van Saun[59] reported that almost 25% of the calves born to mature Holstein cows were more than 45 kg (100 lb). This factor has more of a critical impact on the MP requirement than the ME requirement. Part of the requirement that becomes a reality in the 30+ days before calving is the mammary requirement. With the onset of birth, hormonal changes trigger the rapid development of new mammary tissue in readiness for calving. Also, during this period, cows go through a period of immunosuppression. The maintenance and the enhancement of the immune system are critical. One of the critical aspects of the immune system is meeting the MP requirement not only during the dry period but also in the last 2 months of lactation. Cows giving birth to larger calves are at greater risk for suffering clinical and subclinical issues if not receiving sufficient nutrient intake.

Age and days carried calf

There are 4 different dry cow group scenarios, with different management protocols within the scenarios: 1 group, early dry, close-up, and now more frequently, a heifer group. Each grouping strategy has its own unique challenges. With the 1 dry cow group, there is a mix of all ages and days pregnant. With the 2-group system, there are usually the second calf and older cows in the early dry, and then in the close-up, there are a variable mix of older cows and heifers. It is critical that the distribution of ages and thus frame sizes is sufficiently defined in each of the groups. It is also important within each of these groups that the BCS is carefully assessed as well as changes between groups if more than 1 group. In this figure, the groups being fed need to be carefully considered. It is suggested that 280 days be used for a 1 dry cow group as well as for a springer group. Of course, frame changes for each group type, and if there is a springer group, then the calf birth weight can be reduced to 41 kg (90 lb).

To this point, there has been no discussion about either the late lactation cows before going into the dry period or the cows after calving. There is recognition of the importance of controlling body condition. Many rations are fed to late lactation cows that are marginal on energy and protein. Because of the lower amount of fermentable carbohydrate in the rumen, less microbial protein is produced, which is a high-quality protein. This factor coupled with lower protein rations can result in a negative MP balance. The key is to define the requirements correctly. The cows in late lactation begin to have a significant requirement because of pregnancy. If the cows are going to be dry for 60 days, then, the days pregnant needs to be set at 220 days. If the cows are going to have a 40-day dry period, then, the days pregnant should be set at 240 days. The guidelines for calf birth weight were discussed earlier.

Dry matter intake expectation
One of the challenges is in predicting DMI. It has been observed in many studies that as a cow comes closer to calving, DMI decreases. Our goal is to minimize this change. Part of this decrease is caused by a decrease in rumen volume caused by an increase in conceptus size but also caused by the reduction in intake as a result of a lower nutrient demand when the cow dries off. This situation makes the cow more sensitive to the amount of indigestible NDF in the ration (we now call this uNDF). Because lower digestibility forages are being fed, the uNDF is a higher percentage of the total NDF. uNDF escapes from the rumen when the particle size is reduced to less than 2 mm with a higher density. One of the recent strategies is to feed a high straw ration in the early dry period. This strategy decreases the energy in the ration and also tends to maintain a larger rumen volume, which helps as the cow gets closer to calving relative to degree of intake reduction in the last 2 to 4 weeks before calving.

Dietary Nutrient Specifications

Recommended dry cow dietary nutrient content for a 2-group feeding system based on NRC guidelines is summarized in **Table 4**.

Energy considerations
University of Illinois research has shown that the ME requirement of the cow should not be exceeded.[38,40,53] This goal becomes difficult to achieve without the use of forages with which energy intake can be controlled. This strategy usually means a grass source. On many farms, grasses of appropriate qualities are not available. There are corn silage and alfalfa or legume-grass mixtures. The solution to this situation has been the use of straw, which, relatively speaking, is more consistent than purchasing other forages. Care must be taken not to assume book values for straw, especially mineral content, because some sources have high K. The key is to have forages that control energy intake and have adequate digestibility to minimize the decrease in DMI as the cow approaches calving. Using a grass hay or silage with a 58% to 65% NDF with a 10% to 12% CP usually performs well. If corn silage and alfalfa are the only options, then, the use of straw is the solution. Another key point, if using silages, is to make sure that the fermentation quality is excellent. Moldy and unstable silages should not be fed.

The energy requirement for dry cows is significantly affected by the environment that surrounds her. In the CNCPS platforms, there is the opportunity to make the appropriate adjustments. This situation affects not only the energy requirement but also the predicted DMI. It is important to enter details of the environment that surrounds the cow. This factor affects the rations that are developed to feed the cows. The details of the impact of the environment and the management of the cows within the environment are discussed in other articles by Allen and Piontoni, Oelburg and Stone, and McFarland et al, elsewhere in this issue.

The first 2 to 4 weeks after calving are a critical time. Dr Mike Allen, Michigan State, has proposed that feeding rations during this period that produce high amounts of

Table 4
Recommended dietary nutrient concentrations (DM basis) suggested for pregnant nonlactating dairy cattle

Nutrient	Units	Early Dry[a]	Close-Up Dry[b]
Net energy (NE$_l$)	Mcal/kg	1.10–1.20	1.45–1.55
	Mcal/lb	0.50–0.55	0.65–0.70
CP	% DM	12–13	13–14
MP	% DM	6.0–6.6	7.0–8.0
Soluble CP	% CP	40–50	35–45
Degradable CP	% CP	65–70	62–67
Undegradable CP	% CP	30–35	33–38
Acid detergent fiber	% DM	35–40 (27)[c]	30–35 (21)[c]
NDF	% DM	50–65 (35)[c]	40–55 (30)[c]
Calcium	% DM	0.31–0.35	0.36–0.41
Phosphorus	% DM	0.19–0.21	0.22–0.25
Magnesium[d]	% DM	0.18–0.20	0.22–0.25
Potassium	% DM	0.65–0.75	0.70–0.80
Sodium	% DM	0.10–0.13	0.12–0.15
Chloride	% DM	0.20–0.22	0.24–0.26
Sulfur	% DM	0.16–0.18	0.19–0.21
Cobalt	PPM	0.10	0.12
Copper	PPM	10–15	12–18
Iron	PPM	50	60
Iodine	PPM	0.60	0.70
Manganese	PPM	40	50
Zinc	PPM	40	50
Selenium[e]	PPM	0.3	0.3
Vitamin A	IU/kg	5576	8244
	IU/lb	2530	3747
Vitamin D	IU/kg	1520	2249
	IU/lb	690	1022
Vitamin E	IU/kg	88	120
	IU/lb	40	55

[a] Early dry period is defined as 4–6 weeks after dry-off with suggested nutrient densities based on a DMI of 1.9%–2.1% of BW.
[b] Close-up dry period is defined as 2–4 weeks before calving with suggested nutrient densities based on a DMI of 1.6%–1.8% of body weight.
[c] Mininum recommended dietary fiber levels.
[d] Increase dietary concentrations to 0.35%–0.4% when potassium levels exceed 1.2%–1.5%, respectively.
[e] Maximum intake allowed by the US Food and Drug Administration.
Adapted from National Research Council. Nutrient Requirements of Dairy Cattle. 7th rev. edition. Washington, DC: National Academy Press; 2001. Assuming a thermoneutral environment and 10% activity allowance.

propionate results in potentially lower intake via receptors at the liver that signal satiety.[39,83] This situation can be counterproductive at a time when cows are accelerating in milk output, which accelerates lipid mobilization and results in associated negative consequences. This investigator's suggestion is that we need to reduce the fermentable starch in the first 3 weeks post partum.

Table 5 shows suggestions from Allen's work. This is based on an assay that he developed and suggests is tentative but provides a beginning means for assessing carbohydrate fermentation in the rumen. The grouping is based on Dr Allen's suggestions. Recommendations provided give an opportunity to look first at the starch concentration in the rations. This is a familiar formulation parameter. The next 3 columns are based on the 7-hour starch assay. The higher starch fermentability for the close-up cow is caused by the low starch inclusion level and the need to provide a reasonable microbial protein contribution to MP to reduce the amount of a bypass protein needed in the ration. Fermentable starch as % DM provides a means to place minimums and maximums for optimization of the rations as well as a guideline to examine the ration. The right column expresses the fermentable starch as a percent of total fermentable starch. It is suggested that the total optimum fermentable carbohydrate (CHO) level in the CNCPS system, as it is reflected in the current version, is 40% DM. This factor also includes the fermentable fiber (the other major fermentable CHO source) as well as sugar and soluble fiber.

The recommendation for the cows 0 to 3 weeks post partum is low relative to the next 2 groups. This recommendation can be achieved by feeding a combination of a highly fermentable fiber source, a starch source low in fermentable starch, and a higher fermentable soluble fiber source. This strategy basically results in higher acetate:propionate fermentation in the rumen, resulting in a faster acceleration in DMI during the first 3 weeks post partum. Moving the cows into the next group increases propionate production and provides the glucose needed for lactose synthesis, as well as increasing feed efficiency.

This approach to CHO formulation in the first 3 weeks of lactation moderates microbial protein output to some degree but not as extensively as might be believed because of improved pH control during this period when the cows' eating behavior has not reached equilibrium. It is suggested that attention needs to be paid to the inclusion of a good-quality bypass protein as well as careful formulation for amino acids.

Protein metabolism and supply

Dry cow protein nutrition has been misunderstood and is still a controversial area of investigation. The controlled studies in this area have often been confounded by the method of balancing to meet pregnant cow protein requirement. The NRC recommendations for protein supply were based on research that was limited, and the experimental rations were often formulated inappropriately, providing wrong conclusions.

Table 5
Suggested starch and fermentable carbohydrate (CHO) fractions in formulating transition diets

Group	Starch in Ration (%DM)	Fermentable Starch (%Starch 7-h)	Fermentable Starch (%DM)	Fermentable Starch (% Total Fermentable CHO)[a]
Close-up	16–18	80	12.8–14.4	34
Fresh cows (0–3 wk)	22–25	74	16.3–18.5	43.5
Early to mid lactation, 3 wk to 150 d in milk	25–30	83	20.7–24.9	57
Late lactation >150 d in milk	18–22	74	13.3–16.3	37

[a] Based on a suggested total ration fermentable CHO of 40% DM.

Data from Allen MS. Adjusting concentration and ruminal digestibility of starch through lactation. In: Proc 4-State Dairy Nutr and Manage Conf. Debuque, IA. 2012. p. 24–30.

Further, the recommendations did not recognize the importance of the mammary requirement and protein reserves. The CNCPS system now recognizes the importance of both; however, it does not recognize the importance of labile protein reserves relative to immune function as well as the need in the early postpartum period when cows can mobilize 800 to 1000 g/d.[30] This situation puts greater emphasis on the maintenance of labile protein reserves in the last 60 to 80 days of gestation. This is a period in late lactation and during the dry period when lower-energy rations are being fed, reducing microbial protein output, and MP balance can easily become negative, especially with hay-crop silage-based diets. Field observations suggest that there is a need to exceed the NRC 2001 recommendations for protein and meet and not exceed the ME requirements. This need coupled with variation in DMI within a group of cows being fed a balanced ration dictates that there should be an adequate concentration of MP in the rations being fed during this time to ensure that all cows are able to maintain the protein reserves that were replenished in midlactation. In addition, recent work has suggested that protein quality may be important as well. This theory suggests that it is important to pay attention to the source of MP as well as the amount of MP.

Mineral recommendations

Many studies have reported the need for careful formulation of minerals during the transition period relative to maintaining calcium homeostasis. The metabolic consequences are discussed in an other article by Martin-Tereso and Martens elsewhere in this issue; a formulation approach is discussed in this article. It is important to analyze the forages using wet chemistry and not near-infrared spectroscopy. Balancing of both macrominerals and trace minerals is dependent on knowing the forage mineral contribution. Recommendations for dietary trace mineral supplementation are provided by Swecker elsewhere in this issue (see article on trace minerals). It is essential to know forage K content relative to modifying dietary Mg content and addressing potential for using anionic salt supplementation to manipulate dietary cation-anion difference (DCAD). Recommendations for dietary macrominerals relative to promoting calcium homeostasis are provided in **Table 6**.

Vitamins

Fat-soluble vitamins generally decline in late gestation, a consequence of their transfer to colostrum or declining intake. Vitamin E status as measured by serum α-tocopherol

Table 6
Suggested dietary macromineral content (% of DM) in close-up dry cow diets to maintain calcium homeostasis with or without using anionic salts to manipulate DCAD

Mineral	Without Anionic Salts (%)	Anionic Salt (%)
Calcium[a]	<0.5	0.85–1.1
Phosphorus	0.25–0.33	0.25–0.33
Magnesium	0.35–0.4	0.35–0.4
Potassium	<1.1[b]	1.2–1.8[b]
Sodium	0.1–0.15	0.1–0.15
Chloride	0.3–0.5	0.5–1.3[c]
Sulfur	0.25–0.3	0.3–0.4
DCAD (mEq/kg DM)	<100	−100–0

[a] Need to feed <20 g available Ca to be truly low Ca diet.
[b] Keep as low as possible.
[c] Suggested dietary Cl content = %K − 0.5.

concentration has been related to risk of mastitis and retained fetal membranes.[84,85] Serum vitamin A concentration has been related to mastitis risk in early lactation.[85] Vitamin D is needed to maintain proper calcium homeostasis. Excess intakes of vitamins A and D can have detrimental effects beyond just suppressing DMI. Recommendations for vitamin supplementation during the transition period, as modified from NRC recommendations, are as follows:

- Vitamin A: provide at least NRC recommended amounts (110 IU/kg body weight) through transition (80,000 IU/d for 680 kg cow).[17]
- Vitamin D: provide between 20,000 and 40,000 IU/d through transition. Diets providing more than 60,000 IU/d may predispose to milk fever or result in metastatic calcification of soft tissues.
- Vitamin E: provide at least 1000 IU/d through the dry period. Herds experiencing mastitis or other infectious disease problems may increase prepartum intake to 4000 IU/d and follow this with 2000 IU/d in early lactation.

TRANSITION COW FEEDING MANAGEMENT CONSIDERATIONS
Ensuring Adequate Nutrient Intake

One of the primary challenges of dry cow group management is formulating the diet for an appropriate intake level. Even if a balanced diet for a defined average intake for a given feeding group is provided, statistics show that 50% of the animals in the group consume less than the average intake. French[86] presented summarized prepartum intake data from Phillips and colleagues[61] for multiparous Holstein cows. In this analysis, the average DM intake was 12.3 ± 2.5 kg/d for the last 21 days before calving, with 15% of the cows consuming less than 10 kg/d (1 standard deviation less than group average) and being in a state of negative nutrient balance. A recommendation from this analysis was to formulate the close-up dry diet to 1300 g or 1400 g MP as a safety factor to ensure that an adequate 83% or 95%, respectively, of the cows consume a desired 1080 g MP from the diet.

In another multiparous cow dataset,[59] 21-day prepartum intake was 13.5 ± 2.6 kg/d. In this study, prepartum diets differed in MP content (1100 vs 1350 g/d), but DMI was not different across treatments. The cows consuming the higher-MP diet had less metabolic disease and improved reproductive performance compared with the lower-MP diet. These results seemingly support the concept promoted by French, although a higher-MP requirement is not out of consideration in explaining such responses. Clearly, large variation (higher standard deviation) of DMI within a group results in more cows, and especially heifers in mixed groups, having lower intake and potentially experiencing a negative MP balance.

Matching Diet Formulation to Grouping Strategy

Far-off dry cow group
Fig. 7 shows the ME and MP supply and requirements for an early dry cow. The ME and MP are just met. Even although the average days dry might be 240 days, the

	ME				MP			
	Supply	Requirement	Balance	% Req.	Supply	Requirement	Balance	% Req.
	25.01	24.88	0.13	100.5%	964.8	938.9	26.0	102.8%
Maintenance	25.01	18.31	6.70		964.8	573.5	391.3	
Pregnancy	6.70	5.68	1.03		391.3	334.5	56.8	
Lactation	1.03	0.00	1.03		56.8	0.0	56.8	
Growth	1.03	0.90	0.13		56.8	30.8	26.0	
Reserves	0.13	0.00	0.13		26.0	0.0	26.0	

Fig. 7. Dietary evaluation for properly formulated far-off dry cow described as 655 kg (1443 lb) BW, 259 days pregnant, BCS 3.25, calf birth weight 45 kg (100 lb).

assumption is that the cows are being moved 3 weeks before calving, and the MP requirement for this stage of pregnancy needs to be met. Setting the days pregnant to 259 days with a projected calf weight of 45 kg (100 lb) ensures adequate ME and MP concentrations in the ration to better accommodate the ranges in DMI that occur within a group of early dry cows. A setting at 260 days pregnant activates the mammary requirement. If it is observed that the cows are moved at less than 3 weeks before calving, then, going to a day's pregnant should be considered, which reflects the days that the cows are in the close-up pen before projected calving.

Close-up dry cow group

Fig. 8 shows the ME and MP supply and requirements for a close-up dry cow. The BW has been reduced to 628 kg (1383 lb), assuming that there are also heifers calving for the first time in this group. Care needs to be taken in defining this group. The % of first calving heifers in this group can vary significantly over the year. Even although there are smaller animals in this pen, there are also many cows calving that have calves with weights in excess of 45 kg (100 lb). Also, the growth requirement increased from 31g MP to 270g MP and ME from 0.9 to 3.4 Mcal/d. This increase is to meet the mammary requirement after 260 days pregnant. This is a model set point, but there is not a sudden change but an increasing one over time in the last few weeks of pregnancy. The dairy protocol needs to be known when cows are moved from 1 group to another. The MP and ME requirements can be adjusted if necessary. Field observations suggest a better response when cows are exposed to the close-up diet for 21 days or more; however, research studies suggest that 10 to 14 days is adequate.

The ME requirement for the close-up cow is a requirement based on the cow maintaining body condition. There is a growth requirement as well for springers, which is about 13 g/d (0.3 lb/d). NRC recognized requirements for springers are higher.[17] If these animals do not eat the DM assumed, then, there is not adequate ME or MP. It was recommended earlier to use lower-energy forages for the dry cows. This strategy is positive from an energy standpoint, but if the uNDF is too high, this reduces feed intake, as discussed earlier. The formulated MP is 117% of requirement. This level provides a higher concentration of dietary MP and ensures that cows are not mobilizing protein reserves during the last 3 weeks of pregnancy. This practice also provides additional amino acids, both essential and nonessential, which is not accounted for in the model to account for immune system requirements.

Heifer group

If herd size and housing permits, having a springer group does have the advantage of being able to develop rations for just this group. The additional advantage is that there is little social adjustment as would occur in being introduced into a close-up group with older cows. If these cows are to be moved to a calving area at time of calving that also has older cows, there could be some social adjustments.

	ME				MP			
	Supply	Requirement	Balance	% Req.	Supply	Requirement	Balance	% Req.
	26.84	26.41	0.43	101.6%	1,306.4	1,112.5	193.9	117.4%
Maintenance	26.84	16.87	9.97		1,306.4	463.8	842.6	
Pregnancy	9.97	6.16	3.81		842.6	378.8	463.8	
Lactation	3.81	0.00	3.81		463.8	0.0	463.8	
Growth	3.81	3.39	0.43		463.8	269.9	193.9	
Reserves	0.43	0.00	0.43		193.9	0.0	193.9	

Fig. 8. Dietary evaluation for properly formulated close-up dry cow group described as 628 kg (1383 lb) BW, 280 days pregnant, BCS 3.25. The lower BW accounts for a proportion of springing heifers in the group.

It is important to again obtain the mature frame size in the herd, average month of calving, and the BCS = 3.0 frame size for the springers. It is suggested that a 41 kg (90 lb) birth weight be used as well as 280 days pregnant. With these requirements and the lower DMI, if the ration for the older cows is being used, it is noticed if the ration is not adequate to meet requirements. It is again suggested that the ME requirement be met and about 117% of MP requirements be fed. This strategy reduces the forage being fed and increases the concentrate with changes in the % protein in the ration.

1-group system
A 1-group system is for many smaller dairies the best option as well as for those dairies with limited facilities. It is better to have 1 good facility with proper space and management than 2 facilities with average management. There is another benefit from a 1-group system, and that is that social adjustment is not as much of an issue as it is with shifting cows from an early dry to a close-up group. A 1-group system is also recommended for farms using a 30-day to 45-day dry period.

Feeding for 1 group is labor efficient, but can be a challenge nutritionally. The mix of cows in the group is continuously changing in age and days pregnant. As a consequence, it is best to feed the group as a close-up group in terms of requirements and nutrient concentrations. From a ration cost, this strategy is more expensive than feeding 2 or more groups but a lower cost for labor to feed the cows. There have been concerns in the past if a DCAD ration is being fed that feeding a DCAD ration for the whole dry period can be detrimental. This concern has not proved to be the case. It is suggested that the guidelines on ME and MP suggested earlier for close-up be followed.

Fresh cow group
Fresh cows go through tremendous changes in a short period. Genetic selection has been mainly focused on milk volume, which results in a very rapid increase in milk volume day over day. This situation results in mobilization of both protein and lipid reserves. The cows do not usually come into energy equilibrium until 8 to 10 weeks post partum. This factor is coupled with DMI not reaching maximum until 8 to 10 weeks as well. Cows usually peak in 6 to 8 weeks post partum. Again, definition of the groups during this period is critical. Every dairy has unique protocols for grouping and cow movement between groups. The simplest group is 1 group. Cows calve and go into 1 group and stay in this group until confirmed pregnant. A more complicated scenario can be a fresh cow group, which all cows enter for a defined period, and then they move into a high group, and the heifers move into a first calf heifer group, where they stay for the rest of the lactation. The important issue that needs to be determined is exactly what the protocols are:

- Just before calving
  - Are the cows moved?
    - If so, where?
- Right after calving
  - Are there interventions?
    - Bottles, boluses, and so forth
      - For which group of cows are these interventions used?
  - Is adequate water provided?
- The fresh period in the first 5 to 7 days
- Beyond the transition period

Transition Cow Dietary Supplements

Dietary supplements have been used for many years in an effort to improve transition cow performance.[87] Propylene glycol is the most commonly used and has been for some time. This supplement provides an energy source as a precursor to meet the glucose needs of the cow and promotes insulin secretion. It is most commonly used immediately after calving in liquid form as drench as a means of dealing with ketosis and has been moderately successful as a treatment. It has also been used in the dry form both before and after calving, again with moderate but not always consistent success. It continues to have its place in management practice.

There has also been success with supplements such as yeast products, which provide stimulation to the microbial ecology of the rumen and improve ruminal fermentation, mediating some of the negative responses that occur in the transition from dry to lactating rations.

Another rumen modifier that has been extensively used is ionophores. Rumensin is the most commonly used. This modifier is usually fed to cows in the close-up period to the early lactation period. It provides an increase in propionate, the glucogenic precursor to glucose, reduces the population of bacteria producing lactic acid, and increases the amount of bypass protein. This strategy reduces the risk of acidosis as well as providing additional propionate and glucose as a result. This can be an excellent practice for the prepartum cow.

There has been recent use of B-vitamins like choline and niacin. The challenges with these vitamins is 2-fold: as an added supplement, they are readily degraded in the rumen and often, the assumption that the bacteria produce adequate amounts is not correct. In addition, there are many animal and environmental circumstances that require additional amounts in excess of the supply that can come from microbial synthesis. The problem of being readily degraded has been resolved through the new development of rumen protection technology, which can deliver additional nutrients needed by the cow.

There has been extensive work showing the value of the addition of rumen-protected choline to the prepartum ration. This strategy can be particularly helpful for a group of cows that are overconditioned in the close-up group. The choline is important in enhancing the transport of lipid out of the liver in the early postpartum period.

The use of rumen-protected niacin has received increased interest in recent years. Research has reported than niacin supplementation can reduce NEFA concentrations, and in periods of heat stress it can facilitate cow tolerance to the heat. There has been research to show that poorly ventilated dry cow facilities result in poor postpartum performance. There might be management opportunities for the use of niacin in NEFA and heat management.

It can be concluded that for many herd situations, the use of dietary supplements can be advantageous. There have been many research studies as well as meta-analyses for some of the supplements showing efficacy.[88,89] These transition supplements can help cover some variability issues within a transition program to minimize the number of cows experiencing diseases.

CONFOUNDING ISSUES TO NUTRITIONAL PROGRAMS

Cows calving in many herds are experiencing difficulties with subclinical and clinical problems. Producers have resorted to a host of interventions such as Ca, Mg, dextrose intravenous, subcutaneous, and drenching approaches to mitigate problems. Lately, emphasis has been placed on the mineral nutrition of the cow, which has resulted in moderate success but has been intermingled with many metabolic events in a dairy. Complicating the picture is the management issues of body condition, days dry, grouping, group movement strategy, and quality of facilities. To this end, Drackley asked: "Why do vastly different nutrition and management programs produce similarly good, or similarly poor, transition success?"[3] Overcrowding, exposure to pathogens, changing social organization, among other situations, can induce stress-mediated physiologic and metabolic changes. Animals alter how they use and partition available nutrients in response to these stress situations, which may compromise availability of nutrients to support productive functions. It is thought that the effects of stress are additive, thereby as stress situations accumulate, greater physiologic and metabolic changes occur, resulting in abnormality, seen as metabolic dysfunction or infectious disease. These stress responses are more exaggerated in animals consuming an imbalanced diet, but may also overwhelm an animal consuming an adequate diet.

Body Condition Score

Excessive BCS has historically been associated with poor transition performance.[53,90–93] Adverse transition outcomes associated with cows with high BCS (≥4.0, 1–5 scale) result from reduced DMI or excessive inflammatory mediators impairing hepatic metabolism or impaired insulin regulation.[76,94,95] Cows with low BCS (≤3.0, 1–5 scale) have higher postpartum DMI,[96] but may not support high milk yield.[97,98]

Field observations have suggested that the 1-group low-energy, high-fiber dry cow diet works well even with cows in heavy body condition. A field study of prepartum grouping strategies[99] supported a 2-group system for cows with heavy body condition. This study found a tendency for thinner cows (≤3.0 BCS, 1–5 scale) to perform better post partum. A herd with many overconditioned cows should consider using supplements such as monensin, rumen-protected choline, or niacin, and feeding higher MP in an effort to minimize potential postpartum problems. Efforts should be taken to reduce BCS gain in late lactation. The challenge of body condition variation was indicated by Bell, when he suggested: "Future research should consider why it is that relations between body condition, feed intake, and postpartum health and performance vary so widely among individual cows."[25]

Management Factors

In addressing issues of transition health, Nordlund[100] has moved further from nutritional concerns to focus more on cow management and environment. This investigator identified 5 key nonnutritional factors relative to the risk of periparturient disease. These issues span the realms of management and environmental issues. One concern is adequate feed bunk space in the prefresh and fresh cow groups. These cow groups seem more sensitive to behavioral competition and intimidation, which results in altered feeding behaviors.[101,102] At least 76 cm (30 in) of bunk space is recommended per cow in these groups.[47] Bunk space is most critical in farms where feed availability is limited or where overcrowding occurs. Recommended stocking density for transition feeding groups is 85% based on observational studies, although controlled studies do not show significant alterations in overall feed intake or sorting behaviors.[102,103] In these controlled studies, meal number and feeding rate were more affected in multiparous cows and resulted in greater standing bouts. Patterns of prepartum feed intake have been characterized sufficiently to be used in predicting risk of postpartum disease.[104–107] The question remains, are the feed intakes caused by impending disease, or are the feeding patterns induced and then result in increased disease risk?

A second key factor is the number of pen moves through the transition period. As the social hierarchy is more frequently altered, observational studies suggest a decline in feed intake, with observed higher NEFA concentrations and greater disease prevalence.[47] A recent study of transition cow behavior[108] showed reduced feed intake, more feed bunk evictions, and lower milk production in groups with recent social changes. Overton and Nydam[109] suggested that primiparous cows would benefit to a greater extent from grouping strategies based on parity. In a large herd survey, heifers in comingled transition groups showed a greater prevalence of increased NEFA concentrations compared with herds with separated parity groups. Observational data on pen moves also suggest a greater impact on heifers.[47] An additional concern with comingled groups is the ability to meet the heifer nutritional needs without overfeeding the older cows.

More recently, intense management of the immediately fresh cow (<30 days in milk) has gained significant importance and application on many dairy farms. Cows with more significant disease condition or duration experience greater BW and condition loss, which leads to negative effects on reproductive performance. Immediately fresh cows already have reduced intake and a weakened immune system and thus are more susceptible to problems. The goal of fresh cow programs is to identify potentially sick cows early and intervene in an attempt to limit the adverse effects of disease. Nordlund[100] suggested that the intensity of fresh cow monitoring practices is another key factor in preventing periparturient disease.

In many herds, immediately fresh cows are provided a special group to themselves. Fresh cows are less aggressive at the feed bunk and are easily pushed away by other later lactation cows. These fresh cow groups are generally located close to milking parlors or maternity areas, where cows can be closely monitored. Most large farms have adopted a standardized protocol to manage fresh cows and have identified key personnel who are solely dedicated to fresh cow management. Most fresh cow protocols focus on early disease detection by frequent animal observation and monitoring. Many farms have adopted the practice of monitoring rectal temperature for at least the first 10 days after calving. Depending on the visual appraisal (bright and alert or dull, depressed) and body temperature, further physical evaluation is carried out. Most farms have their fresh cow workers evaluate rumen motility and urinary ketone status. Depending on results of each of the evaluation criteria (ie, body temperature, rumen motility, urine ketones), a set protocol is established for therapeutic applications. Veterinarians play an important role in establishing appropriate criteria and therapeutic strategies.

Environmental Conditions

Two of the 5 key factors for transition success identified by Nordlund[100] are specific to cow comfort issues, namely, stall design and surface cushion. Traditional freestall design has 122-cm-wide (48 in) stalls, which balances well with barn structural design. However, transition cows are typically wider and benefit from wider stalls (127 cm [50 in] recommended). In addition, stalls should be designed to facilitate normal cow lying, resting, and raising behaviors. The need for unimpeded lunge space at the front of the stall to facilitate the cow's ability to stand has been well documented. Stall design and size recommendations are provided in the article by McFarland et al. elsewhere in this issue on nonnutritional factors affecting the nutrition program. The stall surface cushion is recommended to be deep sand, because this provides the best footing anchor for the cow when attempting to stand. Mattresses or sparsely bedded stalls or stalls having wet bedding do not provide sufficient footing and result in altered cow lying/standing times and further accentuate lameness problems.[110,111]

A highly significant environmental factor in transition success is the ability to provide heat abatement.[112] Dry cows not provided with shade have lower birth weight calves and reduced milk yield compared with cows provided with shade.[113] Transition cows exposed to heat stress bouts showed several significant alterations in blood metabolite parameters that indicate lowered DMI, metabolic acidosis, and negative energy balance.[114] In this study, far-off and close-up dry cows as well as fresh cows were equally affected by heat stress, as indicated by the following changes in blood parameters:

- Increased concentrations of NEFA, and chloride in all transition groups and increased BHB and aspartate transaminase levels in fresh cows
- Reduced concentrations of glucose, albumin, cholesterol, calcium, phosphorus, and potassium across all transition groups

Collectively, these changes suggest a state of metabolic acidosis caused by losses of sodium and bicarbonate as a result of drooling. Other parameters reflect a decline in DMI, which predisposes to other metabolic issues. Heat stress also reduces both innate and acquired immune responses in transition cows.[115]

Recent research has shown that heat abatement during transition results in improved milk production, which was mediated through alterations in prolactin concentrations and hepatic gene expression.[116] Recommendations for heat abatement techniques, including fans, sprinklers, and shade, are provided by McFarland et al. elsewhere in this issue.

SUMMARY

Research results have provided further guidance in appropriate issues to address in developing a transition cow management program with expectations for low disease prevalence, high milk production, and efficient reproductive performance. The following are general principles that have been established or suggested.

- Dietary formulation goals:
  - Address intake capacity for grouping strategy and consider the variation in intake within a group to ensure sufficient nutrient intake for a greater percent of the cows within a given group
  - Meet energy needs through appropriately balanced energy density and fiber content to control intake; some additional grain in close-up diet is optional
  - Ensure at least 1100 g MP is consumed by all cows, thus potentially requiring delivery of 1300 g MP to account for DMI variation (more research is needed here relative to amino acid needs)
  - Maintain calcium homeostasis by addressing dietary macromineral content, especially relationships between potassium and magnesium and calcium and phosphorus
  - Provide sufficient dietary vitamins and trace minerals from available sources to meet needs of cow, colostrums, and fetus to minimize negative effects on immune response
- Manage animal grouping strategies and dietary formulations in late lactation and dry period to achieve proper BCS and minimize the number of excessively fat or thin cows (<10% of total group)
- Minimize cow stress response by ensuring adequate cow comfort
  - Proper stall resting area
  - Sufficient feed bunk and watering space
  - Heat abatement and good ventilation
  - Clean, dry bedding of sufficient cushion
- Address behavioral needs of the cow
  - Minimize pen moves resulting in social upheavals
  - Minimize overcrowding in critical groups (85% occupancy)

- ○ Promote the cows' ability to eat and rest collectively as a group
- ○ Provide opportunity for calving cows to isolate themselves from the group
- Establish adequate monitoring system to assess postpartum health status and disease risk parameters

REFERENCES

1. Herdt TH, Sniffen CJ. Dairy nutrition. Vet Clin North Am Food Anim Pract 1991;7(2): 311–628.
2. Van Saun RJ. Dry cow nutrition: the key to improving fresh cow performance. Vet Clin North Am Food Anim Pract 1991;7(2):599–620.
3. Drackley JK. Biology of dairy cows during the transition period: the final frontier? J Dairy Sci 1999;82:2259–73.
4. Kelton DF, Lissemore KD, Martin RE. Recommendations for recording and calculating the incidence of selected clinical diseases of dairy cattle. J Dairy Sci 1998;81:2502–9.
5. Ingvartsen KL. Feeding- and management-related diseases in the transition cow: physiological adaptations around calving and strategies to reduce feeding-related diseases. Anim Feed Sci Technnol 2006;126:175–213.
6. McArt JA, Nydam DV, Oetzel GR. A field trial on the effect of propylene glycol on displaced abomasum, removal from herd, and reproduction in fresh cows diagnosed with subclinical ketosis. J Dairy Sci 2012;95:2505–12.
7. McArt JA, Nydam DV, Oetzel GR. Epidemiology of subclinical ketosis in early lactation dairy cattle. J Dairy Sci 2012;95:5056–66.
8. Gilbert RO, Shin ST, Guard CL, et al. Prevalence of endometritis and its effects on reproductive performance of dairy cows. Theriogenology 2005;64:1879–88.
9. Hernandez JA, Garbarino EJ, Shearer JK, et al. Evaluation of the efficacy of prophylactic hoof health examination and trimming during midlactation in reducing the incidence of lameness during late lactation in dairy cows. J Am Vet Med Assoc 2007;230:89–93.
10. Oeztel GR. Oral calcium supplementation in peripartum dairy cows. Vet Clin North Am Food Anim Pract 2013;29:447–55.
11. Reinhardt TA, Lippolis JD, McCluskey BJ, et al. Prevalence of subclinical hypocalcemia in dairy herds. Vet J 2011;188:122–4.
12. Prior RL, Laster DB. Development of the bovine fetus. J Anim Sci 1979;48:1546–53.
13. Ford SP, Long NM. Evidence for similar changes in offspring phenotype following either maternal undernutrition or overnutrition: potential impact on fetal epigenetic mechanisms. Reprod Fertil Dev 2006;24:105–11.
14. Caton JS, Grazul-Bilska AT, Vonnahme KA, et al. Nutritional management during gestation: impacts on lifelong performance. In: Proc Florida Rumin Nutr Symp. Gainesville, FL. 2007. p. 1–20.
15. National Research Council. Nutrient requirements of dairy cattle. 5th revised edition. Washington, DC: National Academy Press; 1978.
16. National Research Council. Nutrient requirements of dairy cattle. 5th revised edition. Washington, DC: National Academy Press; 1989.
17. National Research Council. Nutrient requirements of dairy cattle. 5th revised edition. Washington, DC: National Academy Press; 2001.
18. National Research Council. Nutrient requirements of beef cattle. 6th edition. Washington, DC: National Academy Press; 1984.
19. National Research Council. Nutrients requirements of beef cattle. 7th revised edition. Washington, DC: National Academy Press; 1996.

20. Bell AW, Slepetis R, Ehrhardt RA. Growth and accretion of energy and protein in the gravid uterus during late pregnancy in Holstein cows. J Dairy Sci 1995;78: 1954–61.
21. Ellenberger HB, Newlander HA, Jones CH. Composition of the bodies of dairy cattle. Burlington (VT): Vermont Agric. Exp. Stn. Bull. 558; 1950.
22. Jakobsen PE. Protein requirement for fetus formation in cattle. In: Proceedings 7th Internat Cong Anim Husb. 1956;6:115.
23. Moe PW, Tyrrell HF. Metabolizable energy requirements of pregnant dairy cows. J Dairy Sci 1972;55:480–3.
24. National Research Council. Ruminant nitrogen usage. Washington, DC: National Academy Press; 1985.
25. Bell AW. Regulation of organic nutrient metabolism during transition from late pregnancy to early lactation. J Anim Sci 1995;73:2804–19.
26. Battaglia FC, Meschia G. Fetal nutrition. Annu Rev Nutr 1988;8:43–61.
27. McNeill DM, Slepetis R, Ehrhardt RA, et al. Protein requirements of sheep in late pregnancy: partitioning of nitrogen between gravid uterus and maternal tissues. J Anim Sci 1997;75:809–16.
28. Fox DG, Sniffen CJ, O'Connor JD, et al. A net carbohydrate and protein system for evaluating cattle diets: III. Cattle requirements and diet adequacy. J Anim Sci 1992;70:3578.
29. VandeHaar MJ, Donkin SS. Protein nutrition of dry cows. In: Proc Tri-State Dairy Nutr Conf. Ft. Wayne, IN. 1999. p. 112–23.
30. Bell AW, Burhans WS, Overton TR. Protein nutrition in late pregnancy, maternal protein reserves and lactation performance in dairy cows. Proc Nutr Soc 2000; 59:119–26.
31. Sniffen CJ. Grouping management and physical facilities. Vet Clin North Am Food Anim Pract 1991;7(2):465–71.
32. Woodward TE, Shepard JB, Graves RR. Feeding management investigations at the United States dairy experiment station at Beltsville, MD. 1930 Report. Beltsville (Maryland): US Dept of Agriculture Miscellaneous Publications; 1932. 130(a).
33. Campbell IL, Flux DS. The relationship between level of nutrition during the dry period and subsequent production of dairy cattle. In: Proc. 8th Ann. Conf., New Zealand Soc. Animal Production. 1948. p. 61.
34. Schmidt GH, Schultz LH. Effect of three levels of grain feeding during the dry period on the incidence of ketosis, severity of udder edema, and subsequent milk production of dairy cows. J Dairy Sci 1959;42:170–9.
35. Coppock CE, Noller CH, Wolfe SA, et al. Effect of forage-concentrate ratio in complete feeds fed ad libitum on feed intake prepartum and the occurrence of abomasal displacement in dairy cows. J Dairy Sci 1972;55:783–9.
36. Minor DJ, Trower SL, Strang BD, et al. Effects of nonfiber carbohydrate and niacin on periparturient metabolic status and lactation of dairy cows. J Dairy Sci 1998;81:189–200.
37. Mashek DG, Beede DK. Peripartum responses of dairy cows fed energy-dense diets for 3 or 6 weeks prepartum. J Dairy Sci 2001;84:115–25.
38. Dann HM, Litherland NB, Underwood JP, et al. Diets during far-off and close-up dry periods affect periparturient metabolism and lactation in multiparous cows. J Dairy Sci 2006;89:3563–77.
39. Allen MS, Piantoni P. Metabolic control of feed intake: implications for metabolic disease of fresh cows. Vet Clin North Am Food Anim Pract 2013;29:279–97.
40. Drackley JK, Janovick-Guretzky NA. Controlled energy diets for dry cows. In: Proceedings Western Dairy Management Conference. Reno, NV. 2007. p. 7–16.

41. Collier RJ, Annen EL, Fitzgerald AC. Prospects for zero days dry. Vet Clin North Am Food Anim Pract 2004;20:687–701.

42. Annen EL, Collier RJ, McGuire MA, et al. Effect of modified dry period lengths and bovine somatotropin on yield and composition of milk from dairy cows. J Dairy Sci 2004;87:3746–61.

43. Grummer RR, Rastani RR. Why reevaluate dry period length? J Dairy Sci 2004; 87(E Suppl):E77–85.

44. van Knegsel AT, van der Drift SG, Čermáková J, et al. Effects of shortening the dry period of dairy cows on milk production, energy balance, health, and fertility: a systematic review. Vet J 2013;198:707–13.

45. Bigras-Poulin M, Meek AH, Martin SW, et al. Health problems in selected Ontario Holstein cows: frequency of occurrences, time to first diagnosis and associations. Prev Vet Med 1990;10:79–89.

46. LeBlanc S. Monitoring metabolic health of dairy cattle in the transition period. J Reprod Dev 2010;56(Suppl):S29–35.

47. Cook NB, Nordlund KV. Behavioral needs of the transition cow and considerations for special needs facility design. Vet Clin North Am Food Anim Pract 2004;20(3):495–520.

48. Ospina PA, Nydam DV, Stokol T, et al. Association between the proportion of sampled transition cows with increased nonesterified fatty acids and β-hydroxybutyrate and disease incidence, pregnancy rate, and milk production at the herd level. J Dairy Sci 2010;93:3595–601.

49. Toni F, Vincenti L, Grigoletto L, et al. Early lactation ratio of fat and protein percentage in milk is associated with health, milk production, and survival. J Dairy Sci 2011;94:1772–83.

50. Nordlund KV. Transition cow index. In: The AABP Proceedings. 2006;39:139–143.

51. Bauman DE, Currie WB. Partitioning of nutrients during pregnancy and lactation: a review of mechanisms involving homeostasis and homeorhesis. J Dairy Sci 1980;63:1514–29.

52. Overton TR, Waldron MR. Nutritional management of transition dairy cows: strategies to optimize metabolic health. J Dairy Sci 2004;87(E Suppl):E105–19.

53. Drackley JK, Dann HM, Douglas GN, et al. Physiological and pathological adaptations in dairy cows that may increase susceptibility to periparturient diseases and disorders. Ital J Anim Sci 2005;4:323–44.

54. Roche JR, Bell AW, Overton TR, et al. Nutritional management of the transition cow in the 21st century–a paradigm shift in thinking. Anim Prod Sci 2013; 53(9):1000–23. http://dx.doi.org/10.1071/AN12293.

55. Xu S, Harrison JH, Chalupa W, et al. The effect of ruminal bypass lysine and methionine on milk yield and composition of lactating cows. J Dairy Sci 1998; 81:1062–77.

56. DeGaris PJ, Lean IJ, Rabiee AR, et al. Effects of increasing days of exposure to pre-partum diets on reproduction and health in dairy cows. Aust Vet J 2010;88: 84–92.

57. Curtis CR, Erb HN, Sniffen CJ, et al. Path analysis of dry period nutrition, postpartum metabolic and reproductive disorders and mastitis in Holstein cows. J Dairy Sci 1985;68:2347–60.

58. Holtenius P, Hjort M. Studies on the pathogenesis of fatty liver in cows. Bov Pract 1990;25:91–4.

59. Van Saun RJ. Effects of undegradable protein fed prepartum on subsequent lactation, reproduction, and health in Holstein dairy cattle. PhD Thesis. Ithaca (New york): Dept. Anim Sci, Cornell University; 1993.

60. van der Drift SG, Houweling M, Schonewille JT, et al. Protein and fat mobilization and associations with serum β-hydroxybutyrate concentrations in dairy cows. J Dairy Sci 2012;95:4911–20.
61. Phillips GJ, Citron TL, Sage JS, et al. Adaptations in body muscle and fat in transition dairy cattle fed differing amounts of protein and methionine hydroxyl analog. J Dairy Sci 2003;86:3634–47.
62. Van Saun RJ. Insulin sensitivity measures in dry dairy cows and relationship to body condition score (Abstr). In: Proceedings 14th International Congress of Production Diseases in Farm Animals. Ghent, Belgium. 2010. p. 43.
63. Van Saun RJ. Insulin sensitivity measures in lactating dairy cows and relationship to body condition score (Abstr 113). 26th World Buiatrics Congress. Santiago, Chile. 2010 (CD proceedings).
64. Canfield RW, Butler WR. Energy balance, first ovulation and the effects of naloxone on LH secretion in early postpartum dairy cows. J Anim Sci 1991; 69:740–6.
65. Van Saun RJ. Production factors influencing overall conception risk in dairy cows (Abstract P 599). In: Proceedings 27th World Buiatrics Congress, Abstract Book. Lisbon, Portugal. 2012. p. 184.
66. Van Saun RJ. Production factors influencing first service conception in dairy cows (Abstract OC 78). In: Proceedings 27th World Buiatrics Congress, Abstract Book. Lisbon, Portugal. 2012. p. 62.
67. Dalbach KF, Larsen M, Raun BM, et al. Effects of supplementation with 2-hydroxy-4-(methylthio)-butanoic acid isopropyl ester on splanchnic amino acid metabolism and essential amino acid mobilization in postpartum transition Holstein cows. J Dairy Sci 2011;94:3913–27.
68. Law RA, Young FJ, Patterson DC, et al. Effect of dietary protein content on animal production and blood metabolites of dairy cows during lactation. J Dairy Sci 2009;92:1001–12.
69. Bertoni G, Trevisi E, Han X, et al. Effects of inflammatory conditions on liver activity in puerperium period and consequences for performance in dairy cows. J Dairy Sci 2008;91:3300–10.
70. Van Saun RJ. Metabolic profiles for evaluation of the transition period. St. Paul (Minnesota): In: Proc 39th Ann Am Assoc Bovine Pract Conv 2006;39:130–8.
71. Burke CR, Meier S, McDougall S, et al. Relationships between endometritis and metabolic state during the transition period in pasture-grazed dairy cows. J Dairy Sci 2010;93:5363–73.
72. Roche JR, Kay JK, Phyn CV, et al. Dietary structural to nonfiber carbohydrate concentration during the transition period in grazing dairy cows. J Dairy Sci 2010;93:3671–83.
73. Overton TR, Burhans WS. Protein metabolism of the transition cow. In: Proc Cornell Nutr Conf. Syracuse, NY. 2013. p. 91–100.
74. Ji P, Dann HM. Negative protein balance: implications for transition cows. In: Proc Cornell Nutr Conf. Syracuse, NY. 2013. p. 101–12.
75. Bertoni G, Trevisi E, Lombardelli R. Some new aspects of nutrition, health conditions and fertility of intensively reared dairy cows. Ital J Anim Sci 2009;8:491–518.
76. Bernabucci U, Ronchi B, Lacetera N, et al. Influence of body condition score on relationships between metabolic status and oxidative stress in periparturient dairy cows. J Dairy Sci 2005;88:2017–26.
77. Ametaj BN, Bradford BJ, Bobe G, et al. Strong relationships between mediators of the acute phase response and fatty liver in dairy cows. Can J Anim Sci 2005; 85(2):165–75.

78. Bionaz M, Trevesi E, Calamari L, et al. Plasma paraoxonase, health, inflammatory conditions, and liver function in transition dairy cows. J Dairy Sci 2007; 90:1740–50.

79. Zebeli Q, Sivaraman S, Dunn SM, et al. Intermittent parental administration of endotoxin triggers metabolic and immunological alterations typically associated with displaced abomasum and retained placenta in periparturient dairy cows. J Dairy Sci 2011;94:4968–83.

80. Bossaert P, Trevisi E, Opsomer G, et al. The association between indicators of inflammation and liver variables during the transition period in high-yielding dairy cows: an observational study. Vet J 2012;192:222–5.

81. Lochmiller RL, Deerenberg C. Trade-offs in evolutionary immunology: just what is the cost of immunity? Oikos 2000;88:87–98.

82. Tylutki TP, Fox DG, Durbal VM, et al. Cornell net carbohydrate and protein system: a model for precision feeding of dairy cattle. Anim Feed Sci Technnol 2008; 143:174–202.

83. Allen MS. Adjusting concentration and ruminal digestibility of starch through lactation. In: Proc 4-State Dairy Nutr and Manage Conf. Debuque, IA. 2012. p. 24–30.

84. Weiss WP, Hogan JS, Todhunter DA, et al. Effect of vitamin E supplementation in diets with a low concentration of selenium on mammary gland health of dairy cows. J Dairy Sci 1997;80:1728–37.

85. LeBlanc SJ, Herdt TH, Seymour WM, et al. Peripartum serum vitamin E, retinol, and beta-carotene in dairy cattle and their associations with disease. J Dairy Sci 2004;87:609–19.

86. French P. How to meet the MP & AA needs of "most" cows. In: Proc Penn State Dairy Cattle Nutr Conf, RP Feed Components Post-Conference session. Grantville, PA. 2012. Available at: http://extension.psu.edu/animals/dairy/courses/dairy-cattle-nutrition-workshop/previous-workshops/2012/rp-feed-components-post-conference/practical-ration-guidelines-for-meeting-the-needs-of-most-transition-cows. Accessed March 29, 2014.

87. Lean IJ, Van Saun RJ, DeGaris PJ. Energy and protein nutrition management of transition dairy cows. Vet Clin North Am Food Anim Pract 2013;29:337–66.

88. Duffield TF, Rabiee AR, Lean IJ. A meta-analysis of the impact of monensin in lactating dairy cattle. Part 3. Health and reproduction. J Dairy Sci 2008;91:2328–41.

89. Sales J, Homolka P, Koukolová V. Effect of dietary rumen-protected choline on milk production of dairy cows: a meta-analysis. J Dairy Sci 2010;93:3746–54.

90. Morrow DA. Fat cow syndrome. J Dairy Sci 1976;59:1625–9.

91. Grummer RR. Etiology of lipid-related metabolic disorders in periparturient dairy cows. J Dairy Sci 1993;76:3882–96.

92. Rukkwamsuk T, Wensing T, Geelen MJ. Effect of overfeeding during the dry period on regulation of adipose tissue metabolism in dairy cows during the periparturient period. J Dairy Sci 1998;81:2904–11.

93. Bobe G, Young JW, Beitz DC. Pathology, etiology, prevention, and treatment of fatty liver in dairy cows. J Dairy Sci 2004;87:3105–24.

94. Hayirli A, Grummer RR, Nordheim EV, et al. Animal and dietary factors affecting feed intake during the prefresh transition period in Holsteins. J Dairy Sci 2002; 85:3430–43.

95. De Koster JD, Opsomer G. Insulin resistance in dairy cows. Vet Clin North Am Food Anim Pract 2013;29:299–322.

96. Garnsworthy PC, Topps JH. The effect of body condition of dairy cows at calving on their food intake and performance when given complete diets. Anim Prod 1982;35:113–9.

97. Waltner SS, McNamara JP, Hillers JK. Relationships of body condition score to production variables in high producing Holstein dairy cattle. J Dairy Sci 1993; 76:3410–9.

98. Domeqc JJ, Skidmore AL, Lloyd JW, et al. Relationship between body condition scores and milk yield in a large dairy herd of high yielding Holstein cows. J Dairy Sci 1997;80:101–12.

99. Contreras LL, Ryan CM, Overton TR. Effects of dry cow grouping strategy and prepartum body condition score on performance and health of transition dairy cows. J Dairy Sci 2004;87:517–23.

100. Nordlund KV. The five key factors in transition cow management of freestall dairy farms. In: Proc 46th Florida Dairy Production Conference. Gainesville, FL. 2009. p. 27–32.

101. Huzzey JM, von Keyserlingk MA, Weary DM. Changes in feeding, drinking, and standing behavior of dairy cows during the transition period. J Dairy Sci 2005; 88:2454–61.

102. Proudfoot KL, Veira DM, Weary DM, et al. Competition at the feed bunk changes the feeding, standing, and social behavior of transition dairy cows. J Dairy Sci 2009;92:3116–23.

103. Hosseinkhani A, DeVries TJ, Proudfoot KL, et al. The effects of feedbunk competition on the feed sorting behavior of close-up dry cows. J Dairy Sci 2008;91:1115–21.

104. Urton G, von Keyserlingk MA, Weary DM. Feeding behavior identifies dairy cows at risk for metritis. J Dairy Sci 2005;88:2843–9.

105. Huzzey JM, DeVries TJ, Valois P, et al. Stocking density and feed barrier design affect the feeding and social behavior of dairy cattle. J Dairy Sci 2006;89:126–33.

106. Gonzalez LA, Tolkamp BJ, Coffey MP, et al. Changes in feeding behavior as possible indicators for the automatic monitoring of health disorders in dairy cows. J Dairy Sci 2008;91:1017–28.

107. Goldhawk C, Chapinal N, Veira DM, et al. Prepartum feeding behavior is an early indicator of subclinical ketosis. J Dairy Sci 2009;92:4971–7.

108. von Keyserlingk MA, Olenick D, Weary DM. Acute behavioral effects of regrouping dairy cows. J Dairy Sci 2008;91:1011–6.

109. Overton TR, Nydam DV. Integrating nutritional and grouping management of transition cows. In: Proc Cornell Nutr Conf. Syracuse, NY. 2009. p. 104–10.

110. Cook NB, Bennett TB, Nordlund KV. Effect of free stall surface on daily activity patterns in dairy cows with relevance to lameness prevalence. J Dairy Sci 2004;87:2912–22.

111. Fregonesi JA, Veira DM, von Keyserlingk MA, et al. Effects of bedding quality on lying behavior of dairy cows. J Dairy Sci 2007;90:5468–72.

112. Tao S, Dahl GE. Heat stress effects during late gestation on dry cows and their calves. J Dairy Sci 2013;96:4079–93.

113. Collier RJ, Doelger SG, Head HH, et al. Effects of heat stress during pregnancy on maternal hormone concentrations, calf birth weight and postpartum milk yield in Holstein cows. J Dairy Sci 1982;54:309–19.

114. Van Saun RJ, Davidek J. Diagnostic use of pooled metabolic profiles in Czech dairy herds (Abstr). In: Proc 41st Ann Am Assoc Bovine Pract Conv. Charlotte, NC. 2008. p. 286.

115. do Amaral BC, Connor EE, Tao S, et al. Heat stress abatement during the dry period influences metabolic gene expression and improves immune status in the transition period of dairy cows. J Dairy Sci 2011;94:86–96.

116. do Amaral BC, Connor EE, Tao S, et al. Heat-stress abatement during the dry period: does cooling improve transition into lactation? J Dairy Sci 2009;92:5988–99.

Monitoring Total Mixed Rations and Feed Delivery Systems

Thomas J. Oelberg, PhD[a],*, William Stone, DVM, PhD[b]

KEYWORDS

- Total mixed ration (TMR) • TMR Audit • Mixing factors
- Penn State Particle Separator (PSPS) • Percent coefficient of variation • Sampling

KEY POINTS

- Total mixed rations (TMRs) are formulated to contain a combination of feedstuffs that provide the right balance of nutrients in every bite consumed.
- Poorly mixed TMRs negatively impact animal performance and health.
- A system has been developed to monitor the feeding process and the consistency of the TMR (TMR Audit is a system developed by Diamond V dairy technical specialist to evaluate TMR consistency. 2008).
- There are 9 main factors in the TMR mixing process that can each create variation in the TMR.
- Facing silage from bunkers and piles and premixing the defaced silage with a loader bucket or mixer wagon makes the silage more consistent in moisture and nutrients and is a key to minimizing variation between formulated and prepared diets.
- Mixing feedstuffs into a uniform TMR requires a lifting and dropping action created by augers, reels, paddles, or a combination of these elements in mixers.
- The Penn State Particle Separator (PSPS) is a useful tool to evaluate particle size variation in a TMR and to evaluate TMR consistency.
- TMR consistency or mix quality can be determined by performing PSPS analysis on 10 equally spaced samples of freshly delivered TMR along the feed bunk.

 Videos of pushing, lifting, and mixing defaced haylage as it is made into a pile; mixing and unloading haylage that was stored in a bag; mixing action of a well-maintained vertical mixer and lack of proper mixing action of a vertical wagon with a wornout kicker plate; 2 fresh cows in the same pen eating hay or grain in a TMR that was poorly mixed with underprocessed alfalfa hay; the influence of unlevel mixer box (left) and level mixer box (right) on distribution and

[a] Diamond V, 59562 414th Lane, New Ulm, MN 56073, USA; [b] Diamond V, 4619 Wyckoff Road, Auburn, NY 13021, USA
* Corresponding author.
E-mail address: toelberg@diamondv.com

Vet Clin Food Anim 30 (2014) 721–744
http://dx.doi.org/10.1016/j.cvfa.2014.08.003
0749-0720/14/$ – see front matter © 2014 Elsevier Inc. All rights reserved.

consistency of the TMR; feeder loading corn silage in the front of a dual-auger vertical mixer wagon; overfilled and normal-filled reel-auger mixer; overfilled 4-auger mixer and overfilled dual-auger vertical mixer; an underfilled dual-auger mixer containing close-up dry cow TMR with mineral remaining on the auger; grain mix does not get mixed into the TMR; liquid dispensed through a single pipe in front of the mixer box accompany this article at http:// www.vetfood.theclinics.com/

THE TOTAL MIXED RATION AUDIT

The TMR Audit is an on-farm evaluation of the following:

- Silage management
- Distribution and levels of feed and sorting across feed bunks
- Feed center organization and feed mixing equipment flow
- Total mixed ration (TMR) loading and mixing process
- TMR delivery
- Evaluation of the TMR particle size consistency within and across loads of TMR

This article focuses on reducing variation in TMRs with silage face management and with TMR loading and mixing.

REDUCING VARIATION IN CORN SILAGE AND HAYLAGE

A key part of the TMR Audit evaluates the feed out management of silages. Key practices that minimize dry matter (DM) and nutrient variation and silage spoilage are as follows:

- Vertical and smooth faces from where the silage is removed each day
- An adequate depth of silage is removed from the face each day to prevent heating and spoilage
- The leading edge of plastic covering the silage is cut back at least twice weekly to minimize spoilage and weighted with a continuous row of tires to prevent air from traveling across the silo beneath the plastic
- Spoiled silage is removed before facing
- Multiple layers of plastic, and the use of oxygen-limiting plastic, help to reduce spoilage
- The mechanically defaced silage is premixed with the loader bucket or mixer wagon before feeding
- Little to no loose silage should remain after feeding is complete

Significant variation in DM and nutrients often exists across the vertical face of haylage and corn silage stored in bunker silos.[1] Similar variation occurs in forages stored in bags and bales. A key management approach to minimizing this variation, and in making "the paper" ration more similar to the prepared TMR, is to premix forages before they are used to make a load of feed. For example, there was a stepwise reduction in the differences between the high and low content of crude protein (**Figs. 1–3**) in haylage sampled directly from the face (F) of a drive-over pile, from haylage mechanically faced into a windrow (WR) and from mechanically faced haylage after it was pushed and lifted into a conical shaped pile (P) as shown by the video (Video 1). **Fig. 4** shows average content and coefficients of variation of selected nutrients in alfalfa haylage sampled from the F, WR, and P. Pushing and lifting haylage into a pile with the pay loader created a mixing action that reduced the nutrient variation

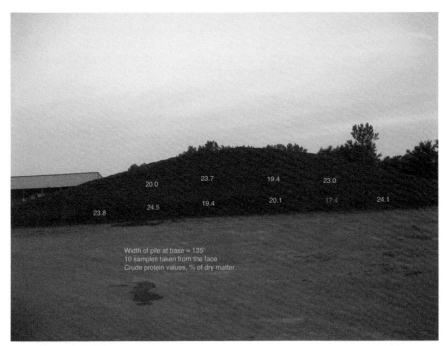

Fig. 1. The crude protein content expressed on a dry matter basis in 10 samples taken from the face of a haylage drive-over pile.

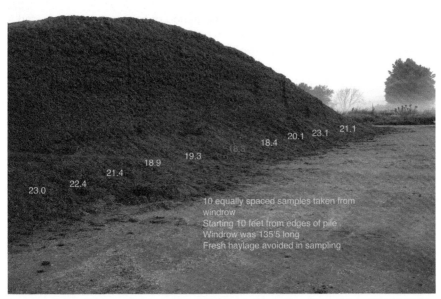

Fig. 2. The crude protein content expressed on a dry matter basis in 10 samples taken from haylage that was mechanically faced from a drive-over pile.

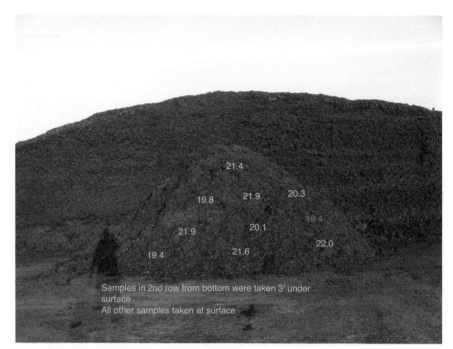

Fig. 3. The crude protein content expressed on a dry matter basis in 10 samples taken from haylage that was mechanically faced and then pushed and lifted into a conical-shaped pile.

in the haylage. This process can be done for corn silage and alfalfa hay bales. Haylage or corn silage stored in bags can vary a lot in moisture and nutrient content as one moves from one end to the other. Video 2 shows how haylage stored in a bag was loaded into a mixer, blended for a short period of time, and then unloaded at the feed center where the loading of TMRs occurred on this particular dairy.

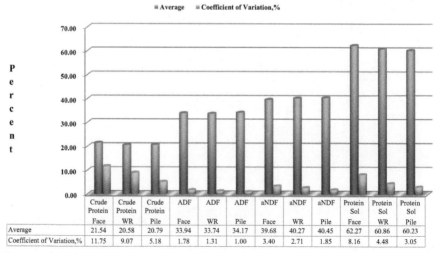

	Crude Protein Face	Crude Protein WR	Crude Protein Pile	ADF Face	ADF WR	ADF Pile	aNDF Face	aNDF WR	aNDF Pile	Protein Sol Face	Protein Sol WR	Protein Sol Pile
Average	21.54	20.58	20.79	33.94	33.74	34.17	39.68	40.27	40.45	62.27	60.86	60.23
Coefficient of Variation,%	11.75	9.07	5.18	1.78	1.31	1.00	3.40	2.71	1.85	8.16	4.48	3.05

Fig. 4. Reducing nutrient variation in alfalfa haylage.

TMR SAMPLING

Ten equally spaced samples of TMR are taken across the feed bunk for each load of TMR that is tested for consistency. Samples are taken immediately after the TMR is delivered and before the cows start eating and disturbing the TMR. Spacing of the samples is determined by counting the number of supporting posts along the feed bunk or along the freestalls and then divide that number by 10 (**Fig. 5**). A scoop (**Fig. 6**) is used to collect enough TMR to fill a quart-sized sample bag that can be sealed shut for subsequent analysis. Alternatively, as suggested in Lammers and colleagues,[2] collect a slightly packed sample with a volume of approximately 1.4 L. It is important that the size of all samples is similar to minimize sample-induced variability in the PSPS results. Collected sample sizes should range from 350 to 550 g depending on the TMR. Quart-sized or larger Ziploc bags are labeled (A–J, for example) with a dark-colored Sharpie with "A" representing the beginning (front of the mixer box) and "J" representing the ending of a load (back of the mixer box) of TMR. The detail on knowing front and back of the mixer box helps determine effects of loading position on the mixer box and unlevel mixer boxes on TMR mix quality (discussed later in this article). Note that the effects of loading position and unlevel boxes cannot be evaluated in wagons (usually triple-auger vertical) that unload from the front and back at the same time or when the feeder backs up several times along the bunk to deliver the TMR. However, variation of the TMR can still be evaluated in these situations by taking the 10 samples.

PENN STATE PARTICLE SEPARATOR PROCEDURE AND DATA ANALYSIS

- Arrange samples in order from A to J for each load
- Use the PSPS procedure on each sample, with a consistent sample size and PSPS technique.[2–4]

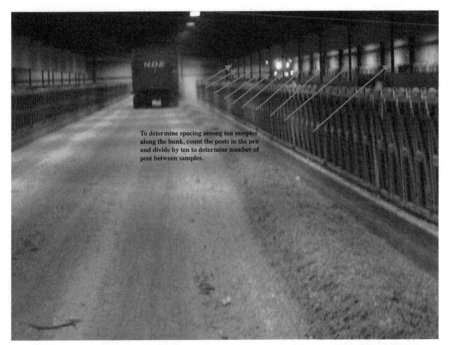

To determine spacing among ten samples along the bunk, count the posts in the pen and divide by ten to determine number of post between samples.

Fig. 5. Counting the posts along the feed bunk help determine the sampling interval.

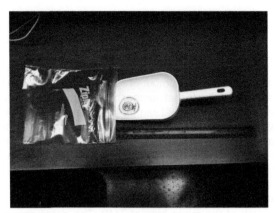

Fig. 6. Plastic scoop (1-pint) used to take TMR samples.

- Record weights for top, middle, and bottom screens
- Use a spreadsheet software to determine the average and SD. The percent co-efficient of variation (CV%) is determined for the top, middle, and bottom screens. The CV% is SD divided by the average times 100. The 4-screen system can be used, but CV artificially increases because percentage levels decrease on the third screen and pan causing the numerator in the CV calculation to become smaller. For the purpose of determining TMR consistency, the 3-screen system works better.
- Use the data from the middle and bottom screens to evaluate particle size consistency of the TMR. The middle and bottom screens are the important screens to use for milking rations.
- Use CV% as the standard for TMR particle size consistency (mix quality) and to test mixer efficiency.[5]
- Goal: 2% CV or less for the middle and bottom screens.
- Plot the data in a line chart and summarize the data as shown in **Table 1**.

Table 1
Penn State Particle Separator results on a total mixed ration along the length of a feedbunk to assess consistency of mixing

Bunk		Penn State Shaker Box, %		
Location	Bunk Sample No.	Top	Middle	Bottom
A Front of load	1	4.5	56.2	39.2
B	2	5.6	55.8	38.6
C	3	5.6	55.5	38.9
D	4	6.8	55.2	38.0
E	5	3.4	57.1	39.5
F	6	3.8	56.6	39.6
G	7	5.0	55.5	39.5
H	8	4.2	55.4	40.4
I	9	2.6	55.9	41.5
J Back of load	10	3.9	54.5	41.5
Average	Ave	4.5	55.8	39.7
Coefficient of variation	% CV	26.96	1.32	2.90

This procedure was adapted from the feed industry standard of testing mixer performance in feed mills.[5]

THE 9 FACTORS CAUSING TOTAL MIXED RATION VARIATION

The goal of the TMR Audit is to help reduce variation of the major ingredients (corn silage, haylage, and hay). The next part of the audit is to evaluate the TMR mixing process and reduce variation in the critical control points of making a TMR. There are 9 factors or critical control points that can contribute to TMR variation individually or in combination. Each of these is discussed in detail. They are as follows:

1. Worn mixer augers, kicker plates, and knives
2. Mix time after the last added ingredient
3. Unlevel mixers
4. Loading position on the mixer box
5. Load size
6. Hay quality and processing
7. Loading sequence
8. Liquid distribution
9. Vertical mixer auger speed

Worn Mixer Augers, Kicker (Deflector) Plates, and Knives

There are 2 major types of TMR mixers, horizontal and vertical, that can be pulled by tractors, mounted on trucks, or mounted as stationary mixers. There are several types of horizontal wagons:

- 4-augers
- Mono-mixer (1 auger)
- 3-augers
- Reel-auger
- Paddle
- Drum mixers

Figs. 7 and **8** are schematics of a 4-auger and reel-auger, respectively. Drum mixers are usually seen on small dairies that are mixing small batches of TMR or are used in larger feedlot operations to mix mineral and protein premixes. The most common horizontal mixers seen on dairies in the United States are 4-auger and reel-auger mixers. Vertical mixers are replacing the horizontal mixers in both the dairy and beef feedlot industries because they can mix larger volumes of wet feeds without getting overfilled too easily.

The vertical mixers are defined as follows:

- Single auger
- Dual auger
- Triple auger

Fig. 9 is a schematic of a dual-auger vertical mixer. Most types and brands of mixers can mix a high-quality TMR if the feeder follows the proper procedures for all 9 critical control areas. However, TMR particle size consistency, as well as moisture and nutrient consistency along the feed bunk (TMR mix quality), can decrease significantly with worn blades, kicker plates, and augers.

Worn augers

Mixers are factory set with specific agitator clearances of 0.3 to 0.9 cm.[6] As these clearances increase because of wear, mixer efficiency is impaired.[6] The easiest way

728

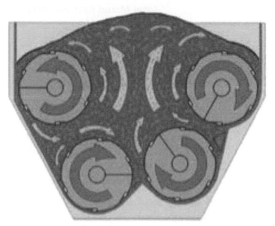

Fig. 7. A 4-auger horizontal mixer. (*Courtesy of* Kuhn North America, Inc., Brodhead, WI; with permission. Available at: http://www.kuhnnorthamerica.com/us/product-tips-tmr-mixer-guide.html.)

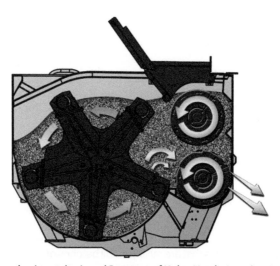

Fig. 8. A reel-auger horizontal mixer. (*Courtesy of* Kuhn North America, Inc., Brodhead, WI; with permission. Available at: http://www.kuhnnorthamerica.com/us/product-tips-tmr-mixer-guide.html.)

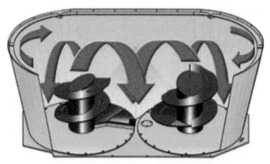

Fig. 9. A dual-auger vertical mixer. (*Courtesy of* Kuhn North America, Inc., Brodhead, WI; with permission. Available at: http://www.kuhnnorthamerica.com/us/product-tips-tmr-mixer-guide.html.)

to evaluate wear on augers is to look for feed under horizontal augers or reels (**Figs. 10** and **11**) and to look for the feed ring inside vertical mixers (**Fig. 12**). **Fig. 13** shows the changes in the levels of TMR in middle and bottom screens of the PSPS from the front (samples 1–5) to the back (samples 6–10) of the reel mixer shown in **Fig. 11**. These changes resulted in significant variation in the TMR particle size due to the malfunctioning part of the reel.

Worn kicker plates

Kicker plates or shoes are welded or bolted to the top and at the leading corner of the bottom piece of flighting on vertical augers. Some brands of mixers will bend part of the leading edge of the bottom flighting down toward the floor of the wagon to create a deflector. When the auger rotates, these devices lift the TMR upward to create a hole or space for the TMR to fall into. Also, these devices direct the feed toward the center of the auger so that the feed can be lifted and dropped into the holes. This action mixes the TMR. Video 3 (left video) is correct mixing action in a new mixer wagon and Video 3 (right video) is poor mixing action in a vertical wagon with a worn kicker plate. Notice in the video (see Video 3, left) how the TMR comes up through the top of the augers and then rolls toward and down the sides of the mixer box. Contrast to the video on the right where there is very little movement of the TMR because of the worn kicker plate. As a result, the TMR will be inconsistent in particle size distribution and chemical analysis. Inconsistent particle size maybe clumps of unprocessed hay, or clumps of haylage, or streaks of grain and/or protein concentrate in the TMR along the bunk. There also can be differences in moisture and nutrients in the TMR along the bunk. In addition to worn augers and kicker plates, rotational speed (rpm) of the auger can also affect movement of the TMR. Slow auger speed will make the TMR move up and down with no rolling action. This type of action will decrease mix quality, which is discussed in the section "Vertical Speed Auger Mixer."

Fig. 14, left, shows a well-conditioned kicker plate and **Fig. 14**, right, is a photo of a worn out kicker plate in Peecon mixer boxes. The arrow in the picture on the left shows a metal plate on top of the metal wedge welded to the flighting, whereas the arrow in the picture on the right shows the metal plate missing. The best way to determine what the kicker plate should look like is to download a photo of the new kicker plate from the Web site of the manufacturer and compare. **Fig. 15** is a photo of a worn deflector in a Trioliet mixer box resulting in feed lying on the floor of the mixer box.

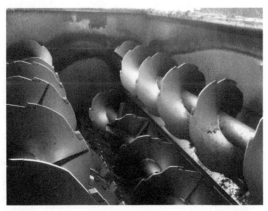

Fig. 10. TMRs under the augers indicate excessive wear, which decreases auger diameter and mixing ability.

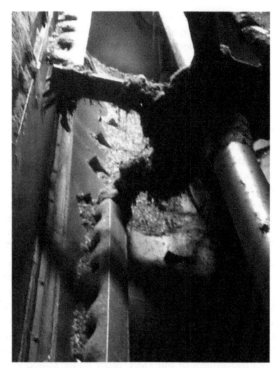

Fig. 11. TMR under the front part of the mixer rail indicating a bent or worn rail.

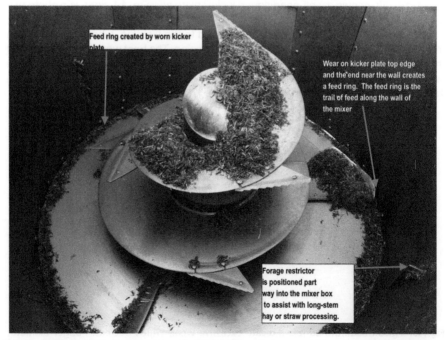

Fig. 12. TMR ring between augers and mixer wall suggests worn kicker plate and/or augers.

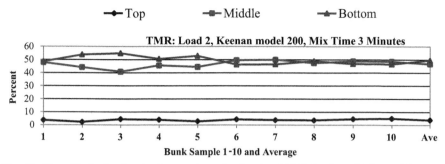

Fig. 13. The effect of a bent mixer reel on the levels of TMR in the middle and bottom screens of the PSPS.

Worn knives

Fig. 16, left, is a photo of a mixer box with sharp knives and **Fig. 16**, right, shows dull knives. Dull knives do not process alfalfa hay or baleage or straw very well, resulting in extra-long pieces or clumps of hay (shown in **Fig. 17**) that are easily sorted against and not eaten by cows. Video 4 is a video of 2 fresh cows eating the same ration at the same time; however, one is eating hay while the other is eating the grain because the forage was not well processed and the TMR not well mixed.

The degree and speed of wear on the augers, kicker plates, and knives depends on the size of the herd, and the amounts of hay, baleage, or straw fed. Routine replacement of blades, kicker plates, and augers is required to keep TMRs consistent. Feed managers should have maintenance programs in which these critical parts are inspected at least monthly.

Mix Time After the Last Added Ingredient

Several investigators have cited mixing time as a critical element to obtain consistent mixes.[6–8] Groesbeck and colleagues[5] showed that the amount of mix time after the last ingredient was added to a swine diet in a horizontal ribbon mixer was important in reducing the variation in the concentration of salt. Salt is an essential nutrient added to the diet and is often used in the feed industry as a marker to measure mixer efficiency.[5]

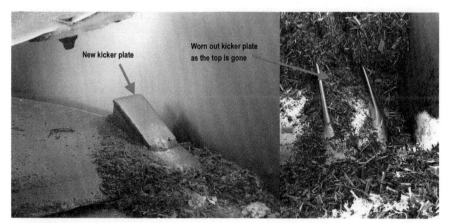

Fig. 14. A good conditioned (new) kicker plate (left photo) and a worn out kicker plate (right photo) in Peecon vertical mixer boxes.

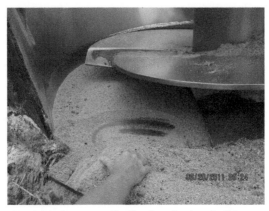

Fig. 15. The deflecting edge is worn off, allowing feed to build up on the floor of this Trioliet mixer box.

Mixer efficiency is defined as the amount of time needed to reach 10% CV or less among 10 samples.[5] One of the most common mistakes in TMR mixing is lack of mix time after the last added ingredient (usually corn silage or liquid supplement). With inadequate mix times, often the corn silage at the top of the load does not get mixed and is delivered toward the end of the load as pure corn silage. This is even more prevalent as mixer boxes are overfilled. Suggested mix times after the last ingredient with tractors/trucks at nearly full power (1700–2000 rpm engine speed) are as follows:

- Horizontal auger mixers: 5 minutes
- Horizontal reel-augers and verticals: 3–5 minutes

Inadequate mix times result in inconsistent TMRs, as shown in **Table 2** comparing 3.5 versus 5.0 minutes of mix time in a 4-auger horizontal mixer on CVs.

Unlevel Mixers

Video 5 is a video of a dual-auger vertical mixer on the left that has an improper hitch mount causing the wagon to be lower in front than in back. As a result, whole

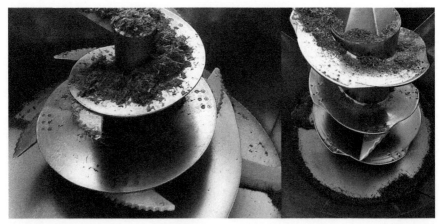

Fig. 16. Sharp knives in a vertical mixer box (left photo), and a vertical mixer with completely worn out knives (right photo).

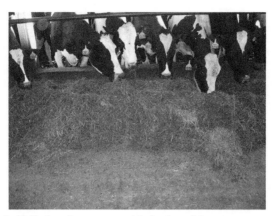

Fig. 17. Clumps of alfalfa hay from a round bale that did not get processed in a vertical mixer with dull knives.

cottonseed builds up at the front of the wagon due to poor distribution. The video on the right shows the very same mixer with the hitch adjusted to make it level. There is even distribution of ingredients, including whole cottonseed. **Fig. 18** shows the TMR from the unlevel load (left) and level load (right), respectively. The unlevel load of TMR was very inconsistent due to the grain-concentrate and whole cottonseed migrating to the lower part of the wagon during loading and mixing. **Fig. 19** shows PSPS analysis of 10 samples taken from a triple-auger vertical that was parked in a ramp that was too short. This caused the grain-concentrate portion of the TMR to migrate to the lower part of the wagon, which was the back end in this case. Notice how the amount of relatively more dense material in the bottom screen increases from sample 1 (front) to sample 10 (back), and the opposite trend is observed for the middle screen. The middle screen typically contains less dense feedstuffs, such

Table 2
Influence of mix time after the last added ingredient on total mixed ration mix quality (percent coefficient of variation [CV%])

| | Penn State Shaker Box Results | | | | | |
| | 3.5 min | | | 5 min | | |
Bunk Sample No.	Top	Middle	Bottom	Top	Middle	Bottom
1 Front	10.9	38.2	50.8	14.9	38.8	46.3
2	8.6	38.8	52.6	12.6	41.5	45.9
3	11.6	38.4	50.0	12.5	40.0	47.5
4	15.6	37.8	46.7	14.3	39.3	46.5
5	13.9	39.1	47.0	13.1	39.8	47.1
6	10.8	38.2	51.0	11.7	39.5	48.8
7	9.2	39.1	51.7	12.6	38.8	48.6
8	12.2	41.7	46.0	12.4	38.7	48.9
9	14.1	38.1	47.7	13.0	40.2	46.9
10 Back	11.6	37.3	51.1	11.4	39.3	49.3
Average, %	**11.8**	**38.7**	**49.5**	**12.8**	**39.6**	**47.6**
CV%	**18.52**	**3.11**	**4.81**	**8.15**	**2.12**	**2.56**

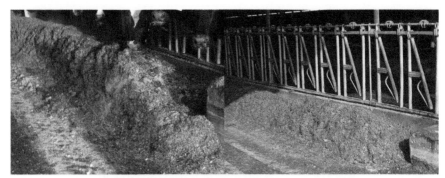

Fig. 18. The influence of unlevel mixer box (left photo) and of a level mixer box (right photo) on TMR consistency at the feed bunk.

as haylage and corn silage and small particles of hay. This is a typical pattern in the PSPS analysis for both unlevel mixer boxes and for improper loading position on vertical wagons.

Loading Position on the Mixer Box

Loading position refers to the location on the mixer box where the feeder is dumping ingredients. Improper loading position on the mixer box will create a poorly mixed TMR. The correct loading positions on mixer boxes are as follows:

- Reel with a horizontal auger should to be loaded over the augers in the center of the wagon
- Single-auger, dual-auger, triple-auger, and 4-auger horizontal mixers need to be loaded in the center of the box
- Single-auger verticals can be loaded from either side of the box
- Dual-auger verticals need to be loaded between the augers and can be loaded from either side
- Triple-auger verticals need to be loaded over the middle auger and can be loaded from either side
- One exception to loading position on the verticals is that the feeder needs to drop large round or square bales of forage directly on top and center of the augers to avoid bending the auger flighting

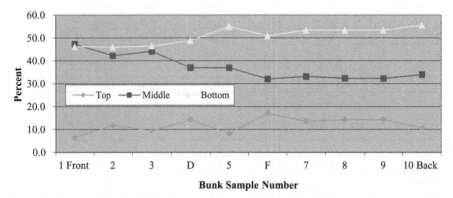

Fig. 19. Influence of unlevel mixer box on TMR particle size distribution on the PSPS screens.

Fig. 20 shows a feeder loading out of position on a dual-auger vertical mixer. This particular brand of mixer has placed a red dot on the side of the mixer denoting the proper loading spot. **Fig. 21** shows the influence of loading liquid in the front versus the middle of a dual-auger vertical mixer on TMR distribution in the middle and bottom screens of the PSPS. The liquid was a whey product that bound more of the small feed particles in the bottom screen to the larger particles in the middle screen at the front of the wagon. There was a continuous increase in the amount in the bottom screen as the load was discharged and more of the feed came from the back of the wagon. The opposite trend was seen for the middle screen. The mixer was moved ahead approximately 4 feet so that the liquid whey could be loaded between both augers or in the center of the mixer box. This resulted in the very consistent TMR shown by the dotted lines (see **Fig. 21**). **Fig. 22** shows the influence of loading a liquid protein supplement in the back of a dual-auger vertical wagon on moisture and protein content in the TMR. Both moisture and protein increase linearly as you move from the front to back of the wagon. This resulted in a very inconsistent TMR along the feed bunk. Because cows are quite territorial within the pen, an inconsistent TMR like this will result in cows consuming variable diets. This potentially leads to differences in rumen health and digestion, rumination patterns, and manure consistency among cows within the pen fed this ration. Video 6 shows a feeder dumping corn silage over the front auger of a dual-auger mixer wagon and **Fig. 23** shows the increased particle distribution in the middle screen of the PSPS for samples representing the front part of the wagon. As the amount of corn silage decreased on the middle screen, the particle amount in the top screen increased as the load was discharged from the front to the back of the wagon. Most dual-auger and triple-auger vertical wagons move feed back and forth in the wagon, but it takes time. These results show that feed dumped in either end of these wagons does not completely mix during routine mixing. If mixing time is increased so that the TMR is completely mixed, then there is increased risk of decreasing effective particle size in the TMR. The increased mixing time would also increase fuel and labor cost. Load all mixers at the proper position as designated by the manufacturer for best performance. Most of the examples on loading position were vertical wagons. However, the same effects of loading position (especially liquid supplements) on TMR mix quality have been observed in horizontal wagons.

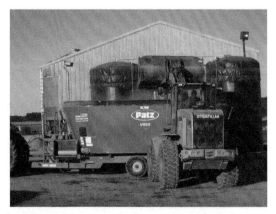

Fig. 20. Improper loading position on a dual-auger vertical mixer.

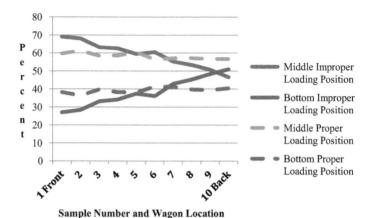

Sample Number and Wagon Location

Fig. 21. The influence of loading liquid whey in the front versus center of a dual-auger vertical mixer on levels of TMR in the middle and bottom screens of the PSPS.

Load Size

Overfilling of mixer wagons

Load capacity can be exceeded on all types of mixer wagons, resulting in a poorly mixed load of feed. This is a common TMR mixing error on many dairies and feedlots. Overfilling is a key cause of shrink during TMR loading and mixing. Shrink from overfilling is the loss of feed spilled on the ground. Overfilling occurs for several reasons:

- Undersizing the mixer box for the dairy
- Inaccurate pen counts
- Changes in forage moisture levels (ie, drier silages take up more space)
- Too large of an increase in bunk calls where the mixer box is already at full capacity

The videos in Video 7 show an overfilled reel-auger (left video) and one that is not overfilled (right video). Video 8 shows an overfilled horizontal mono-mixer (left video) and an overfilled dual-auger vertical (right video). Reducing the load size in the mono-mixer shown in Video 8 by 5000 pounds effectively decreased the CV

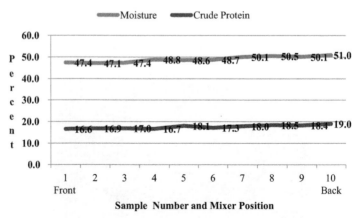

Sample Number and Mixer Position

Fig. 22. The influence of loading a liquid protein supplement in the back of a dual-auger wagon on moisture and crude protein levels in the TMR.

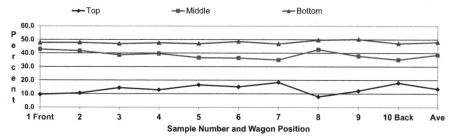

Fig. 23. Influence of loading corn silage in the front of a dual-auger vertical mixer wagon on the level of TMR in the middle and top screens of the PSPS.

(**Table 3**) for TMR particle size distribution in all 3 PSPS trays and improved TMR mix quality. Recommendations for filling mixer boxes are as follows:

- Reel-auger: allow 4 to 6 inches between the TMR and the rails on the reel (see Video 7 on the right)
- 3-auger and 4-auger horizontal: top of the metal side walls or where you can see good movement of the TMR
- Mono-mixer horizontal: where you can see good movement of the TMR and below the top of the metal side walls
- Vertical mixers: a good rule of thumb is 2 feet above the top of the augers for most brands and types of augers.

Underfilling vertical mixers

Underfilling of vertical mixers occurs when the TMR does not reach the top of the augers so that all of the ingredients are pushed off the augers and mixed. This happens often on smaller dairies that mix rations for smaller pens, such as fresh cow and close-

Table 3
Influence of load size in a mono-mixer horizontal mixer on total mixed ration mix quality (percent coefficient of variation [CV%])

| | Penn State Shaker Box Results | | | | | |
| | Overfilled[a] | | | Normal Filled[b] | | |
Bunk Sample No.	Top	Middle	Bottom	Top	Middle	Bottom
1 Front	4.9	45.9	49.2	5.6	44.8	49.6
2	2.9	46.3	50.7	6.0	46.0	48.0
3	2.3	44.2	53.5	4.7	46.2	49.1
4	3.8	44.0	52.2	7.4	45.9	46.7
5	4.8	43.8	51.4	5.5	44.5	50.0
6	3.4	47.7	48.9	8.8	42.8	48.5
7	4.3	44.6	51.1	7.0	46.5	46.5
8	3.8	44.2	51.9	8.1	44.1	47.8
9	7.0	37.3	55.7	7.2	43.9	48.9
10 Back	3.6	38.8	57.6	5.9	44.1	50.0
Average, %	4.1	43.7	52.2	6.6	44.9	48.5
CV%	31.58	7.39	5.22	19.35	2.72	2.58

[a] Total mixed ration was overflowing the sides of the mixer box and falling onto the ground.
[b] Load size was reduced by 5000 lb so that feed would not flow out of the mixer. The top of the feed was approximately 2 feet below the top of mixer box.

up dry cow pens. Video 9 shows a dual-auger mixer with close-up dry cow mineral remaining on the auger after loading is complete. Sometimes smaller loads like this can still mix properly if the augers are run at a higher speed.

Hay Quality and Processing

Most nutritionists and dairy producers prefer to have alfalfa hay in the TMR processed so that the maximum length is 3 to 4 inches. Straw should be processed shorter, with few particles longer than 2 inches. These particle lengths are recommended to provide good mixing and to prevent cattle from sorting against the forage. Sorting is a major problem on many dairies throughout the United States. Forage processing is best achieved with commercial grinders that are fitted with screens of defined pore sizes depending on whether alfalfa hay, grass hay, or straw is being ground. The screens used to grind alfalfa hay, grass hay, and straw usually have pore size diameters of 8, 6, and 4 inches, respectively, to grind these forages to desired length. Oftentimes, the same screen is used to process hay and straw by changing the rotational speed of the grinder. Slower speeds are used to process alfalfa hay and higher speeds are used to process straw. The nutritionist often works with the dairy to get the desired length of chop on the forages by experimenting with the grinder pore sizes and rotational speed on the grinder. However, many smaller dairies in United States process hay and straw through mixer wagons equipped with knives. The quality of the forage processing in mixer wagons is highly dependent on the number of knives, auger speed, and condition of the knives (see section on worn mixers, augers, and knives). If clumps of hay or long pieces of hay or straw are observed in the TMR, it usually means dull mixer knives or an inadequate amount of time that the forage was processed in the mixer. It could also be an ingredient mix order problem in which the forage was added later in the mix and was not given enough time to process. Poor hay quality and inadequate processing make TMRs very inconsistent and can affect both variation and level of milk components in a herd (**Fig. 24**).

Loading Sequence

Several investigators have addressed loading sequence as a factor contributing to TMR mix quality.[6–9] The loading sequence will depend on:

- Mixer wagon type (auger-reel vs 4-auger or vertical)
- Ingredient type (density, particle size, and shape and moisture level and flowability)

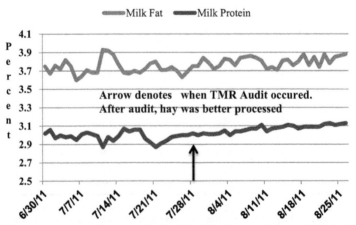

Fig. 24. Milk fat and protein levels in the bulk tank before and after a TMR Audit.

- Inclusion level[6]
- Convenience of loading based on where ingredients are stored at the feed center and time available to the feeder (not the most ideal situation on many dairies)

Generally, lower density and large particle feeds are loaded first, followed by dry more dense feeds followed by wet feeds and last with liquid. With the dry feeds of higher densities, the lower inclusion-level feeds are added first so that they can be blended properly.[6] Use the ratio of 50:1 to blend lower inclusion dry feeds, such as rumen bypass fats and vitamin/mineral premixes. Example, if 50 lb of rumen bypass fat is being added, then the load size should be no more than 2500 lb. The mixer should be running to allow the lower inclusion feed to mix.

An example of a dairy lactation TMR loading sequence in vertical and 4-auger mixers would be as follows:

1. Long-stem or chopped hay or straw
2. Dry grain (use as a carrier for blending low-inclusion dry feeds)
3. Low-inclusion dry ingredients
4. Protein mix
5. Wet by-products
6. Haylage
7. Corn silage
8. Liquid

If loading a reel-auger mixer, grain has to be added before hay or straw to prevent breaking or bending of the reel. Then follow the rest of the sequence shown previously. Sometimes, the order has to be adjusted to get a better TMR mix quality. An example is loading wet alfalfa haylage first or second so as to break down chunks of the haylage that may be frozen or simply clumped together.

Figs. 25 and **26** show the results of the PSPS on a lactating cow TMR with haylage added second to last and second, respectively, in a 4-auger horizontal mixer. Loading the haylage second behind the alfalfa hay with this particle type of wagon allowed the haylage and hay to blend and break down the forage chunks. The CVs for the middle and bottom screens decreased on an average from 7.8% to 1.8% with the change in mix order.

Fig. 27 is another example in which TMR mix quality was improved dramatically by increasing mix time from 2 to 4 minutes after the last added ingredient and then changing mix order to further improve the mix quality. This TMR was mixed with a dual-auger

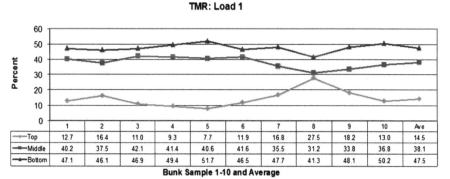

TMR: Load 1

	1	2	3	4	5	6	7	8	9	10	Ave
Top	12.7	16.4	11.0	9.3	7.7	11.9	16.8	27.5	18.2	13.0	14.5
Middle	40.2	37.5	42.1	41.4	40.6	41.6	35.5	31.2	33.8	36.8	38.1
Bottom	47.1	46.1	46.9	49.4	51.7	46.5	47.7	41.3	48.1	50.2	47.5

Bunk Sample 1-10 and Average

Fig. 25. PSPS results of a lactation TMR in which haylage was added second to last in a 4-auger horizontal mixer wagon.

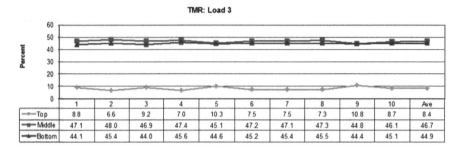

Fig. 26. PSPS results of a lactation TMR in which haylage was added second behind alfalfa hay in a 4-auger horizontal mixer.

vertical that was in excellent condition, was level, was not overfilled, the hay was well processed, and the liquid was well distributed.

Many farms load ingredients out of the proper order because of the daily routine of mixing and the convenience of where ingredients are stored on the dairy. Video 10 shows how the grain mix does not get mixed into the TMR when added last in combination with a worn out mixer. It is clearly evident that the grain does not mix appropriately.

Liquid Distribution

Liquids, such as water, whey, and cane molasses, are routinely added to the TMR to add moisture, sugar, or are used as a carrier for micro-ingredients as in the case for some commercial supplements of cane molasses. Another important reason liquids are added to the TMR is to help reduce sorting by cattle. The liquids, especially cane molasses and liquid whey, are sticky and they help bind the smaller particles to the larger forage particles. As a result, the levels on the bottom pan of the PSPS will shift to the middle and top screens by as much 5% to 7% units depending on type and level of liquid added directly to the TMR.

It is usually best to add the liquid last to the TMR to prevent any balling or clumping of the drier ingredients.[6] There are 2 challenges of adding liquid directly to the TMR: time and distribution. Depending on the amount of liquid added to the TMR and the sizes of the pumps and pipes to load the liquid, the amount of time it takes to add liquid can range from 2 to 10 minutes per load and sometimes even longer. This can create a

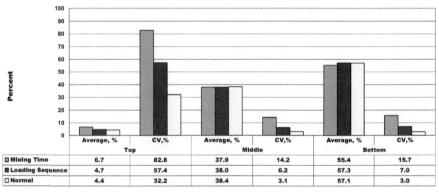

Fig. 27. Influencing of mixing time after the last added ingredient and loading sequence on TMR variation.

bottleneck in getting cattle fed on time for larger operations. Many dairy operations are adding the liquid to the on-farm commodity blend. The on-farm commodity blend is often a mixture of alfalfa hay and/or straw, protein, dry by-product feeds, and grain. The key advantages of the on-farm blend are *reduced feed shrink* and *less time to load the TMR*. It is best to make the blend fresh each day after all the cattle are all fed so that there is no interference with the feeding schedule.

Adding the liquid directly to the on-farm blend instead of the TMR decreases TMR loading time and helps feeders stay on time with respect to feeding pens of cows. Instead of loading 8 to 12 ingredients per load of TMR, the on-farm blend can reduce the number ingredients to 4, (example: on-farm blend, wet by-product, haylage, and corn silage).

Improper distribution of the liquid can make the TMR very inconsistent along the feed bunk. Video 11 shows liquid dispensed through a single pipe in front of the mixer box. Notice the difference in the distance from the top of the TMR and the top of the wagon between the front where the liquid is loading and the back of the wagon where there is no liquid. There is no mixing action between the wetter and drier TMR in this video because of poor distribution of the applied liquid. **Fig. 28** (photo) is a great example of how liquid should be added to a TMR or to an on-farm commodity blend.

Vertical Mixer Auger Speed

Vertical mixer augers lift feed upward from the bottom of the mixer to the top of the auger and then the feed rolls away from the top of the auger toward the mixer walls. As the feed approaches the walls, it falls to the bottom of the mixer to repeat the mixing process. Each revolution of the auger lifts the feed several inches and the amount of lift depends on the type of auger and brand of mixer box. The speed at which the auger rotates is critical to getting good mixing action, good clean out, and smooth delivery of the TMR along the feed bunk.

The following discussion is a case study on the apparent effects of vertical auger rotational speed on TMR mix quality and milk production for a large dairy herd. The mixer was a triple-auger mixer box with an initial auger speed of 42 rpm. The dairy replaced the 2-speed gearbox with a 3-speed gearbox for maintenance purposes. The feeder continued to mix in the lowest gear with the new gear box generating only 28 rpm on auger speed. There was a decrease in TMR mix quality with the lower

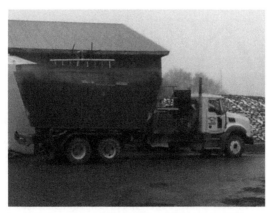

Fig. 28. A spray system to properly load liquid into a TMR or an on-farm commodity blend.

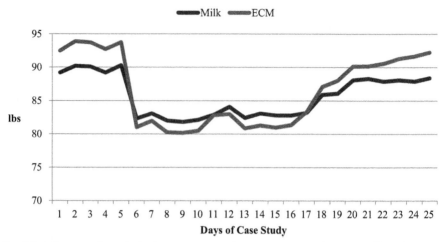

Fig. 29. Influence of vertical mixer auger speed on TMR mix quality and milk and energy corrected milk production.

auger speed and at the same time there were substantial decreases in energy-corrected milk (**Fig. 29**), fat and protein percentages, and a large increase in milk urea nitrogen (**Fig. 30**). Changing to second gear in the new gearbox increased auger speed to 38 rpm, improved TMR mix quality back to its original level, and improved milk production and components within 1 to 2 days after the change.

Table 4 is a list of several brands of vertical mixers with CVs of TMR mixed at low and higher auger speeds. The data in **Table 4** show better mix quality with higher auger speeds. Most brands of vertical mixers can make very uniform TMRs with co-efficients of variation approaching 2% for averages observed on the middle and bottom screens of the PSPS.

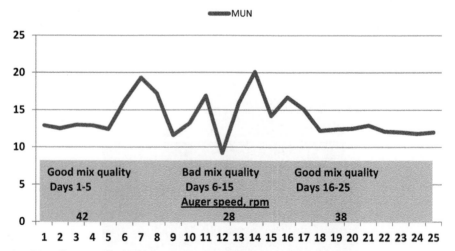

Fig. 30. Influence of vertical mixer auger speed on TMR mix quality and milk urea nitrogen.

Table 4
A summary of different brands of vertical mixers with slow and fast auger speeds on the average percent coefficient of variation of shaker box levels in the middle and bottom screens for lactation total mixed rations

Vertical Mixer	Auger Speed	
	Slow	Fast
Kuhn VTC 1100, dual auger (Kuhn North America, Brohead, WI)	3.50	2.00
Peecon, 3-auger (Peeters Landbouwmachines, The Netherlands)	5.00	1.78
Penta 1420 HD, dual auger (Penta TMR Inc, Canada)	6.13	2.19
Roto Mix 1355, dual auger (Roto-Mix, Dodge City, KS, USA)	5.00	3.24
Supreme 1600 with Forage Auger, dual auger (Supreme International Ltd, Canada)	8.53	2.45
Supreme with Feedlot Auger 1200T, dual auger (Supreme International Ltd, Canada)	—	2.11
Trioliet (Trioliet, The Netherlands)	4.83	2.81
Average	5.50	2.37

SUMMARY

A system to test TMR consistency along the feed bunk and to evaluate mixer performance has been developed. Implementation of this system has improved TMR consistency on many dairies across the United States. The standard for TMR particle size consistency determined on 10 samples is 2% or less CV for the average levels on middle and bottom screens of the PSPS.

ACKNOWLEDGMENTS

The authors thank the following Diamond V colleagues for their many contributions to this article: David Greene, Mark Tegeler, Dr Jeff Mikus, Dr Brian Perkins, Mitch Deimund, Kristy Pagel, Todd Franz, Kyle Moos, Dr Kristy Dorton, Don Martel, John Miller, Mark Anderson, and Nick Nickerson.

SUPPLEMENTARY DATA

Supplementary data related to this article can be found online at http://dx.doi.org/10.1016/j.cvfa.2014.08.003.

REFERENCES

1. Stone WC. Nutritional approaches to minimize subacute ruminal acidosis and laminitis in dairy cattle. J Dairy Sci 2004;87(E Suppl):E13–26.
2. Lammers BP, Buckmaster DR, Heinrichs AJ. A simplified method for the analysis of particle sizes of forages and total mixed rations. J Dairy Sci 1996;79:922–8.
3. Kononoff PJ, Heinrichs AJ, Buckmaster DR. Modification of the Penn State forage and total mixed ration particle size separator and the effects of moisture content on its measurements. J Dairy Sci 2003;86:1858–63.
4. Kononoff PJ, Heinrichs AJ, Lehman HA. The effect of corn silage particle size on eating behavior, chewing activities, and rumen fermentation in lactating dairy cows. J Dairy Sci 2003;86:3343–53.

5. Groesbeck CN, Goodband RD, Tokach MD, et al. Effects of salt particle and sample preparation on results of mixer-efficiency testing. Swine Day. 2004. p. 177–81. Available at: http://krex.k-state.edu/dspace/handle/2097/1909.

6. Zinn RA. A guide to feed mixing. 2004. U of CA, Davis. Available at: http://animalscience.ucdavis.edu/faculty/zinn/pdf/04.pdf.

7. Behnke KC. Mixing and uniformity issues in ruminant diets. Penn State Dairy Cattle Nutrition Workshop. Grantville, PA. Nov 9-10, 2005. p. 39–45.

8. Biermann S. Mixing integrity for ruminant diets containing by-products. Minnesota Nutrition Conf. Owatonna, MN. September 16-17, 2009. p. 145–59. Available at: http://spac.adsa.org/showpdf.asp?file=proceedings+of+the+2008+minnesota+nutrition+conference%5C0145%2Epdf.

9. Barmore J. Fine-tuning the ration mixing and feeding of high producing herds. Tri-State Nutrition Conf. 2002. p. 103–26. Available at: http://spac.adsa.org/showpdf.asp?file=proceedings+of+tri-state+dairy+nutrition+conference+2002%5C0103%2Epdf#search=%22barmore+AND+CONFERENCE+IS+Tri%2DState+Dairy+Nutrition+Conference%22&.

Nonnutritional Factors Influencing Response to the Nutritional Program

Dan F. McFarland, MS[a],*, John T. Tyson, MS[b],
Robert J. Van Saun, DVM, MS, PhD[c]

KEYWORDS

• Facilities • Dairy shelter • Heat abatement • Feed bunk • Feeding area

KEY POINTS

- The design and management of each animal shelter component (feeding, resting, drinking, floor surface, ventilation) can influence the willingness and ability for dairy cows to consume an adequate amount of dry matter.
- The design of the feeding area should provide a comfortable feeding experience for cows and convenient management for the caretaker.
- Good animal shelter and feeding area design cannot make up for poor (or varying) feed quality or poor management.
- Existing facility components that influence feed consumption can usually be improved.
- Heat stress can adversely affect feed intake, rumination, and metabolic status, resulting in greater predisposition to disease conditions.
- Heat abatement strategies should first focus on cooling cows in stalls, then address the feeding area.

ANIMAL SHELTER DESIGN BASICS

Clean, healthy, productive dairy cows require at least 5 basic elements from a dairy shelter. They include:

- Excellent air quality
- A clean, dry, comfortable resting area

Funding Sources: Nil (D.F. McFarland and J.T. Tyson); Pennsylvania Department of Agriculture Grant #44123907, Zoetis Unrestricted funds grant (Dr R.J. Van Saun).
Conflict of Interest: Nil.
[a] Penn State Extension York County, 112 Pleasant Acres Road, York, PA 17402-9041, USA; [b] Penn State Extension Mifflin County, 152 East Market Street, Suite 100, Lewistown, PA 17044-2125, USA; [c] Department of Veterinary & Biomedical Sciences, College of Agricultural Sciences, Pennsylvania State University, 115 W.L. Henning Building, University Park, PA 16802-3500, USA
* Corresponding author.
E-mail address: dfm6@psu.edu

- Convenient access to (and supply of) good-quality feed
- Convenient access to (and supply of) good-quality water
- Confident footing

These elements provide the opportunity for cows to be productive and must not be compromised in dairy shelter design. Proper design and management of a dairy shelter (not just the feeding area) is necessary for dairy cows to take full advantage of a ration that has been carefully balanced, formulated, prepared, and delivered. Altered feeding behavior pre partum is associated with greater risk for metritis[1] and subclinical ketosis,[2] although cows experiencing a range of postpartum diseases showed lower prepartum intake compared with healthy cows.[3,4] Competition for feed bunk space, because of overcrowding or poor design, may result in sorting[5] or altered animal behavioral responses,[6] predisposing primiparous or submissive cows to diseases. In many ways, facility design can make or break the quality of a nutritional program. In this article, some design considerations for the feeding and drinking water areas are described, as well as other factors that may influence feed intake and animal health in freestall shelters.

FACTORS INFLUENCING FEED INTAKE

Although good design of the feeding and drinking water areas is important, it is not the only factor that may prevent or discourage dairy cows from consuming a desired (or expected) amount of dry matter. The following factors contribute to reduced feed intake:

1. Feed not available to cows
2. Cows not able to feed
3. Poor or varying feed quality
4. Undesirable eating area
5. Feed not within reach
6. Sick cows
7. Injured cows
8. Lame cows
9. Hot cows
10. Thirsty cows
11. Submissive cows
12. Feeding area difficult to get to
13. Cows associate pain with feeding
14. Not enough feeding space

For items 1 to 5, feeding area management has more influence than design. These items may seem obvious or trivial but are often overlooked. How many farms have you visited where the feed table was empty or feed not pushed within cow reach? Timely feed delivery, feed push-back, and feed area cleaning are high-priority tasks on dairy farms achieving high milk production levels. The amount of time cows spend away from feed (eg, milking center, exercise lot) should also be considered. Many producers, dairy scientists, and nutritionists suggest that cows should not be away from feed more than 3 hours per day. The more time cows spend away from the feeding area, the more critical adequate feeding space becomes, because the entire group may want to eat at the same time.

Healthy, mobile cows are more likely to visit the feeding area regularly. The environment surrounding the cows and herd health management influence items 6 to 9. Air quality, resting area comfort and cleanliness, and the floor surface all affect cow health and well-being. Ventilation system design and management should provide an adequate air exchange and good air mixing during all seasons. The resting area needs to provide comfort, promote cleanliness, and reduce chance of injury. The floor surface should be cleaned regularly (especially in cold weather), provide good traction, and not injure the cows' feet. Provide space to isolate sick, injured, or lame cows that need to be separated from the group to receive special care and recover.

Heat stress can significantly affect feed intake.[7] If a cow cannot adequately get rid of the heat she is producing, why create more? Good ventilation and heat stress abatement methods (circulation fans, spray cooling, or evaporative cooling) can help cows maintain dry matter intake and milk production during hot weather.

THE FEEDING AREA: GROUP HOUSING

The remaining items listed influence the feeding area design. Proper design considers cow dimensions, typical bovine feeding behavior, method of feed delivery, and feeding area management. The feeding area should[8,9]:

- Encourage and allow each cow to consume an adequate amount of feed dry matter during each feeding episode and throughout the day.
- Provide a comfortable feeding experience for the cow.
- Facilitate 24-hour availability of high-quality feed.
- Be clean and easy to clean.

Basic design guidelines for construction and management of modern group feeding systems include[8]:

- Cows are fed at a fence line, not a walk-around feed bunk.
- Facing fence lines are far enough apart to negate feeling of confrontation.
- Cow alleys wide enough to allow cows and caretakers to pass behind feeding cows without disturbing them.
  - Minimum 3.7 m (12 ft) clearance allows for 2 cows to pass behind cows at feed line
  - 3.96 to 4.26 m (13 to 14 ft) clear if rear curb of freestalls located along opposite edge of feeding alley
- Cows eat in normal head down (grazing) position: eating surface (feed table) located 5.08 to 15.2 cm (2 to 6 in) above cow alley.
- Flat feed table to encourage easy mechanical clean-out and feed push-back.
- Smooth, nonporous, easy-to-clean eating surface (feed table) that is 81.3 to 91.4 cm (32 to 36 in) wide.
- A hard surface area at same elevation as eating surface where feed is stored after delivery or where cows may push feed away during eating.
  - Approximately 61 cm (24 in) wide
  - Surface beyond feed table should slope away 0.318 cm per 30.5 cm (1/8 in per ft)
- Feed should be pushed or scraped back to the eating surface, toward the cow, without becoming contaminated with gravel or mud from unpaved driveway or vehicle track in.
- Driveway is wide enough to allow delivery vehicle to pass without driving where feed is to be delivered or on previously delivered feed.
  - Feed delivery alleys with feeding fence line on both sides should provide a minimum 4.88 m (16 ft) clear, with 5.5 to 6.1 m (18 to 29 ft) preferred.
  - Feed delivery alleys with feeding fence line on 1 side should provide a minimum 3.7 m (12 ft) clear, with 3.96 to 4.26 m clear preferred.
- Door openings should be wide and high enough to allow largest expected feeding equipment to pass without damage.

- o 4.3 m (14 ft) high typical
- o Door width should be at least 0.3 to 0.6 m (1 to 2 ft) wider than feeding unit with discharge chute in feeding position
- Separation device, or feed barrier, allows cows convenient access to feed table without undue twisting, turning, or repositioning of the head and neck.
- Expected contact points between cow and separation device are shaped and located to prevent abrasion, penetration, or bruising.

Feeding space per cow is calculated by dividing the total length feeding space provided along the fence line by the number of cows that have access to it. Approximately 68.6 to 76.2 cm (27 to 30 in) of feeding space per cow is needed for entire group to stand and eat comfortably at the fence line at the same time. Well-designed 2-row and 4-row freestall shelter layouts can provide enough fence line length for all cows in a group to eat at once, if the group is not overpopulated.

Properly designed 3-row and 6-row freestall shelters provide approximately 48.3 cm (19 in) of feeding space per cow, which is not enough for all cows in the group to eat at once. Overpopulating a group further reduces the available feeding space per cow. **Table 1** shows the effect of various overpopulation rates on available feeding space per cow. The importance for all cows to eat at the same time is a management decision, not an engineering decision.[8]

A study of feed bunk length requirements for Holstein dairy heifers found that limited feed bunk length did not affect group growth rates, but significantly affected individual growth rates.[10] Perhaps, the same is true with respect to individual dry matter intake and milk production of lactating dairy cows. Continued research on feeding space for high-producing dairy cows is necessary.

To allow better access and more uniform feed consumption along the feeding area, crossover lanes between the feeding and resting areas should be provided every 18.3 to 24.4 m (60 to 80 ft).[9] This is especially important in freestall arrangements, in which feeding area access for 67% to 100% of the stalls is located in a cow alley opposite the feeding alley.

The feed barrier must allow each cow convenient, injury-free access for eating and prevent her from walking onto the feeding area. She should be allowed to consume feed in a natural way, with a minimum of annoyance or obstruction by the feed barrier or separation device. The separation device should also protect feed from contamination by manure and minimize feed spillage into the standing area.[8] Two feed barriers types commonly found in modern freestall shelters are the post and rail design and self-locking stanchions (**Fig. 1**).

Table 1
Effect of various group population rates on approximate feeding space per cow in typical freestall shelters

| Overpopulation Rate (%) | Approximate Feeding Space per Cow, cm (in) | |
	2-Row Barn	3-Row Barn
0	76.2 (30)	48.3 (19)
10	71.1 (28)	44.7 (17.6)
20	66.0 (26)	40.6 (16.2)
30	61.0 (24)	37.8 (14.9)
40	55.9 (22)	35.3 (13.9)
50	52.1 (20.5)	33.0 (13)

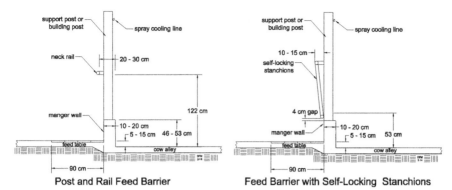

Fig. 1. Typical feed barrier types and dimensions for mature Holstein cows (1400 lb).

The post and rail feed barrier provides excellent access to the feed table for cows and is inexpensive to construct. Proper placement of the upper rail allows the cow good access to feed with a minimum of interference. The neck of the cow should nudge the rail only slightly as she reaches for and consumes feed.

Self-locking stanchions, often called head-locks, allow a group of cows, or a single cow, to be restrained for observation, treatment, or other herd management activities. They are often mounted on a slant so that the cows can reach further into the feeding area more comfortably.[11]

It is important to select a stanchion design that allows each cow to insert her head and neck easily and comfortably through the access opening, without excessive head twisting and turning. Some manufacturers have overlooked this important design consideration, perhaps intending to provide more openings in a given length, simplifying assembly, or saving material. Designs are available that allow the lower portion to open wide to aid cow release if a cow falls while her head is in the stanchion.

The feed table eating surface must be smooth, clean, and free of leftover feed and debris to encourage good feed intake and aid in disease control.[12] The low pH of silage can etch the manger surface, exposing the cow's tongue and mouth to rough edges.[13] High-strength concrete and admixtures are used to improve the durability of feeding surfaces. Properly installing tile along the feed table provides a durable, smooth surface. Epoxy coatings are also used but must be applied properly to allow good adhesion.[9]

Without proper care and management, any feeding area design can fail. Feed should be readily available to the cows, and cows should be able to feed. This point is especially important in feeding areas with limited feeding space or overpopulated groups. Cows tend to work feed away from feed barrier and out of reach as they eat. Feedstuffs should be pushed back regularly so it is readily available when cows approach the feeding area. Debris and unconsumed feed should be removed daily, so fresh feed may be put in its place. The feeding area should be well ventilated, and the cow alley cleaned frequently so cows do not stand in an accumulation of manure and urine.

Elevated Feed Bunks

The feed table height on older elevated feed bunks is commonly 50.8 cm (20 in) or more above the cow standing surface. This specification most likely came from their use in loose housing systems before 1950, in which the elevated design accommodated bedded manure packs. As the level of the pack increased, the relationship of the cow to the feed table changed. Some recommendations suggested adequate manger guards be installed to prevent cows from falling into the manger.[12]

Elevated bunks with feeding access on both sides, also known as H-bunks, are generally 1.2 to 1.5 m (4 to 5 ft) wide. Cows eating at 1 side of the bunk tend to push feed within reach of cows on the other side. Some dairy managers rely on this back-and-forth action for emptying the bunk, because entering it to clean it is difficult, especially if a mechanical bunk feeder is used. Splitting the elevated bunk to allow different rations to be fed along each side often creates a dark, poorly ventilated feeding area, which becomes even more difficult to clean.

Sanitary steps, 30.5 to 40.6 cm (12 to 16 in) wide and 15.2 cm (6 in) high, are commonly found at the base of elevated feed bunks. These steps discourage cows from defecating or urinating into the bunk, further reducing the need to clean the feed table. Observation indicates that cows avoid the step until they can no longer reach feed, and when they do, their eating posture seems awkward.

Renovating Elevated Feed Bunks

The cow standing area adjacent to the feeding area is regularly cleaned in modern freestall and loose housing dairy systems, and therefore, the need for an elevated feed table is unnecessary. Many producers have noticed improved feed intake when an elevated feed bunk is replaced with a unit that incorporates features described earlier that allow a more natural cow feeding posture and a smooth clean surface.

Fig. 2 shows how a more desirable feeding area can be created in the same space occupied by an elevated feed bunk using a mechanical feeder.

Systems in which feed is delivered by a mobile unit require a clear opening between the top of the feed manger wall and the feed barrier neck rail. One method to accomplish this goal is by suspending a horizontal rail supported from the opposite side, as shown in **Fig. 3**. Securing the rail at each end of the feed bunk helps limit its movement.

GOOD ACCESS TO WATER

Water plays an important role in milk production, temperature control, and body functions for dairy cattle. Cows may consume 2.2 to 2.3 kg of water, from drinking and feed, per pound of milk produced.[14] Providing the opportunity for dairy cows to consume a large quantity of clean, fresh water is essential.

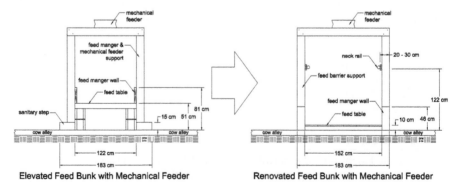

Elevated Feed Bunk with Mechanical Feeder   Renovated Feed Bunk with Mechanical Feeder

Fig. 2. Elevated feed bunk with mechanical feeder (*left*) refitted using modern feeding area guidelines (*right*).

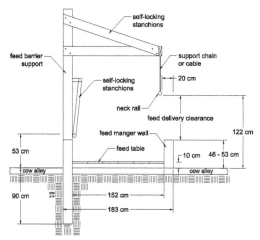

Renovated Feed Bunk for Drive-By Feed Delivery

Fig. 3. Refitted feed bunk to allow drive-by feeding with mobile feeder.

Drinking water satisfies 80% to 90% (**Table 2**) of the dairy cow's total water needs.[15] Plenty of good-quality, frost-free drinking water must be conveniently located in areas where cows spend most of their time and offered from watering units that allow cows to easily drink. Mature cows can consume up to 19.25 L (5 gallons) of water per minute. Water system must be size and design must allow each station to keep up with peak demand. Water station must also be easy to clean and must be cleaned regularly.

Periods of highest water intake occur when feed intake is greatest. Given the opportunity, cows alternately consume feed and drink water. Fresh, clean water should be available whenever cows consume feed.[16] Cows also tend to seek drinking water soon after being milked. Cows experience heat stress in areas of the United States that have extended periods of hot weather. Having sufficient drinking water available, and even adding additional water stations, during warm weather is desirable.

Basic water station design guidelines:

- Provide at least 2 water stations per group to reduce effect of dominant cows.[17]
- Provide adequate water vessel space per cow within a group.
  - Ensure that a minimum of 5% to 7% of a group can drink at the same time.[18] Needed trough length is calculated as 3.0 to 4.1 cm (1.2 to 1.6 in) of accessible linear space times cow number in the group.

Table 2
Drinking water intake by dairy cattle

	Daily Milk Production, kg/d (lb/d)	Daily Drinking Water Intake[a], L/d (gallons/d)
Lactating cows[b]	13.6 (30)	69.3-84.7 (18-22)
	22.7 (50)	88.6-104.0 (23.27)
	36.3 (80)	115.5-138.6 (30-36)
	45.4 (100)	134.8-157.9 (35-41)
Dry cows	Pregnant (6–9 mo)	27.0-50.1 (7-13)

[a] Higher water intakes apply to higher dry matter rations.
[b] Cattle under heat stress may require 1–1.2 times more water per day.
Adapted from Adams RS. Calculating drinking water intake for lactating cows. In: Walker K, editor. Dairy reference manual. 3rd edition. Ithaca (NY): NRAES; 1995. p. 145.

- For milking parlor water access or heat stress conditions, allow for 15% to 20% of the group to drink at the same time (Dennis Armstrong, MS, personal communication, 1998, Tucson, AZ). Needed trough length is calculated as 3.5 to 4.8 in of accessible linear space times cow number in the group.
- Place water stations in crossovers (**Fig. 4**).[19]
  - Minimum 3.4 m (11ft) clear for single-file travel behind cows at waterer.
  - Minimum 4.6 m (15 ft) clear for 2-direction travel behind cows at waterer.
- Provide minimum water supply of 22.7 to 37.8 L (6–10 gallons) per minute per waterer.
- Place water vessel at proper height (**Fig. 5**).
  - Top edge 61.0 to 81.3 cm (24 to 32 in) from cow alley for large-framed cows. Reduce 5.1 to 7.6 cm (2 to 3 in) for smaller framed cows.
  - Water level 5.1 to 10.2 cm (2 to 4 in) below top edge.
  - Shallow water depths 10.2 - 20.3 cm (4–8 in) preferred.
- Place guard rail directly above watering unit top edge 121.9 to 152.4 cm (48 to 60 in) from floor surface.
  - Provide 61 cm (24 in) clear vertical opening from top edge of waterer.
- Provide concrete support base that provides a 5.1 cm (2 in) ledge beyond the perimeter of watering unit.

THE RESTING AREA

Dairy cows spend a significant portion of their day resting and ruminating. When cows lie down, they take pressure off their feet and legs, which can reduce lameness. Several studies indicate that cows tend to lie down 10 to 14 hours per day. The type of housing, stall or resting area comfort, type of diet, pregnancy, and climatic factors all have an effect on resting time of lactating dairy cows.[20] Cows prefer dry bedding, and stand for greater lengths if only wet bedded stalls are available.[21] Stall surface can influence usage and cow preference, which can influence prevalence of leg lesions and lameness risk or recovery.[22,23]

Properly designed freestalls provide a clean, dry, comfortable resting area with good air circulation, protection from other animals, and do not cause injury or entrapment. Ease of maintenance is also important, but animal comfort and cleanliness should be the primary factors to consider when selecting a freestall structure, resting surface, bedding, and management combination.

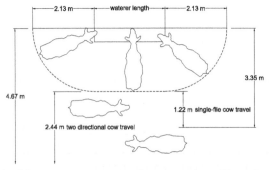

Fig. 4. Space required for mature cows around water stations. (*From* Graves RE, McFarland DF, Tyson JT, et al. Idea plan watering locations for dairy cattle, IP 723-49. University Park (PA): Pennsylvania State University; 1997.)

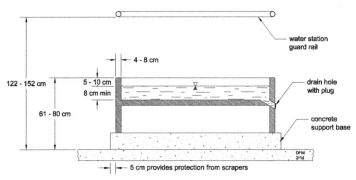

Fig. 5. Cross section of concrete or polyethylene water trough. (*From* Graves RE, McFarland DF, Tyson JT, et al. Idea plan watering locations for dairy cattle, IP 723-49. University Park (PA): Pennsylvania State University; 1997.)

Freestall dimensions and structural features must allow each cow to enter stall, recline easily, rest comfortably, rise easily, and exit the stall. Total required stall length is determined by the space needed for cows to rise and recline. As cows rise (recline) they lunge forward, shifting their weight ahead, allowing them to raise (lower) their hind quarters more easily. Designers and builders need accurate information concerning cow size and grouping to select the proper dimensions. **Fig. 6** shows typical freestall dimensions for mature Holstein cows (635 kg [1400 lb]), using mattresses and generously bedded stall beds. Stall dimensions should accommodate the largest cows in the group.

The resting surface should be resilient to conform to the shape of resting cows, provide cushion when rising and reclining, and traction so they can enter and exit the resting area easily. There are many satisfactory stall bed alternatives to consider. Generous amounts of inorganic (eg, sand, limestone tailings) and organic (eg, sawdust, straw, shavings) bedding can provide a suitable surface. Another alternative, often referred to as mattresses, typically uses a fabric cover to secure a layer of resilient material such as crumb rubber, molded rubber, gel, or foam. Another resilient stall bed alternative uses 1 or more bladders filled with water as the resting surface.

There are several alternatives that can provide a suitable resting surface; each has advantages and disadvantages. Select an alternative that provides best benefit for the cows and the disadvantages that good management can overcome.

- Generously bedded: a 10.2 cm (4 in) minimum of inorganic or organic bedding material. Generally best accepted by dairy cows, but require good stall maintenance and grooming to be successful.

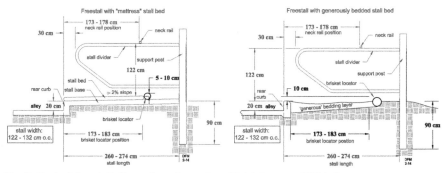

Fig. 6. Typical freestall dimensions for mature Holstein cows (635 kg).

- Fabric-covered mattresses: popular alternatives contain crumb rubber, foam, gel, or water filler material. These alternatives do not replace bedding but can reduce the total amount needed compared with generously bedded stalls.
- Soft resilient mats: the best choices provide a suitable degree of comfort with adequate bedding. With use, most soft mats tend to expand in width and length. Therefore, proper installation and trimming may be necessary at times.

Bedding should be added regularly to help keep surface dry, provide additional comfort, and reduce abrasions.

- Inorganic bedding materials, such as sand and ground limestone, can provide an excellent resting surface for dairy cows. These materials tend to drain moisture away from the resting surface and may not support pathogen growth, reducing the chance of udder infection. However, inorganic materials can be difficult to handle, increase wear on equipment and floor surfaces, present a manure handling challenge, and can be a concern in cold weather, because they have little insulating value and can draw heat away from the resting cow.
- Organic bedding materials, such as sawdust, straw, shavings, paper, and dried manure solids, absorb moisture to help dry the stall surface. These materials can support pathogens growth, so diligent handling, storage, and management are required.

While the cow is resting, the udder and teats contact the resting surface. Therefore, the resting surface must be clean and dry. This factor requires not only good stall design but diligent stall and bedding management, which includes regular bedding intervals and frequent stall surface grooming. Manure and soiled areas should be removed from the stall surface at least 3 times per day.

Bedding amount, frequency, and management must to be determined by cow cleanliness and condition, not the calendar. The bedding application interval varies with the material used and season. Bedding material is typically added to generously bedded sand stalls 1 to 2 times per week and may use 11.3 to 22.7 kg (25 to 50 lb) per stall per day. Organic bedding is usually used on top of mattress stall beds. It is more difficult to keep bedding on mattress stall beds, so fresh bedding should be added every 1 to 2 days. More bedding and more frequent application is typically required during cold and wet weather to maintain a desirable level of cow cleanliness and comfort.

Existing freestalls can be improved to better meet the needs of productive dairy cows. Some require minor adjustments, whereas others need major structural modification. In either case, time spent studying cow needs, observing successful examples, and making necessary changes is worth the effort.

Improving Existing Freestall Dimensions

Suggested freestall dimensions, stall structure details, and preferred stall bed alternatives are based on several years of experience, observation, and evaluation of freestall success and failure. However, cows are the best evaluators of freestall performance. Regular observation of stall acceptance and use is necessary. Adjustments to the stall structure or stall management may be necessary to realize desired results.

- Periods of high stall use are typically observed in early morning and approximately 2 hours after returning from the milking area. Acceptance of 90% or more at these times is desired.
- Perching (standing half in/half out) usually indicates improper neck rail placement.

- Standing in stall with head above neck rail usually indicates improper neck rail placement.
- Diagonal resting is often caused by improper neck rail or brisket locator placement.
- Hock injuries generally result from inadequate body space on stall bed, a hard stall surface, or inadequate bedding.

Adding length

Stalls need to be long enough to allow comfortable resting postures and adequate space for forward lunging when rising and reclining. Dairy cows require approximately 76.2 to 111.8 cm (30 to 44 in) of space ahead of their front knee location to lunge.

- For stall rows along outside stalls:
  - Remove lunging obstacles at wall below 81.3 cm (32 in) and above 20.3 cm (8 in).
  - Construct a sloping adjustable sidewall curtain support beyond the outside wall line that provides necessary additional length at stall level to allow forward lunging (**Fig. 7**).
  - Extend stall bed to achieve desired stall length. However, do not reduce cow alley width to less than 2.4 m (8 ft).
  - If sidewall obstruction cannot be removed, install wide-span dividers that provide a 206.5 cm² (32 in²) opening at stall front to allow side lunging.
- For head-to-head and inside stall rows:
  - Remove lunge barriers and modify stall support structure at stall front so there are no obstacles higher than 15.2 cm (6 in) above the stall surface, and provide a minimum vertical clearance of 81.3 cm (32 in).
  - Extend stall bed into scrape alleys.

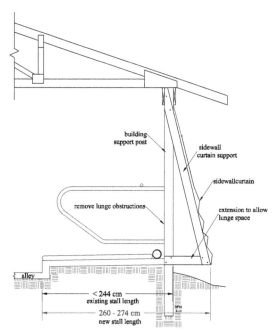

Fig. 7. Adding length to a freestall row along an outside wall using a sloping sidewall curtain support.

Adding width
Stall dividers should be spaced to encourage cows to enter, recline, rest, rise, and exit without striking them abruptly.

- Reposition narrow stall dividers to recommended width
  - 121.9 to 132.1 cm (48 to 52 in) on center for large-framed cows
  - 111.8 to 121.9 cm (44 to 48 in) on center for large-framed cows
  - Dry cows may require 5.1 to 10.2 cm (2 to 4 in) additional width during gestation

Improving stall dividers
There seems to be an infinite number of types and configurations available. The best designs encourage cows to lie parallel to the stall length, and allow both forward and side lunging.

Improving neck rail position
Positioned properly, the neck rail allows the largest cow in a group to stand on the stall surface with her back level, legs squarely placed beneath her, and gently touching the neck rail.

- Typical neck rail location for large-framed dairy cattle:
  - Provide vertical clearance from stall bed to bottom of neck rail 116.8 to 127.0 cm (46 to 50 in)
  - Provide horizontal location from alley side of rear curb 172.7 to 177.8 cm (68 to 70 in)
- If the neck rail is too low, moving the neck rail forward to allow approximately 208.3 to 213.4 cm (82 to 84 in) measured diagonally between neck rail and top of alley side of rear curb
  - Note: ensure neck rail position is not too far forward to weaken lateral stall divider support
- Existing neck rail can be raised to recommended height without moving the stall divider using box steel, welded pipe fixtures, or clamps

Improving brisket locator position
If the brisket locator is located properly, the largest cow in a group should rest comfortably on the stall surface. It must also allow cows to extend their front legs forward when resting and step forward when rising.

- Typical brisket locator position for large-framed dairy cattle
  - Horizontal dimension to cow side of brisket locator
    - Mattress or mat stall base: measure from rear edge of mattress or mat: 172.7 to 182.9 cm (68 to 72 in)
    - Generously bedded stalls: measure from cow side of rear curb: 172.7 to 182.9 cm (68 to 72 in)
  - Brisket locator height: 10.2 to 15.2 cm (4 to 6 in) above stall surface

GOOD VENTILATION

The importance of good air quality cannot be understated. Fresh, dry air is essential to the health and well-being of cows and caretakers. Good ventilation provides the necessary air exchange to remove excess moisture, gases, pollutants, and heat produced by the animals, manure, bedding material, and feedstuffs. Moisture control is the primary concern. A significant amount of moisture is added to air as cows breathe

(11.6-27 L/cow/d [3-7 gallons/cow/d]), and evaporation from cow alleys, which must be removed from the building to ensure good cow health.

Natural ventilation is often the most economical and practical system used in free-stall shelters. The primary goal of natural ventilation is to provide similar inside air quality, with respect to moisture level, gas concentrations, and pollutants, as outside air. During cold weather, temperature is not the primary concern. If the cows are protected from cold winds, kept dry, and fed properly, they can be healthy and productive. During hot weather, a rapid air exchange also helps remove excess heat from the building. Circulation fans located over the resting and feeding areas help reduce heat stress. Further heat stress can be abated by adding spray cooling along the feeding area or high-pressure misting in the entire animal area.

Basic natural ventilation design guidelines:

- Proper building orientation is important
  - Position building length 45° to 90° to predominant prevailing winds
    - Allows ridge opening to draw air more uniformly
    - Breezes blow across the width of the building
  - East-west orientation favors summer shading patterns
    - Minimal sunlight intrusion into animal area
- Provide adequate separation
  - 15.2 m (50 ft) minimum from obstructions that block air flow (eg, buildings, trees, silos)
  - 22.9 m (75 ft) preferred to allow firefighting equipment to maneuver
  - Wind shadow created by long or tall obstructions increases necessary separation distance
- Sidewall height 3.7 to 4.9 m (12 to 16 ft)
  - Adds building volume
  - Moves roof further away from animal level (reduces heat stress)
  - Allows opportunity for more air to enter and exit building
- Adjustable sidewall and end wall openings
  - Minimum sidewall opening half-ridge opening (each side)
  - Open side and end walls as much as possible in warm weather, especially at cow level
  - Block cold winds and precipitation as needed
  - Automatic control of sidewall openings preferred with proper adjustment and management
- Ridge opening
  - 5.1 to 7.6 cm (2 to 3 in) continuous ridge width opening per 3 m (10 ft) of building width

HEAT STRESS ABATEMENT

A common problem in dairy housing facilities is providing the necessary heat abatement during the hot summer months. St-Pierre and colleagues[7] estimated that the US livestock industry could lose approximately $2.4 billion annually in production because of heat stress without the use of some type of heat abatement. Heat stress adversely affects reproduction, milk production, and immunity.[7,24,25] Nutritional consequences of heat stress stem from reduced feed intake (approximately 20%), decreased rumination, and altered metabolic status, thus predisposing cows to reduced milk yield, decreased feed efficiency, and greater risk of metabolic and nutritional diseases.[26,27]

Heat stress occurs when the animal's heat gain is greater than its heat loss. The animal produces body heat through metabolism, physical activity, and performance. Heat can also be gained from the environment through radiation from other bodies of higher temperature, convection from the air if at a higher temperature, and conduction from a surface if at a higher temperature. Heat can be lost from the animal through radiation to a body of lower temperature, convection to surrounding air of a lesser temperature, conduction to a resting surface if at a lesser temperature, or through evaporation when heat is lost because of the phase change of water from liquid to vapor.[28]

The 4 modes of energy transfer represented (radiation, convection, evaporation, and conduction) are governed by physical law (**Fig. 8**). For the animal to maintain a homoeothermic state, energy gains from transfer modes and from internal metabolic processes must equal energy losses.[29]

Heat abatement is provided in dairy facilities using 4 basic procedures:

- Shade is provided for the animals by the shelter to remove the direct radiation heat load.
- Air exchange of the facility is optimized with the use of natural or mechanical ventilation to remove the animal heat and solar gain from the shelter, to maintain the inside temperature at or less than outside temperature to maximize convective cooling.
- Air velocity within the facility is optimized, at animal level, with mechanical means to further enhance convective cooling of the cow.
- Additional cooling may then be provided by using evaporative cooling to remove heat from the air or animals within the facility.

Shade

Shade is considered to be essential to reduce loss of milk production and reproduction efficiency and may be necessary for survival.[30] Shades change the radiation balance of an animal but do not affect air temperature or humidity. The shade structure should provide at least 4.2 m² (45 ft²) of floor space per cow and preferably 5.6 m² (60 ft²) or more. To achieve maximum benefits from a shade structure, the cows must have access to feed and water under the shade.[31]

Shelter orientation has an effect on shading. Shelters with a north-south orientation have greater solar radiation exposure than shelters with an east-west orientation. Sunlight can directly enter north-south–oriented shelters in both morning and afternoon.

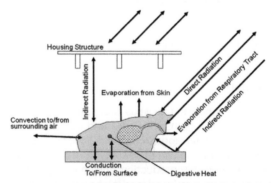

Fig. 8. Energy exchanges between the animal and its surroundings. (*Modified from* Graves RE. Heat stress. 2002. Available at: http://www.powershow.com/view1/6701a-ZDc1Z/Robert_E_Graves_powerpoint_ppt_presentation. Accessed May 20, 2014; and Hahn GL. Management and housing of farm animals in hot environments. In: Yousef MK, editor. Stress physiology in livestock. vol. II. Boca Raton (FL): CRC Press; 1985. p. 151–74.)

Because cows seek shade during hot weather, usage of stalls located on east and west outside walls is greatly affected when in direct sunlight. Protection from direct sunlight is vital for effective heat stress abatement.[32]

Increased Air Exchange and Air Velocity

The 2 most common ways of increasing air exchange and speed in dairy housing are (1) tunnel ventilation (a specific type of mechanical ventilation) and (2) natural ventilation with increased local airspeed at animal level with the use of axial circulation fans or high-volume low-speed (HVLS) fans.

Tunnel ventilation

Tunnel ventilation is a system composed of exhaust fans at 1 end of the shelter, an airflow path over the cows, inlets for fresh air entry at the other end of the shelter, and some control for the transition into and out of tunnel ventilation mode. Sidewall and ridge openings of natural ventilated shelters must be closed during operation of the tunnel ventilation system. The shelter may be mechanically or naturally ventilated in times that tunnel ventilation is not used. Tunnel ventilation is most often a separate ventilation system from the one that is used during cold and mild weather.

Gooch and Stowell[33] reported a slight overall advantage in mean inside air temperature and temperature-humidity index of tunnel-ventilated freestalls over naturally ventilated barns with circulation fans. However, airspeeds were not uniform along the lengths and widths of barns. Measured airspeeds within the lower portion of many tunnel-ventilated barns were noticeably lower than the design airspeed. Measured airspeeds in the central areas, like drive-through alleys, and higher off the floors were usually greater than in the corresponding freestall areas and other occupied cow spaces. This finding shows that airflow naturally channels toward those areas with least resistance to air movement and away from areas offering more resistance as a result of blockage (cows or freestalls). Longer barns seem to have a more pronounced airflow-channeling effect, resulting in little air movement at cow level. Also noted was a change in animal behavior. In 2 of the 3 tunnel-ventilated barns, the tendency observed was that more cows were on their feet (standing at a bunk, in cow alleys, or in stalls) within upwind quadrants, to expose their bodies to higher levels of airflow.

Tunnel ventilation airflow capacity is based on the cross-sectional area (height × width) of the shelter and a desired airspeed through that shelter. For a freestall shelter, the design airspeed should be 2.5 to 3.0 m/s (500–600 ft/min), whereas in tiestall facilities, the design airspeed minimum is 1.5 m/s (300 ft/min). The reason for the higher airspeed in freestall shelters is that the air channels or escapes the cow-occupied area more easily because of the higher ceiling height and wider, more open alleys than in tiestall facilities. An alternative method is to provide a 45-second air exchange of the shelter. The larger of these 2 methods should be used for the design.

The inlet area provided should be a minimum of 0.25 m² (2.5 ft²) per 28 m³/min (1000 ft³/min) of fan capacity. In large freestall shelters where the design airspeed exceeds 2 m/s (400 ft/min), the inlet area should be equal to the cross-sectional area of the shelter plus 10% to 20% to account for obstruction to airflow within the inlet area (eg, structural posts, bird netting, curtain hardware).

Natural ventilation with increased airspeed

In this system, the natural ventilation of the shelter is first maximized to increase air exchange. In an evaluation of several naturally ventilated freestall barns, Stowell and Bickert[34] found that those exposing large amounts of open wall area to cows (on a per cow basis) provided a more suitable environment, with less interior variation.

The target opening for summer natural ventilation is 1 m² (11 ft²) of windward sidewall and end wall per animal within the shelter. An open ridge vent should also be provided.[35]

Exposure of the barn to local winds is also critical to successful natural ventilation. Naturally ventilated barns are best located on high ground, with open space around them. When allowed to choose, cows avoid areas downwind of objects during hot weather.[34] A minimum of at least 15 m (50 ft) from trees, silos, and other small buildings is recommended. Recommended separation between large freestall buildings is greater than 23 m (75 ft).

Axial circulation fans

The objective with circulation fans is to increase the convective cooling capacity of the cow. An airspeed of at least 2.2 m/s (440 ft/min or 5 miles/h) is desired at animal level. To achieve airspeed, fans are placed in rows perpendicular to the stalls and, in freestall shelters, may in addition be added along the feed line. Mounting height is most often 2.1 to 2.4 m (7–8 ft) above the stall surface or floor. Fans can be mounted higher if needed to allow equipment clearance; however, fans need to be tilted more to force the air down. Fan spacing should be no more than 10 to 12 times the fan diameter. If fans are located too far apart, dead spots with little or no air movement develop between fans. A tilt angle of 15° to 20° from vertical is needed to push the air down to animal level. The goal is to have the airstream from the first fan strike the freestall surface or floor under the second fan and so on down the length of the barn.

In freestall shelters, although fans over both stalls and feed line are preferred, priority should be given to locating fans over the stalls if only a limited number of fans are going to be used. Because cows spend twice as much time during a 24-hour period lying as they do eating, locating fans over the stalls provides cooling where cows spend most of their time. Although locating fans at the feed line may encourage animals to come to the bunk, it may also encourage them to stand for long periods rather than lie down.

Whether in a freestall or tiestall shelter, fans should be placed so the center of the airstream is traveling over the center of the cow. In an effort to maximize convective cooling, the airspeed must be maximized over the largest surface of the cow, which is the area between the front shoulders and the rear hips.

Circulation fans can also be staged by ambient temperature to reduce operational costs. One method is to turn one-third of the fans on at 16°C (60°F), two-thirds of fans by 18°C (65°F), and all fans by 20°C (68°F). Fans in the center of the shelter over the stalls should be turned on first, and then, fans at the feed bunk, and in the outer areas of the shelter second and third, respectively.

High-volume low-speed circulation fans

The goal with HVLS fans is the same as the axial fan objective: to increase cow level air velocity and thus increase convective cooling of the animals. These fans have been shown to achieve an airspeed of 1.0 to 1.5 m/s (200–300 ft/min) over an area of approximately 2 times their diameter at a height of 1.5 m (5 ft) above the floor.[36] Although this airspeed is less than desired, some benefit may be seen. Thus, location and spacing of HVLS fans are critical to their success. Fans need to be located so the downward air column is over the stall area where cows are going to be located most of the day. These fans do little to aid in convective cooling of the cows when located over the center driveway of a large drive-through freestall shelter. Spacing should be approximately 2 times the HVLS fan diameter. If HVLS fans are being considered in a new structure, the ceiling height must be sufficient. As per manufacturer's recommendations, a minimum ceiling height of 4.5 m (15 ft) and blade clearance to ceiling/roof of 0.6 m (2 ft) are preferred for mounting these fans. Before installation of HVLS fans, it is recommended that a structural engineer be consulted about the impact of the additional load(s) of the fan(s) on the structure.

Evaporative Cooling

Evaporative cooling can be broken down into 2 main categories: indirect and direct. With indirect evaporative cooling, a system is used to lower the ambient air temperature by evaporating water into the air and then circulate that cooler air around the cow to increase convective cooling. This cooling can be achieved with evaporative pads, in which ambient outside air is drawn though the pad while water is circulated over the pad. Heat contained in the entering air is used to evaporate the water. Thus, the dry bulb temperature is decreased, but the relative humidity is increased.[37] This same principle can be followed with high-pressure misters or foggers, in which the water is injected directly into the air stream. The water particles are of small enough diameter that they are evaporated before falling to the surface.

Direct evaporative cooling wets the cow to the skin and then uses cow body heat to evaporate that water to provide cooling of the cow. The evaporation of 0.45 kg (1 lb) of water requires approximately 1055 kJ (1000 Btu) of energy. Most of that heat is acquired from the cow's body in direct cooling systems. For cooling to be achieved, the cow needs to be wetted with a system that produces a droplet size large enough to penetrate the hair coat in a short period, and then, the sprinkler system needs to shut off and allow the cow to dry before the next wetting cycle is started. The animal's hair should be dried to a point at which no more free water is present. This drying time is typically 5 to 10 minutes dependent on ambient temperature, humidity, and air velocity at animal level. Sufficient air exchange for the shelter and air velocity at cow level is needed to aid in evaporation of the water from the cow and removal from the shelter.

The major difference between direct and indirect evaporative cooling is whether the cow's skin is wetted or not. Care must be taken to not cover the animal with a fine layer of water on top of the hair coat, trapping a layer of air between the skin and the water film. This layer acts as an insulator and may increase the severity of heat stress by reducing convective cooling.[30] Also, because the fine droplets cling to the animal's outer hair coat, the heat for evaporation comes from the air rather than from the body.[29]

A comprehensive heat abatement system consists of:

- Increased air exchange
- Increased air velocity
- Evaporative cooling

The components used to develop the system for a specific facility depend on that facility's design, construction, and management.

CONFIDENT FOOTING

All surfaces that cows come in contact with should provide a confident, nonskid footing. A floor surface that provides confident footing reduces the chance of serious injury caused by slipping and falling. Cows are more likely to mount and show signs of estrus in an area providing a good, nonskid footing.

Basic cattle flooring construction guidelines:

- Use 24.1 MPa air entrained concrete
- Well-drained compacted subgrade

- Floor thickness 10.2 to 15.2 cm (4 to 6 in) depending on vehicle traffic
- Groove patterns
  - Parallel: 5.1 to 10.2 cm (2 to 4 in) on center in direction of scraper travel
  - Diamond: 10.2 to 15.2 cm (4 to 6 in) on center each direction
- Groove size: 9.5 to 12.7 mm (3/8 to $^1/_2$ in) wide
- Form grooves before curing or saw in later (sawn grooves create cleaner edge)
- Remove sharp edges and exposed aggregate before allowing cows access; wash or sweep debris away

Resilient flooring materials (eg, rubber belting, rubber mats, ethylene vinyl acetate mats) have become popular in dairy freestall shelters, especially in holding areas and cow alleys along the feeding area. Limited information is available as to the short-term and long-term benefits of these materials. Observation indicates that cows prefer to walk and stand on resilient flooring rather than concrete. However, some resilient flooring materials become slippery when wet, whereas durability has been a problem others.

SUMMARY

Feed, water, and air are essential elements in animal well-being and the production of quality milk. The design and management of each component in a dairy shelter, including the feeding and drinking water areas, resting areas, floor surfaces, and ventilation system, influences each cow's willingness and ability to express typical behaviors and consume an adequate amount of dry matter. Dairy system designers need to pay close attention to the needs of cows and all aspects of the animal area when developing designs and recommendations. Dairy cows should be able to consume large volumes of fresh, good-quality feed and water, easily, comfortably, and without injury. The design of the feeding and watering areas should also allow the caretaker to perform the tasks of feed delivery, observation, maintenance, and cleaning easily and safely. Access to feed and water must not limit the production and profit potential of a modern dairy enterprise.

DAIRY FACILITY DESIGN RESOURCES

Penn State Agricultural and Biologic Engineering Dairy Plans: http://abe.psu.edu/extension/idea-plans/dairy

The Dairyland Initiative (University of Wisconsin): https://thedairylandinitiative.vetmed.wisc.edu/index.htm

REFERENCES

1. Huzzey JM, Veira DM, Weary DM, et al. Prepartum behavior and dry matter intake identify dairy cows at risk for metritis. J Dairy Sci 2007;90:3220–33.
2. Goldhawk C, Chapinal N, Veira DM, et al. Prepartum feeding behavior is an early indicator of subclinical ketosis. J Dairy Sci 2009;92:4971–7.
3. Zamet CN, Colebrander WF, Callahan CJ, et al. Variables associated with peripartum traits in dairy cows. I. Effect of dietary forages and disorders on voluntary intake of feed, body weight and milk yield. Theriogenology 1979;11:229–44.
4. Zamet CN, Colenbrander VF, Erb RE, et al. Variables associated with peripartum traits in dairy cows. II. Interrelationships among disorders and their effects on intake of feed and on reproductive efficiency. Theriogenology 1979;11:245–60.

5. Hosseinkhani A, DeVries TJ, Proudfoot KL, et al. The effects of feed bunk competition on the feed sorting behavior of close-up dry cows. J Dairy Sci 2008;91:1115–21.

6. Proudfoot KL, Veira DM, Weary DM, et al. Competition at the feed bunk changes the feeding, standing, and social behavior of transition dairy cows. J Dairy Sci 2009;92:3116–23.

7. St-Pierre NR, Cobanov B, Schnitkey G. Economic losses from heat stress by US livestock industries. J Dairy Sci 2003;86(E Suppl):E52–77.

8. Graves RE. Design configurations for feeding spaces. In: Proceedings from the Dairy Feeding Systems Management Components, and Nutrients Conference. Camp Hill (PA): NRAES; 1998. p. 153–66.

9. McFarland DF. Designing dairy housing for convenient animal handling, feed delivery, and manure collection. In: Proceedings of the Third International Dairy Housing Conference. Orlando (FL): ASAE; 1994. p. 509.

10. Longenbach JI, Heinrichs AJ, Graves RE. Feed bunk length requirements for Holstein dairy heifers. J Dairy Sci 1999;82(1):99–109.

11. Dumelow J, Sharples T. Developing improved designs of feeding barriers and mangers for cattle from data collected from an instrumented test rig. In: Proceedings ASAE International Livestock Symposium. St Joseph (MO): ASAE; 1998. p. 155–62.

12. Bickert WG. Feed manager and barrier design. In: Proceedings from the Dairy Feeding Systems Symposium. Harrisburg (PA): NRAES; 1990. p. 199–206.

13. Albright JL. Putting together the facility, the worker and the cow. In: Dairy housing II. Proceedings of the Second National Dairy Housing Conference. Madison (WI): ASAE; 1983. p. 15–22.

14. Graves RE, McCarty TR. Guidelines for potable water on dairy farms DPC-30. Keyport (NJ): The Dairy Practices Council; 2006. p. 33.

15. Ishler VA. Don't forget about water. Dairy and Animal Science Dairy Digest (DAS 98–12). University Park (PA): Pennsylvania State University; 1998.

16. Grant R. Water quality and requirements for dairy cattle. Lincoln (NE): NebGuide; 1993. p. 1.

17. Graves RE. Guideline for planning dairy freestall barns, DPC-1. Barre (VT): Dairy Practice Council; 2009. p. 9.

18. Bickert WG, Holmes B, Janni K, et al. Dairy freestall housing and equipment. 7th edition. Ames (IA): MWPS; 2000. p. 136.

19. Graves RE, McFarland DF, Tyson JT, et al. Idea plan watering locations for dairy cattle, IP. University Park (PA): Pennsylvania State University; 1997. p. 723–49.

20. Albright JL, Arave CW. The behavior of cattle. 1st edition. Wallingford (United Kingdom); New York: CAB International; 1997. p. 306.

21. Fregonesi JA, Veira DM, von Keyserlingk MAG, et al. Effects of bedding quality on lying behavior of dairy cows. J Dairy Sci 2007;90:5468–72.

22. Tucker CB, Weary DM, Fraser D. Effects of three types of free-stall surfaces on preferences and stall usage by dairy cows. J Dairy Sci 2003;86:521–9.

23. Drissler M, Gaworski M, Tucker CB, et al. Freestall maintenance: effects on lying behavior of dairy cattle. J Dairy Sci 2005;88:2381–7.

24. Ealy AD, Drost M, Hansen PJ. Developmental changes in embryonic resistance to adverse effects of maternal heat stress in cows. J Dairy Sci 1993;76:2899–905.

25. do Amaral BC, Connor EE, Tao S, et al. Heat stress abatement during the dry period influences metabolic gene expression and improve immune status in the transition period of dairy cows. J Dairy Sci 2011;94:86–96.

26. Soriani N, Panella G, Calamari L. Rumination time during the summer season and its relationships with metabolic conditions and milk production. J Dairy Sci 2013; 96:5082–94.

27. Van Saun RJ, Davidek J. Diagnostic use of pooled metabolic profiles in Czech dairy herds (Abstract). In: Proceedings of the Annual American Association of Bovine Practitioners Conference. 2008;41:286.

28. Graves RE. Heat stress. 2002. Available at: http://www.powershow.com/view1/6701a-ZDc1Z/Robert_E_Graves_powerpoint_ppt_presentation. Accessed May 20, 2014.

29. Hahn GL. Management and housing of farm animals in hot environments. In: Yousef MK, editor. Stress physiology in livestock, vol. II. Boca Raton (FL): CRC Press; 1985. p. 151–74.

30. Armstrong DV. Heat stress interaction with shade and cooling. J Dairy Sci 1994; 77:2044–50.

31. Buffington DE, Collier RJ, Canton GH. Shade management systems to reduce heat stress for dairy cows in hot, humid climates. Trans ASAE 1983;26(6):1798–802.

32. Brouk MJ, Smith JF, Harner JP III. Heat stress abatement in four-row freestall barns. In: Proceedings of the 5th Western Dairy Management Conference. Reno (NV): 2001. p. 161–6.

33. Gooch CA, Stowell RR. Tunnel ventilation for freestall facilities: design, environmental conditions, cow behavior, and economics. In: Proceedings of the Fifth International Dairy Housing Conference. St Joseph (MI): 2003. p. 227–34.

34. Stowell RR, Bickert WG. Environmental variation in naturally ventilated free stall barns during the warm season. In: Dairy systems for the 21st century. Proceedings 3rd International Dairy Housing Conference. St Joseph (MI): ASAE; 1994. p. 569–78.

35. Graves RE, McFarland DF, Tyson JT, et al. Penn State housing plans for milking and special-needs cows: NRAES-200. Ithaca (NY): NRAES; 2006.

36. Kammel DW, Raabe ME, Kappelman JJ. Design of high volume low speed fan supplemental cooling system in dairy freestall barns. In: Proceedings of the Fifth International Dairy Housing Conference. St Joseph (MI): ASAE; 2003. p. 243–54.

37. Wheeler EF. Psychometric chart use. Ag. and Bio. engineering fact sheet G-83. University Park (PA): Penn State University; 1996. Available at: http://pubs.cas.psu.edu/freepubs/pdfs/G83.pdf.

Undertaking Nutritional Diagnostic Investigations

Garrett R. Oetzel, DVM, MS

KEYWORDS

- Dairy cows • Nutrition diagnostic investigations • Nutrition troubleshooting
- Diet evaluation

KEY POINTS

- A dairy herd nutritional diagnostic investigation is a comprehensive exercise that evaluates herd production records, disease rates, the cow environment, feed ingredient characteristics, estimates of nutrient intake, evaluations of feed delivery, and evaluations of the cows, such as body condition score, cud chewing activity, manure characteristics, locomotion score, and blood testing results.
- Important aspects of an evaluation of the cow's environment include access to or restrictions from eating and resting space, access to quality water, cleanliness, and ventilation. These factors interact with nutrient intake to determine cow health and productivity.
- Tools that can be used to evaluate feed ingredient quality include visual inspection, analysis for nutrient content, pH, organic acid content, forage particle length, and grain particle size.
- Bunk samples of total mixed rations can be evaluated for nutrient analysis, particle length, and sortability.
- Conclusions from a herd nutritional diagnostic investigation are most plausible when they are supported by more than 1 finding from the investigation.

INTRODUCTION

Nutrition is a crucial determinant of dairy cow health and productivity. Veterinarians can work with dairy nutritionists to solve nutritional problems in dairy herds. It is useful to follow a systematic pattern of data gathering when conducting nutritional investigations.

INITIAL HERD NUTRITIONAL INVESTIGATION DATABASE
Herd Signalment

A herd nutritional diagnostic investigation starts with the herd signalment. A useful herd signalment is the herd size, breed of cows, herd milk production (usually rolling

Disclosures: Nil.
Food Animal Production Medicine Section, Department of Medical Sciences, School of Veterinary Medicine, University of Wisconsin-Madison, 2015 Linden Drive, Madison, WI 53706, USA
E-mail address: groetzel@wisc.edu

herd average), and feeding system (ie, whether the herd is fed a total mixed ration [TMR] or is component-fed). Clearly establishing the herd signalment at the start creates a proper frame of reference for the rest of the herd investigation.

Herd Problem Definition

It is essential that the herd's nutrition-related problems be thoroughly understood and carefully quantified. A producer's view of the herd's problems may be biased. For example, a complaint that "too many fresh cows are dying" might be overstated. The investigator should not accept this information at face value but should evaluate the herd records (as much as they exist) to determine how many cows have died in the last year, what their days in milk were at death, what treatments were given, what diagnoses were made (ante or post mortem), and what laboratory information is available for each case.

As self-evident as the need to carefully and objectively define a herd's problem may seem, it is common for veterinarians to ignore this step and to immediately delve into the details of the diets being fed to the cows. Many herd investigations are redirected by carefully and objectively defining the herd's problems.

Herd Production Records

A thorough review of the herd's production records should be performed as a part of a herd nutritional investigation. In many cases, this review shows that the initial client complaint is not the most important herd problem.

Dairy record systems vary considerably and may consist of paper records, dairy herd improvement (DHI) records, bulk tank information, or on-farm herd management software. It is hoped that the herd investigator can obtain access to reasonable herd production information from 1 or more of these sources. If the herd is enrolled in DHI testing, the herd summary report from the previous month's test is a good starting point. Depending on the DHI processing center involved, there may be additional options for more detailed herd historical information. Examples of these options include DHI-Plus (DHI-Provo, Utah), PCDART (Dairy Records Management Systems, Raleigh, NC), and WisGraph (AgSource Cooperative Services, Verona, WI).

A good minimum database for herd production records consists of the following:

- Current rolling herd average (**Fig. 1**)
- Mature equivalent (ME) milk production for the last year for the herd and by lactation group (usually first lactation vs ≥second lactation groups, see **Fig. 1**)
- Peak milk production by lactation group (**Fig. 2**)
- Milk production by month (**Fig. 3**)
- Milk components (fat and protein) by month (**Fig. 4**)

If cow health problems are part of the client's concerns, it is helpful to plot herd removals (sold and died cows) for the last year by days in milk at removal. It is normal for herds to have more herd removals in early lactation; however, removals in the first 30 days in milk should not exceed about 4% of herd size, and removals between 30 and 60 days in milk should not exceed about 2% of herd size. An example of this report is presented in **Fig. 5**.

If the herd is neither enrolled in DHI nor uses on-farm dairy management software, then it becomes difficult to obtain relevant herd data and accurately define herd problems. Whatever records exist can be used. For example, it may be possible to access

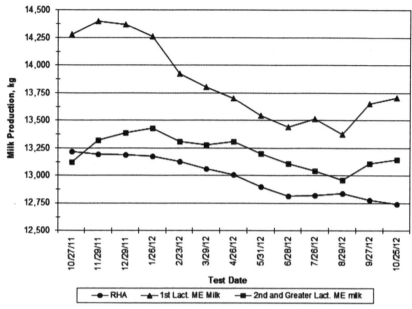

Fig. 1. Rolling herd average (RHA) and mature equivalent (ME) milk production by lactation group for a 1-year period before a herd nutritional investigation. Current values are annotated onto the chart. For this example, the herd has lost about 1000 lb of RHA milk in the last year. The decline has been dominantly in the first lactation animals. (*Data from* DHI records.)

paper records for herd removals and electronic records from the herd's milk processor for bulk tank milk production and milk components.

Disease Rates

It is useful to include disease incidence data in a herd nutritional investigation, even if increased disease incidence is not a part of the initial herd complaint. The clinical diseases most related to nutritional management are milk fever, retained placenta, metritis, ketosis, displaced abomasum, and lameness. Death loss should also be considered at the same time that diseases are evaluated. The definitions for these diseases (and even for death loss) may vary considerably from herd to herd. **Table 1** lists suggested disease definitions, average rates of these diseases, and general alarm levels for disease conditions and for death loss. For sake of convenience, disease rates are typically evaluated as crude incidence rates (the number of cases in a 1-year period divided by the average herd size for the same 1-year period). There are situations in which it may be appropriate to use more detailed evaluations of disease rates. These evaluations could include evaluation of disease rates by parity group, for different periods than the last year, or by specifically evaluating at-risk groups of cows. Evaluating herd disease data may expose previously undetected or unappreciated herd problems and redirect the herd investigation.

EVALUATING THE COW ENVIRONMENT
Basic Evaluation of the Cow Environment

Basic aspects of cow comfort profoundly interact with nutritional management to affect cow health and productivity. Observations of the cow environment should be

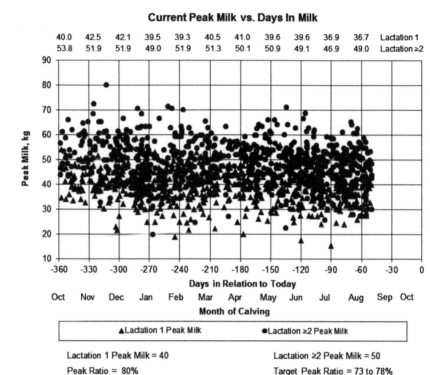

Fig. 2. Scatterplot of peak milk production by lactation group for a 1-year period before a herd nutritional investigation. Monthly averages by lactation group are annotated along the top of the chart. For this example, peak milk yields have decreased about 10% in the past year for both lactation groups, and peak milk yield for the first lactation group is slightly higher than expected compared with the second and greater lactation group. (*Data from* DHI records.)

included in a dairy herd nutritional evaluation. These observations should include the following:

- Amount of eating space available to the cows
- Time cows have access to feed bunks
- Type and cleanliness of the feed bunks
- Size and type of stalls available to the cows
- Type and amounts of bedding provided
- Overall cleanliness of the cows
- Ventilation system in place for the cows

Detailed aspects of evaluating a cow's environment have been reviewed elsewhere.[1] Cow environmental evaluations are particularly relevant for the prevention of laminitis, but are applicable to more general herd nutritional investigations as well. Key criteria are:

- Adequate eating space ($\geq$76 cm (30 in) of bunk space per cow); and
- Adequate resting space ($\geq$1 free stall per cow or $\geq$7 m^2 (75 ft^2) of resting space in loose housing).

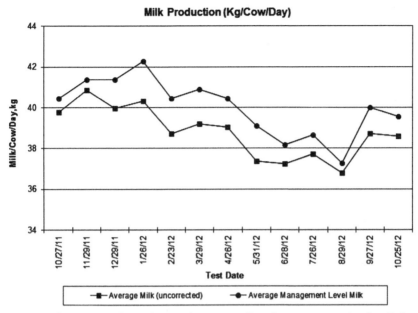

Fig. 3. Plot of average milk production (uncorrected) and management level milk (MLM) production for the last year. For this example, both uncorrected milk yield and MLM have declined about 10% in the last 7 months. Production has increased slightly in the last 2 months; this could in part be normal seasonal change after the summer heat. Average MLM is higher than uncorrected milk production; this is normal and expected, because MLM corrects milk yield to 150 days in milk, and most herds have greater than 150 days in milk. (*Data from* DHI records.)

Failure to provide adequate eating and resting space (particularly in the transition period) greatly impairs cow health and production. Failure of ventilation systems to adequately remove heat in the summer months and moisture in the winter months also impairs cow health, dry matter intakes, and milk production.

Table 2 presents an example summary of the available resting and eating space by pen for a dairy herd.

Access to Quality Water

An evaluation of the water sources, availability, and cleanliness is crucial. Key criteria are:

- ≥10 cm (4 in) of linear waterer space per cow in the pens (year-round)
- 0.6 m (2.0 feet) of linear waterer space per milking parlor stall in the return alleys during the summer months
- A minimum of 2 waterers per pen (for pens containing >10 cows).

Waterers should generally be located close to feed bunks (but not in the bunk itself) and should be protected from direct sunlight, which promotes algae growth. Water contained within waterers should be clear, and waterers should be regularly cleaned. A water sample can be collected and submitted to a laboratory for analysis if there are concerns about water quality. Water quality standards have been reviewed in detail elsewhere.[2]

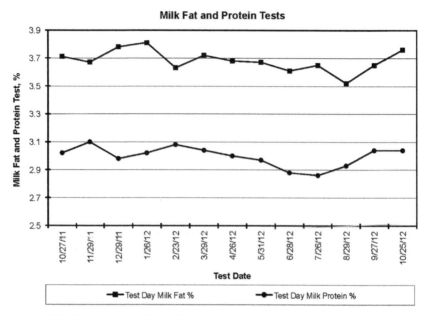

Fig. 4. Plot of test day average milk fat and protein percentages for the last year. For this example, both milk fat and milk protein percentages were normal. A slight reduction in milk fat and milk protein percentage in the summer months is normal. (*Data from* DHI records.)

EVALUATING INDIVIDUAL FEED INGREDIENTS
Initial Evaluation of Feed Ingredients

Before evaluating the diets fed to cows, it is important to carefully evaluate the individual feed ingredients that make up those diets. Nutritionists may overlook the importance of characteristics of individual feed ingredients, especially subjective characteristics such as feed ingredient preservation and palatability.

A part of the standard routine for dairy herd nutritional assessments is to ask to see all of the feed ingredients on the farm, to understand how each ingredient is delivered to the cows, and to perform a quick visual appraisal of each ingredient. It is also important to evaluate the smell of fermented feeds; exercise caution if the feed is moldy or if you have allergies.

Butyric Acid in Silages

It is common to find a butyric acid smell in silages that no one else has yet noticed. The ingestion of butyric acid from silages is a strong risk factor for ketosis. So, it is particularly important that this problem be identified if it is present.

Butyric acid has the strong odor of rancid butter, and most nutritionists and dairy producers believe that they can easily detect its presence. However, it takes some experience to be able to recognize this odor. It is easier to appreciate the butyric acid smell if the feed is at room temperature and in a clean place. Sometimes, other odors on the farm mask the butyric smell.

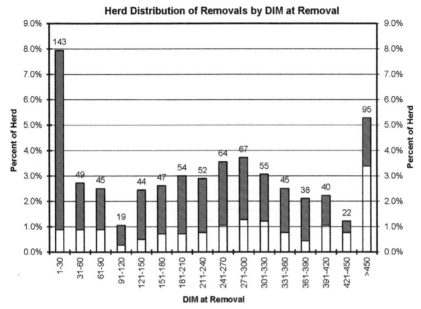

Fig. 5. Plot of herd removals (sold or died cows) by days in milk (DIM) at removal and by lactation group. The number of cows removed per month is annotated on the top of each month's bar. In this example, the number of removals is extremely high in the first month after calving. Second and greater lactation cows make up most of the herd removals, which is typical. (*Data from* DHI records.)

Silages containing butyric acid have an elevated pH (almost always >4.8 and usually between 5.2 and 6.0). Therefore, a check of the silage pH can be helpful if butyric acid is suspected. Silage pH can be easily determined by adding about 1 tablespoon of silage to about 50 mL distilled water, mixing, and then checking the pH of the solution on a calibrated pH meter.

Submit a sample of forages suspected to contain butyric acid to a forage laboratory for a silage organic acid analysis; this analysis quantifies the amount of butyric acid present. Silage organic acid analyses cost about US$20 each and are worth it if there is any concern at all that butyric acid might be present in the silage. No butyric acid should be fed to prefresh or postfresh dairy cows; these cows have the highest risk for ketosis. Small amounts of butyric acid (≤50 g per cow per day) can be fed to dairy cattle that are not in the prefresh or postfresh groups.

Feed Ingredient Dry Matter

A current dry matter content of ensiled feeds should be a standard part of a nutritional investigation. A sample can be sent to a feeds laboratory for dry matter determination, or the feed can be checked using a simple drying oven set at 60°C for 48 hours. Other drying protocols can also be used, but they are less accurate.[3]

The dry matter content of an ensiled feed is the major determinant of the quality of its fermentation. **Table 3** lists recommended dry matter content at harvest for different feeds and different silo types. It is crucial that feed ingredients be harvested at the proper dry matter content. Nothing can be done to alter feed dry matter content once the ingredient is harvested and ensiled. Dairy producers often need assistance

Table 1
Suggested disease definitions, average rates, and alarm levels for common nutrition-related diseases and for death in dairy cattle

Disease	Typical Disease Definition	Average Incidence (%)[a]	Alarm Level Incidence (%)[a]
Clinical milk fever	Sternal or lateral recumbency typically within 48 h of calving; some cases are recognized before recumbency based on other clinical signs such as weakness, ataxia, cold extremities, hypothermia, fine muscle tremors, or loss of anal tone; cases are usually confirmed by response to intravenous calcium treatment or by low blood calcium concentration	5[b]	>2
Retained placenta	Retention of fetal membranes for ≥24 h after calving	8[b]	>8
Metritis	Cows between about 5 and 10 d in milk with a brown, serous, or foul-smelling vaginal discharge, plus 1 or more of the following: fever (≥39.4°C or 103°F), decreased appetite, or decreased milk yield	12	>12
Clinical ketosis	Early lactation cows with decreased appetite, decreased milk yield, or rapid body condition loss; confirmed by a positive cowside ketosis test	10	>15
Displaced abomasum	Early lactation cows with decreased appetite, decreased frequency or strength of ruminal contractions, decreased rumen fill, rumen pushed away from the left body well; characteristic high-pitched ping	4[b]	>4
Lameness	Apparent clinical lameness (locomotion score ≥3 on a 4-point scale or ≥4 on a 5-point scale), which typically results in presentation of the cow for trimming	14[b]	>10
Death	Any cow involuntarily removed from the herd for less than full slaughter value; includes spontaneous death on the farm, euthanasia on the farm, cows condemned at slaughter, or cows with obvious disease problems sold for less than full slaughter value	6[b]	>4

[a] All incidence rates are reported as crude incidence rates: the number of cases in a 1-year period divided by the average herd size for the same 1-year period.
[b] *Data from* USDA, Dairy 2007 Part I: reference of dairy cattle health and management practices in the United States. Available at: http://wwwaphisusdagov/animal_health/nahms/dairy/downloads/dairy07/Dairy07_dr_Partlpdf. Accessed March 3, 2014. Data for other means are from the author's experience in dairy herds in the Upper Midwest, USA.

and access to rapid forage dry matter testing to help them harvest forages at the correct dry matter content. Some dairy producers routinely harvest forages that are either too wet or too dry; this has a profoundly negative effect on cow health and performance.

It is important to accurately represent the dry matter content of a feed ingredient during feed-out so that the correct amount of dry matter from that ingredient can be

Table 2
Summary of resting and eating space by pen for a dairy herd

Pen	Pen Name	Cows	Pen Type	Rows of Stalls	Resting Space				Eating Space		
					Stalls	Pen Width (m)	Pen Length (m)	% Stalls or m²/Cow	Head-Locks	Bunk (m)	cm/Cow
1	Postfresh	147	Free stall	2	167	—	—	88	157	96	65
2	High group lactation 1	190	Free stall	2	176	—	—	108	179	109	57
3	High group lactation ≥2	177	Free stall	2	176	—	—	101	179	109	62
4	Old or lame cows, lactation ≥2	179	Free stall	2 or 3	170	—	—	105	151	92	51
5	Pregnant cows, all lactations	178	Free stall	3	172	—	—	103	121	74	42
6	Pregnant cows, all lactations	192	Free stall	3	172	—	—	112	121	74	39
7	Pregnant cows, all lactations	189	Free stall	3	172	—	—	110	121	74	39
8	Late lactation or culls, all lactations	176	Free stall	3	172	—	—	102	121	74	42
9	High somatic cell count cows	174	Free stall	3	202	—	—	86	—	91	45
17	Far-off dry cows	115	Bedded pack	—	—	15	73	9.5 m²/cow	—	73	63
10	Prefresh dry cows	119	Free stall	2	152	—	—	78	—	109	92
15	Just fresh or nonsaleable milk	29	Free stall	1	36	—	—	81	—	38	131

In this example, there were many pens with insufficient resting space (ie, >100% of stalls) and with insufficient eating space (<76 cm of bunk space per cow).

Table 3
Suggested dry matter and moisture content of various ensiled feed ingredients at harvest

Feed Ingredient	Storage Form	Dry Matter (%)	Moisture (%)
Corn silage	Oxygen-limiting silo[a]	40–45	55–60
	Vertical, open-top silo[b]	30–35	65–70
	Horizontal silo (eg, bunker)	28–33	67–72
Alfalfa silage	Oxygen-limiting silo[a]	50–55	45–50
	Vertical, open-top silo[b]	35–45	55–65
	Horizontal silo (eg, bunker)	35–40	65–70
Grass silage	Oxygen-limiting silo[a]	50–55	45–50
	Vertical, open-top silo[b]	35–45	55–65
	Horizontal silo (eg, bunker)	35–40	65–70
High-moisture shelled corn	Oxygen-limiting silo[a]	75–80	20–25
	Vertical, open-top silo[b]	65–70	30–35

[a] Oxygen-limiting silos include sealed upright silos that unload from the bottom, bagged silage, and wrapped bales.
[b] Open-top silos are upright silos that are not sealed and that unload from the top.

added to the mixer. A part of the nutritional evaluation is determining whether or not this process is being carried out. The needed frequency of dry matter testing depends on the type of feed and the structure in which it is stored. By their nature, corn silage and high-moisture corn have fairly consistent dry matter content at harvest. Weekly or monthly dry matter testing may be sufficient for these crops.

In contrast, hay crop silages have inherently inconsistent dry matter content at harvest. This situation occurs because hay crop dry matter varies depending on location within the field at harvest. Dry matter variations at harvest can carry through to feed-out if hay crop silage is stored in a narrow-diameter silo, such as a bag or a small, top-unloading vertical silo. Feed from 1 load to the next is minimally mixed in narrow-diameter silos; these variations at harvest persist at feed-out. Thus, daily dry matter monitoring may be necessary for hay crop silages being fed from a narrow silo.

Hay crop silages stored in bunker silos have relatively consistent dry matter content at feed-out, because feed from many different loads is layered in the silo and removed simultaneously. Weekly monitoring of dry matter content of hay crop silage from a bunker silo may be sufficient.

Proactive, scheduled monitoring of forage dry matter content is the best approach to ensuring that the correct amounts of feed ingredient dry matter are delivered to the cows. Some producers check forage dry matter only when feed refusals change noticeably or when the feed visibly changes. This practice is better than no dry matter testing at all, but is generally inadequate.

Forage Particle Length

Forage particle length is a critical determinant of dairy cow health and productivity, because it determines whether or not a cow forms an adequate ruminal mat layer. It also influences packing density in silos and sortability of TMR after feed-out. The importance of adequate forage particle length in dairy cattle diets has been reviewed in detail elsewhere.[4]

Visual appraisal of forage particle length is generally unreliable, except for identifying feeds with either very short or very long particle lengths. Some quantitative means of assessing forage particle length is typically necessary when conducting a dairy nutritional investigation. The Penn State Particle Separator (PSPS) is a practical on-farm tool for evaluating forage particle length and has been described in detail elsewhere.[5,6] Some forage laboratories also offer forage particle length evaluations.

A basic dairy herd nutritional investigation should include an evaluation of the particle length of the individual forages in the diet and of each TMR fed to the herd. **Table 4** presents suggested guidelines for forage particle length.

Total Mixed Ration Sorting Analysis

An especially useful application of forage particle length determination is a comparison of the particle length of the TMR offered to the cows with refusals from the same TMR. Ideally, the appearance and particle length of both the TMR offered and the TMR refused should be nearly identical. In reality, modest increases in long particles in the refusals (≤5% points) seem to cause no problems. For example, if the TMR offered to a group of cows contained 7% long particles, it would be acceptable for the refusals to be up to 12% long particles. An increase of 5% to 10% long particles from the TMR offered to the TMR refused is considered moderate sorting. More than a 10% increase in long particles represents a severe sorting problem.

It is ideal (but time consuming) to evaluate TMR particle length in the bunk throughout the feeding period. This exercise can clearly show when the sorting is occurring during the day. However, for most nutritional evaluations, it is sufficient to compare the feed offered with the feed refused at the end of the day. A compromise is to add 1 extra sample during the middle of the day to the TMR sorting analysis. An example of a TMR sorting evaluation with middle of the day and refusal samples is presented in **Table 5**.

Excessive TMR sorting is typically caused by dry forage particles (especially coarse dry hay or straw) that are chopped longer than about 6.4 cm (2.5 in) long. Sorting is also increased if the TMR is too dry (>50% dry matter). When rations are sorted, high-rank cows and cows with the ability to sort can select diets that are too low in effective fiber, whereas low-rank cows are left with diets that are too high in effective fiber. Both groups suffer as a result; the cows that sort may contract ruminal acidosis, and the cows that do not sort lack energy and soluble carbohydrates to support optimal ruminal fermentation.

Most sorting problems can be solved by using 1 or more of the following approaches:

- Process dry hay or straw finer (ie, all particles <6.4 cm) before adding to the mixer
- Feeding more frequently during the day
- Adding extra water or a wet by-product feed (goal of 40%–45% TMR dry matter)
- Adding liquid molasses to the TMR
- Providing ample bunk space so that all cows can eat at the same time

Table 4
Suggested particle lengths for ensiled feeds, TMRs, and feed refusals using 3 boxes on the PSPS

Feed Ingredient	Processing Method	Top Screen (%)	Middle Screen	Pan
Corn silage	Conventional chop	3–8	> Pan	< Middle
	Kernel processed	8–20	≫ Pan	≪ Middle
Hay crop silage	Conventional chop	15–25	> Pan	< Middle
TMR	As offered	7–12	> Pan	< Middle
	Refusals	<5 different from the TMR offered		

Table 5
An example of a TMR sorting analysis conducted on a postfresh group TMR

Screen or Pan (on the PSPS)	TMR Offered (AM)	Midpoint TMR (3 PM)	TMR Refusal (the Next AM)
Top screen	18	22	31
Middle screen	50	51	47
Pan	32	27	22

For this example, minimal sorting was evident by the middle of the TMR feeding period (only 4% more coarse particles on the top screen compared with the TMR offered). However, by the end of the feeding period (the TMR refusal), there was evidence for severe sorting, with 13% more coarse particles compared with the TMR offered.

Adding water or molasses to TMR mixes shortens bunk life during hot weather, because it increases heating of the TMR after feed-out. Feeding more frequently reduces the risk that the TMR heats and also decreases sortability.

Grain Particle Size

If corn is the major grain component of the diets, then, grain particle size evaluation should be included in the nutritional investigation. The goal of processing corn is to create a physical form that has the proper rate and extent of ruminal fermentation, regardless of the dry matter or method of storing the corn. To accomplish this goal, drier corn should be ground more finely, and wetter (ensiled) corn should be ground more coarsely. Using a series of grain screens allows the investigator to quantitatively evaluate the effectiveness of the corn grain processing. The equipment needed for grain particle size evaluation and the methods used have been reviewed elsewhere.[7]

Table 6 presents goals for grain processing different types of corn. There are 2 common errors in corn grain processing. The first is overly coarse grinding of dry shelled corn or relatively dry high-moisture shelled corn (>77% dry matter); this results in incomplete ruminal fermentation, possible hindgut fermentation of the corn, and excessive amounts of corn in the manure. Hindgut fermentation of grains is undesirable and may lead to enteritis, diarrhea, and the appearance of mucosal casts in the manure. The other common error is too finely grinding relatively wet high-moisture shelled corn (<70% dry matter); this results in rapid ruminal fermentation of the corn and increased risk for ruminal acidosis.

Presenting Feed Ingredient Test Results

Table 7 summarizes the feed ingredient test results from a dairy herd nutritional investigation. It is helpful to summarize this information on a single form. Dairy nutritionists may not routinely gather this information themselves and are typically eager to view and discuss these results.

Table 6
Suggested grain particle sizes for ground corn at different dry matter content

Corn Form	Dry Matter (%)	Grain Sieve				
		Number 4	Number 8	Number 16	Number 30	Pan
High-moisture shelled corn	<70	65	20	5	5	5
	70–73	20	50	20	5	5
	74–77	10	25	30	25	10
	>77	0	0	30	50	20
Dry shelled corn	—	0	0	30	50	20

Table 7
Example summary table of feed ingredient and TMR forage particle length, grain particle size, dry matter, and pH

| Feed Ingredient | Penn State Particle Length (%) | | | Dry Matter (%) | | | |
	Top	Middle	Bottom	Actual[a]	Assumed[b]	Error[c]	pH
Alfalfa silage	34	52	14	29.7	37.7	27.1	4.7
Goal	15–25	> Bottom	< Middle	38–42		±5	4.2–4.8
Corn silage	25	58	17	39.3	39.3	0.0	3.8
Goal	8–20	≫ Bottom	≪ Middle	30–35		±5	3.5–4.0
Far-off dry TMR offered	21	53	26	43.8	41.5	−5.2	—
Goal	7–12	> Bottom	< Middle	40–50		±5	—
Far-off TMR refused	22	55	23	—	—	—	—
Goal	<5 different from the TMR offered			—	—	—	—
Prefresh TMR offered	9	41	50	51.5	53.7	4.2	—
Goal	7–12	> Bottom	< Middle	40–50		±5	—
Prefresh TMR refused	9	37	55	—	—	—	—
Goal	<5 different than the TMR offered			—	—	—	—
Postfresh TMR offered	27	30	42	63.3	57.3	−9.6	—
Goal	7–12	> Bottom	< Middle	40–50		±5	—
Postfresh TMR refused	29	37	34	—	—	—	—
Goal	<5 different from the TMR offered			—	—	—	—
Lactation TMR offered	12	38	50	55.9	55.9	−0.1	—
Goal	7–12	> Bottom	< Middle	40–50		±5	—
Lactation TMR refused	11	40	49	—	—	—	—
Goal	<5 different from the TMR offered			—	—	—	—

| Grain Ingredient | Grain Sieve Particle Sizes | | | | | Dry Matter (%) | | | |
	Number 4	Number 8	Number 16	Number 30	Pan	Actual	Assumed	Error	pH
High-moisture shelled corn	1	22	47	12	18	85.1	79.2	−7.0	4.6
Goal	0	0	30	50	20	75–78		±5	4.0–4.8

Key problems noted in these evaluations were wetter alfalfa silage than expected, high-moisture shelled corn that was ground too coarsely, and drier high-moisture shelled corn than expected. The alfalfa silage and corn silage were chopped longer than necessary, but there was no evidence of poor ensiling quality or sorting of the TMR in the bunks.

[a] Actual dry matter values were from the day of the herd investigation and were determined in a drying oven (60°C for 48 hours).

[b] Assumed dry matter values were those used by the producer to mix the TMR on the day of the herd investigation.

[c] Error was the percentage difference between the actual and assumed dry matter values.

DIET EVALUATION

The main element of a dairy herd nutritional investigation is a thorough evaluation of the ration being consumed by the cows. Veterinarians may not be familiar with the process of gathering and summarizing detailed diet information. Yet, it is the most effective means of identifying issues. The challenge is the effort needed to gather and analyze the needed information. There is usually little diagnostic challenge to solving nutritional problems if good data are available. A thorough evaluation of the diet also promotes constructive dialogue with the herd nutritionist about the potential solutions.

Estimating Amounts of Feed Ingredients Eaten

A determination of accurate feed amounts eaten by the cow is the final goal of this portion of the nutritional evaluation. Do not assume that the feeding amounts on the formulated ration sheets are what the cows are eating.

Evaluating the diet eaten by the cows can be time consuming (usually, ≥2 hours for each herd). The amounts of nutrients consumed by the cows may be different from the diet formulated by the nutritionist. For example, the nutrient composition of feed ingredients (especially their dry matter content) might be different from the assumptions used by the nutritionist. Or, the producer may be feeding different ingredients from those listed on the formulated ration (without the nutritionist's awareness). Or, the cows may be selectively consuming portions of the diet offered.

The inputs needed for a thorough diet evaluation are mostly intuitive and include the following:

- Amounts of feed offered to individual cows (or groups of cows if the herd is fed a TMR)
- Nutrient composition of the feed ingredients
- Amount of feed refused by the cows
- Composition of the feed refused by the cows (if the refusals seem to be visually different from the TMR offered)

Obtaining this information is usually not difficult, although at times some questions must be repeated in varying fashions before the feeding program can be thoroughly understood. Start by asking to see all of the feed ingredients and how they are delivered to the cows. On some farms, the feeding system is simple, but on other farms, the feeding system is complicated. In general, simpler feeding systems give better results. Ask about the daily feeding schedule and as much detail as possible about the time of day in which different things happen in the feeding program. It is ideal if you can schedule the investigation to include the direct observation of mixing and delivering some of the TMR, or watching 1 entire feeding in a component-fed herd. This strategy may not always be practical, but it is often revealing.

As individual feed ingredients are encountered during this exercise, perform a simple visual appraisal of them on the spot. Take a handful or 2 of each feed ingredient or mix and qualitatively separate it into some of its different components on a flat surface (eg, the back of a clipboard). Inappropriate processing of feed ingredients or inadvertent errors in feed mixes can often be spotted this way. Samples can then be submitted for wet chemistry analysis or feed microscopy to confirm the problem.

For TMR-fed herds, determine feeding amounts offered from the load sheets being used by the feeder. Do not rely on load sheets provided to you directly by the nutritionist; ask to see the load sheets being used by the feeder. If the herd is using software to monitor TMR mixing and delivery, ask to see the direct data in the software program and print out copies of the key sheets.

For component-fed herds, determine the numbers of scoops, shovels, handfuls, and so forth being offered to the cows. Careful determination of feed weight in each of these measures is critical. Many seemingly difficult nutritional problems in component-fed herds have been solved by carefully determining the weights of each feed measure.

The weights of feed measures used on a dairy are best estimated by weighing multiple numbers of each feed measure in a bucket set on top of an electronic scale. Ask the feeder to place multiple numbers of each feed measure into the bucket. Always involve the feeder in evaluating the weights of feed measures; the fullness of each feed ingredient measure varies considerably from person to person. Adding enough feed measures to fill a 20L (about 5-gallon) bucket is usually sufficient. Then, calculate the average weight for each feed measure. If hay bales are being fed as a separate feed ingredient, weigh at least 5 bales on a scale and then calculate the average bale weight.

Estimating the Nutrient Analysis of Feed Ingredients

Conducting a diet evaluation requires an estimate of the nutrient analysis of each feed ingredient used on the farm. It is not practical or cost-effective to submit a sample of every feed ingredient for a full wet chemistry analysis. Book values can be used for most standard concentrate ingredients. However, many by-product or unusual waste feeds have an inconsistent nutrient profile; each delivery of these to the farm could require a new nutrient analysis. The corn fed on the farm should be sampled at least once for each crop year.

Feed tags for commercial mineral feed ingredients are often complete and may be used as the sole source of nutrient analysis. However, if the feed tag is incomplete, it is necessary to obtain more detailed nutrient analysis information from the manufacturer. If the manufacturer cannot or will not provide this information, then, submit a representative sample of the mineral mix for full wet chemistry analysis.

Obtaining a reliable nutrient analysis for forages can be challenging. Forages vary in nutrition composition; book values are not reliable for forages. If the nutritionist has a current forage analysis that was collected in a representative fashion, then, this analysis may be sufficient for the herd investigation. If there is any question about the reliability of the current forage analysis, do not hesitate to collect representative forage samples and submit them for laboratory analysis.

Either wet chemistry procedures or near-infrared reflectance spectroscopy (NIRS) procedures can be used to analyze the nutrient composition of forages. Wet chemistry is more accurate, but is also more costly, and results are not available for several days. Analysis by NIRS can be performed the same day that the feed sample is received by the laboratory and is typically about one-third the cost of wet chemistry procedures.

In general, NIRS analyses are sufficient for determining the nutrient composition of typical feed ingredients. Forage laboratories usually have good calibration sets for these feed ingredients. Unusual or atypical feed ingredients should always be analyzed by wet chemistry procedures. There may not even be a NIRS calibration set available for some feeds.

NIRS always has modest accuracy at best for evaluating the mineral content of feed ingredients. Wet chemistry analysis is the only choice when a precise knowledge of the mineral content of feed ingredients is critical (such as for prefresh dry cow diets when balancing carefully for dietary cation-anion difference). Analyzing the organic nutrients by NIRS and inorganic (mineral) nutrients by wet chemistry procedures is a common and reasonable approach.

Estimating Total Nutrient Intake by the Cows

Once the data on feeding amounts and feed ingredient nutrient composition have been gathered, this information must be entered into a dairy ration evaluation program to calculate total nutrient intakes. The choice of dairy ration evaluation program is not critical, but the accuracy of the feed ingredient amounts and analyses entered into the program is.

Nutritionists may make errors in estimating the nutrient composition of custom feed mixtures; a part of the nutritional investigation is to detect these errors. So, do not enter the composite nutrient analysis of a feed mixture into the dairy ration evaluation program. Instead, determine the recipe used to make the mix and then enter each feed ingredient within the mix into the program. This process requires obtaining a valid estimate of the nutrient composition of each ingredient within a mix.

Most nutrient intake computations are arithmetical and could be accomplished within a simple spreadsheet program. However, dairy ration software programs have considerable advantages over using spreadsheets alone. These programs do more than just the needed arithmetic. They also provide libraries of typical feed ingredient analyses and have the capability of running sophisticated models of nutrient flows. This modeling cannot be performed casually. Modeling is particularly useful for estimating ruminal undegradability of protein, for evaluating ruminal fermentation of carbohydrates, and for estimating energy intakes based on specific digestibility estimates of individual feed ingredients.

EVALUATING THE ACCURACY OF TOTAL MIXED RATION MIXING
Initial Evaluation of Mixing Accuracy

Error in the accuracy of TMR mixing could cause changes in nutrient intake in the cows that are difficult to detect. Thus, an evaluation of the accuracy of TMR mixing should be included in the nutritional investigation. Start this evaluation by observing mixing. Watch the mixer scale weights as feed ingredients are added and compare the scale weights with the weights called for on the TMR load sheets. Also, evaluate whether or not the TMR mixer scales provide consistent weights. Malfunctioning mixer scales sometimes give erratic readings or different readings when the mixer is moved to a different location or is on a slope (also see article on TMR audit elsewhere in this issue for further discussion).

Inquire about the frequency of checking the accuracy of the TMR mixer scales. Routine servicing of mixer scales (usually by the dealer) is recommended at least once annually. Quantitatively evaluate the accuracy of the mixer scales if there is any concern at all about mixer scale accuracy. This evaluation be made by weighing the mixer on a platform scale at different times during the mixing process. If no scale is available on or near the farm, bags of feed ingredients with known weights can be placed on the mixer at different times during the mixing process.

After observing TMR mixing, follow the mixer as new feed is delivered and visually inspect the TMR as it is discharged from the mixer. The TMR should appear the same from the start to the finish of unloading. Long hay particles should be evenly distributed through the mix, and there should be no unprocessed, large chunks of hay that are distinct from the rest of the TMR.

Whole cottonseeds, if included in the TMR, should be easy to see and evaluate. They should be evenly distributed throughout the TMR load, and they should retain their white, fluffy appearance. Overmixing causes whole cottonseeds to appear brown and matted. If corn silage or hay crop silage is included in the TMR, these forage particles should not appear mashed or pulverized.

Total Mixed Ration Bunk Sampling

Some errors in feed mixing or delivery can be discovered only by sampling the TMR from the bunk and evaluating the nutrient composition of this bunk sample. Examples of these types of errors include errors in TMR scale weights or inadvertent inclusion of the wrong feed ingredient in a mix. Properly applied TMR bunk sampling and testing can be invaluable in these situations.

The best time to sample a TMR for analysis is immediately after it is fed, and before the cows have a chance to sort it. It is important that the TMR bunk sample be as representative as possible of the entire TMR batch. Collect about 12 handfuls of TMR from the start to the end of discharge of the TMR from the mixer. Put these hand-fuls of feed into a 20L (about 5-gallon) bucket as you collect them. The bucket should be full by the last handful. Collect the handfuls by scooping upwards; grabbing a TMR sample from the top of the bunk and pulling it away could result in the selective loss of finer particles from the TMR sample.

After collecting about 20L of the TMR, dump the contents of the bucket onto a flat surface (preferably a smooth, clean table) and mix them gently. Then, separate the TMR into 4 distinct quarters. Decide randomly which two-quarters to discard. Then, remix the remaining two-quarters of TMR and repeat the quartering and random dis-carding procedures. Continue mixing, quartering, and discarding until you have reduced the sample to the needed volume. For particle length analysis in the PSPS, the correct sample volume is 6 cups of TMR.

The correct amount of TMR to submit to a laboratory for nutrient analysis is about 3 cups (200–250 g). The nutrient analysis of a TMR sample should be conducted by wet chemistry procedures and not by NIRS. In addition, it is important that the lab-oratory does not further subsample the TMR bunk sample that was already carefully subsampled before submission to the laboratory. Samples of TMR may separate considerably during shipping and handling, especially if they are fairly dry. This fac-tor makes further subsampling difficult. Therefore, it is best to submit only a small quantity of feed (as described earlier) and to then request that the laboratory dry and grind the entire sample submitted. Most feeds laboratories comply with this request.

A TMR bunk sample is not a perfect representation of what the cows are eating. Laboratory results for TMR bunk samples should be interpreted broadly and not strictly. The expected TMR composition and the TMR bunk sampling results are acceptably close if they are within about 5% of each other (on a total nutrient basis). For instance, if the expected calcium content of a TMR was 1.00%, then TMR bunk sampling results between 0.95% and 1.05% would be acceptable.

There are many possible explanations for discrepancies discovered between the calculated, expected nutrient composition of the TMR and the TMR bunk sample re-sults. These explanations include the following:

- Undetected changes in feed ingredient analyses (especially forages)
- Undetected inconsistencies in adding feed ingredients to the mixer wagon
- Errors in the TMR mixer scales
- Mistakes in communication about which feed ingredients were intended to be added to a feed mix or the TMR

These issues all indicate problems that require prompt intervention.

Other explanations for discrepancies between expected nutrient composition and TMR bunk sample analyses are inherent errors in this process, such as the collection of poorly representative bunk samples or laboratory error in the wet chemistry ana-lyses. Determining the source of discrepancies discovered by TMR bunk sampling can be difficult.

The greatest value in TMR bunk sampling is to identify gross errors in feed analysis, mixing, or delivery. For example, omitting the salt from a custom protein mix results in a TMR bunk sample with unexpectedly low sodium and chloride content. Omitting the trace mineral/vitamin premix from the ration results in unexpectedly low trace mineral concentrations.

It is helpful to summarize the diet evaluation on a single-page form. This summary should include nutrient requirements, a summary of the formulated diet, the dry matter content of the feed ingredients, a summary of the expected diet, and the TMR bunk sample results. Most dairy ration software programs do not have outputs that integrate all this information. They also commonly require multiple pages to summarize a diet. **Table 8** presents an example of a single-page diet evaluation worksheet.

Evaluating Consistency of Feed Delivery

It is difficult to completely evaluate the consistency of feed delivery on a farm, but a few questions may provide most of the needed information. If the farm uses TMR monitoring software, the nutritional investigation can include not only the accuracy of weights of feed ingredients added to the mixer but also an evaluation of the consistency of when that feed is delivered to each pen.

The timing of feed deliveries to the cows on a dairy should be fanatically consistent. Cows seem to have the ability to learn to control their meal patterns (meal frequency and meal size) to self-regulate their ruminal pH. However, if the delivery of feed to the bunks is erratic, the cows fail to accomplish this self-regulation. It seems to be particularly dangerous if cows receive their TMR later than usual, because hungry cows may overeat when feed is offered. Problems with an inconsistent feeding schedule are magnified by shortages in bunk space, a shortage in free stalls (cows may be more concerned about securing a place to lie down rather than regulating their ruminal pH), or inadequate availability of water immediately after milking.

It is helpful if feeding times are consistently synchronized with milking times. The first feeding of the day should coincide with the cows returning from the parlor after the first milking. This meal is likely the biggest of the day for most cows. The consistency and timing of the first milking and feeding are particularly crucial.

Evaluating Frequency of Feed Delivery

It is common practice to offer TMR once daily to most groups of cows. However, it is best to feed TMR at least twice daily. Twice-daily TMR feeding is often mandatory in the summer months, because of the potential heating of the TMR in the bunk. Feeding more than once daily also increases overall dry matter intakes and decreases TMR sorting. Increased feeding frequency is particularly important if the TMR is susceptible to sorting, such as relatively dry TMR (>50% dry matter) or TMR with excessive amounts of coarse forage particles more than about 6.4 cm (2.5 in) long.

Frequently pushing up the TMR in the bunk throughout the day is beneficial but does not fully compensate for infrequent feeding frequency. Pushing the feed up likely stimulates some additional intake but does not reduce the potential for sorting.

Evaluating the Amount of Feed Offered

A dairy producer must decide each day how much feed to offer each group of cows on the farm. Feeding the ideal amount to a pen results in keeping cows from becoming too hungry (and potentially overeating), with the smallest possible amount of feed refusal. The amount of feed offered at the start of each day should be based on the appearance of the bunk at the end of the previous feeding day. A typical goal is to offer enough feed each day so that there is about a 5% daily feed refusal. More feed refusal than this (about 10% per day) is needed for pens with dynamic populations, such as transition cows in the prefresh and postfresh pens. Midlactation and late lactation pens can be fed to lower feed refusal, because their populations are more stable.

Table 8
Example dairy diet evaluation worksheet

Diet Group: Lactating Cows

Feed Ingredients	Formulated Ration				Estimated Ration			
	As-Fed (kg)	DM (%)	DM (kg)	% of Ration (DM Basis)	As-Fed (kg)	DM (%)	DM (kg)	% of Ration (DM Basis)
Alfalfa silage	15.23	38.8	5.91	23.3	15.40	29.7	4.57	19.0
Corn silage	13.64	39.3	5.36	21.1	13.40	39.3	5.27	21.8
High-moisture shelled corn	7.73	79.2	6.12	24.1	7.60	85.1	6.46	26.8
Whole cottonseed	1.82	90.0	1.64	6.5	1.79	90.1	1.61	6.7
Soybean meal, heated	4.80	89.1	4.27	16.8	4.68	89.0	4.17	17.3
Soy hulls	1.36	91.0	1.24	4.9	1.34	90.8	1.22	5.0
Mineral mix	0.84	97.8	0.82	3.2	0.84	98.4	0.82	3.4
Totals	45.41		25.36	100.0	45.04		24.12	100.0

Nutrient Analysis (DM Basis)	Amount Required	Formulated Ration	Estimated Ration	Laboratory Analysis
Dry matter (%)	>40	55.9	53.6	54.2
NEL (Mcal/kg)	>1.67	1.72	1.72	1.72
Ether extract (%)	3.5–5.5	4.0	4.7	4.9
Crude protein (%)	16–17	18.0	17.8	19.0
RUP (% of CP)	>32	44.3	47.8	—
ADF (%)	19–22	18.7	18.0	19.4
NDF (%)	30–32	29.9	27.1	27.7
NFC (%)	35–40	40.1	42.0	41.4
Starch (%)	22–26	28.3	28.8	—
Sugar (%)	3.5–5.5	4.0	3.8	—
Ash (%)	—	8.0	8.4	7.0
Calcium (%)	>0.80	0.96	0.95	0.88
Phosphorus (%)	0.35–0.40	0.41	0.38	0.42
Magnesium (%)	>0.35	0.33	0.33	0.34
Potassium (%)	>1.00	1.43	1.51	1.61
Sodium (%)	>0.18	0.46	0.43	0.46
Chlorine (%)	>0.25	0.41	0.48	0.56
Sulfur (%)	>0.25	0.24	0.22	0.29
DCAD (mEq/kg)	>250	300	301	272
Cobalt (ppm)	>0.10	0.87	1.10	—
Copper (ppm)	>10	16	15	30
Iron (ppm)	>100	161	110	179
Iodine (ppm)	>0.60	0.74	0.81	—
Manganese (ppm)	>40	51	63	76
Zinc (ppm)	>50	72	79	—
Se (ppm)	0.30	0.28	0.28	—

(continued on next page)

Nutrient Analysis (DM Basis)	Amount Required	Formulated Ration	Estimated Ration	Laboratory Analysis
Monensin (mg/d)	~300	419	365	—
Vitamin A (kIU/kg)	>3.30	7.19	7.00	
Vitamin D (kIU/kg)	>1.65	1.43	1.39	
Vitamin E (IU/kg)	>15.4	40.5	46.2	

Table 8 (continued)

Key problems identified were slightly higher than necessary CP formulation and low ADF and NDF values in both the formulated and estimated diets. Starch and NFC were correspondingly higher than recommended.

Abbreviations: ADF, acid detergent fiber; CP, crude protein; DCAD, dietary cation-anion difference (calculated as meq of [Na + K] − [Cl + S]); NDF, neutral detergent fiber; NEL, net energy for lactation; NFC, nonfiber carbohydrate (calculated as 100 − ether extract − CP − NDF − ash); RUP, ruminally undegradable protein.

Some dairy herds consistently feed to zero daily feed refusals. However, this strategy works well only if feeding management is exceptionally consistent. Cows may be able to self-regulate intakes and ruminal pH if the bunks are empty the same time each day, and if new feed is offered at the same time each day. Most dairies cannot manage their feed bunks this well and should target about 5% daily refusals.

How much daily TMR refusal a dairy producer targets depends greatly on the ability of the farm to use TMR refusals. The ideal use for TMR refusals is to feed them to beef feedlot animals or to cull animals that need time to heal and recondition before sale. Some dairies have this option within their own farm enterprise or are able to sell their TMR refusals to beef feedlot producers. If these options do not exist, the next most logical animals on a dairy to receive TMR refusals are the pregnant heifers. Varying amounts of TMR refusal can be added to the TMR mix for these animals, if the amounts are known and the other ingredients added to the mix are adjusted accordingly. Pregnant heifers may become too fat if they consume too much of their diet as TMR refusal or if their TMR is not properly adjusted for the amount of TMR refusal that it contains.

Dairy producers should be encouraged to record the amount of feed offered and feed refused for each pen each day. The refusals do not have to be weighed daily; an estimation of the amount refused (usually as a fraction of a loader bucket) is usually sufficient, if the weight of a full loader bucket is reasonably well determined.

The amount of feed offered to each pen each day should be calculated by adjusting the amount of each feed ingredient included in the TMR. Dairy producers should not lock most of the ingredients in the TMR and then alter just 1 ingredient (usually a forage) to deliver the desired amount of TMR to the bunk. If only 1 ingredient in the TMR is altered, severe nutrient imbalances may occur. If dairy producers monitor forage dry matter regularly and adjust feeding weights accordingly, they can have the confidence to adjust the amount of each ingredient in the TMR up or down each day.

EVALUATION OF THE COWS

Detailed diet information, collected as described earlier, can be complemented by data that come directly from the cows. There is always potential error in our ability to accurately evaluate nutrient intake. The cows' biological response to their diet is always correct, but our ability to evaluate these responses is imperfect. These realities point to the need to evaluate both the diet and the cows' responses to it.

Body Condition Scoring

Body condition of the herd is an indirect measure of energy nutrition and is a useful component of a herd investigation.[8] Body condition scores can be recorded for the entire adult cow herd or a representative portion of the adult cows in the herd. Body condition scores can then be plotted by days in milk (**Fig. 6** shows an example plot). A practical difficulty of this approach to body condition score evaluation is that cows must be individually identified so that their days in milk can be determined.

When evaluating herd body condition scores, pay special attention to the degree of body condition score loss in early lactation. Cows should lose no more than 0.5 units of body condition score in about the first 50 days in milk. It is ideal to score individual cows at calving and at about 50 days in milk to assess this loss; however, even a 1-time session of body condition scoring for the whole herd gives some indication of the general extent of early lactation body condition loss.

Recording the proportion of cows that are either too thin or too fat is an alternative to recording discrete body condition scores for individual cows in the herd. **Table 9** presents an example of body condition scores summarized as the proportion of cows that are either too fat or too thin. This approach is more practical in larger herds. The most useful body condition score information is for the cows in the prefresh group, because this is the most critical time for body condition score to be correct. The body condition

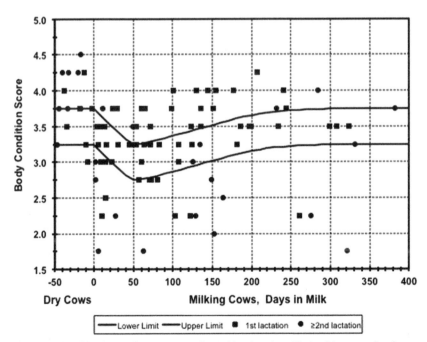

Fig. 6. Example of body condition scores plotted by days in milk. In this example, there was poor overall control of body condition score in the herd. Many of the dry cows were too fat, body condition score loss in early lactation cows appeared to be excessive, a high proportion of the lactating cows were too thin, and a high proportion of the middle to later lactation cows were too fat.

Table 9
Body condition scores (BCS) summarized by numbers of cows that were too thin or too fat

Group Name	Total Cows Scored	Cows ≤2.5 BCS (n) (%)	Cows ≥4.0 BCS (n) (%)
Milk cows, ≥ second lactation	49	8 (16)	1 (2)
Milk cows, first lactation	42	1 (2)	1 (2)
Dry cows	29	0 (0)	11 (38)
Bred heifers	18	1 (6)	4 (22)

Goals: are less than 10% of cows scored either too thin (≤2.5 BCS) and less than 10% of cows too fat (≥4.0 BCS)? The body condition scoring system used has been previously described.[14] In this example, there were too many overconditioned dry cows and bred heifers, plus too many thin lactating cows in the ≥second lactation group.

that a cow has at calving is an important determinant of her health and productivity after calving.

Cud Chewing Activity

Cud chewing activity can be evaluated as part of a herd nutritional investigation. A minimum of 40% of the cows that are not eating should be chewing their cud at any given time. A lack of cud chewing activity could be an indicator of low effective fiber intake and poor ruminal mat layer formation. Cows experiencing stress or health problems may also have reduced cud chewing.

Manure Evaluation

Dairy herd nutritional investigations should include an evaluation of manure characteristics. The presence of undigested corn particles in the manure may indicate that the grain is ground too coarsely. Dry, coarsely chopped corn silage (not kernel processed) may also result in excessive amounts of undigested corn in the manure. Loose manure consistency or an acidic smell to the manure may indicate ruminal acidosis, with excessive amounts of starch reaching the large intestine. A putrid odor to the manure may indicate protein overfeeding with excessive amounts of undigested protein reaching the large intestine.

If problems are seen in the general appearance of the manure, it may be helpful to screen manure samples to more definitively evaluate the number of undigested feed particles. A simple manure screening protocol is to evaluate about 1 cup of manure from 6 or more early lactation to midlactation cows. Gently wash the manure over a grain screen with 6 to 8 squares per inch. There should be few undigested grain particles or forage particles more than 1 in long in a 1-cup manure sample. Finding undigested, long forage particles suggests possible ruminal acidosis, with poor fiber digestion. The presence of undigested grain particles (particularly with white starch remaining inside the grain pieces) suggests that the grains were not processing finely enough before feeding. Kernel processed corn silage harvested with the kernel processing rollers too far apart may also contribute to undigested corn in the manure. The presence of whole cottonseeds in the manure suggests either overfeeding of the cottonseeds or ruminal maldigestion because of inadequate mat layer formation. Visible pieces of roasted soybeans may be present in the manure if the roasted soybeans were not processed finely enough before feeding (they should be broken into fourths or eighths). Manure screening protocols have been described in detail elsewhere.[9]

Locomotion Scoring

In herds with concerns about lameness, it is helpful to conduct a simple lameness scoring of the entire herd (or representative portions of large herds). Watch each cow walk and record a lameness score of 1 for no visible lameness, 2 for slight lameness, 3 for moderate lameness, and 4 for severe lameness.[10]

Less than 10% of the herd should have a score of 3, and there should be no cows with a score of 4. Herds with severe lameness problems may have 50% of the herd or more scored as a 3 or 4.

A practical problem with locomotion scoring is the need to score all milking and dry cows in the herd before interpreting the results. Lame cows may be concentrated in certain pens (eg, older cow pens, lame cow groups), so it is not practical to score a representative portion of the herd. An alternative approach is to conduct locomotion scoring for high-risk animals such as the prefresh cows. All cows in the herd must go through the prefresh pen, and lameness status just before calving is a particularly important determinant of fresh cow health and productivity.

Examination of Affected Cows

If cows showing typical clinical signs of a peripartum disease are present in the herd, they should be given complete physical examinations as part of the herd nutritional investigation. Depending on the disease, appropriate blood samples should also be collected. Inaccurate or inconclusive diagnostic information at this stage of an investigation can set the wrong course for your entire herd workup. Try to conclusively document cow health problems; do not take the dairy producer's diagnosis at face value.

If the client complaint includes cow deaths, then, try to make the best possible postmortem diagnosis for as many cows as possible. In some extreme situations, it could be appropriate to identify an animal with clinical signs typical of the herd problem, euthanize this animal, and conduct a fresh postmortem evaluation.

Good diagnostic information from affected cows often shows that herd health problems are typically not caused by a single type of metabolic or infectious disease, but rather to a combination of problems. The challenge is to uncover the underlying causes of these problems.

HERD-BASED BIOLOGICAL TESTING PROCEDURES

Biological testing results are most useful in supporting a diagnosis already made from the diet evaluation. Biological testing results do not stand alone and must be corroborated by other findings from the herd nutritional investigation.

The most useful biological tests in herd nutritional investigations are ruminal pH, serum β-hydroxybutyric acid, plasma nonesterified fatty acids, urinary pH, and milk or blood urea nitrogen. These tests have been reviewed in detail elsewhere.[11–13]

COMBINING HERD DATA TO MAKE FINAL RECOMMENDATIONS

Final herd nutritional recommendations must integrate information obtained from all aspects of the investigation. None of the data collected during a herd investigation are perfectly reliable; all contain some inherent error. The most reliable diagnostic conclusions are those supported by more than 1 source of data, thus offsetting limitations of inherent error in each piece of data.

It is common to identify numerous problems as part of a herd nutritional investigation. However, not all problems are of equal importance or are even important at all.

Recommendations should focus on correcting the causes of the most pressing herd problems. Some of the herd problems identified during the investigation should wait for a more opportune time to discuss with the client. The initial client complaint that was the cause for the investigation must also be thoroughly addressed in the final recommendations, even if it did not rank as one of the most important overall herd problems.

REFERENCES

1. Cook NB, Nordlund KV, Oetzel GR. Environmental influences on claw horn lesions associated with laminitis and subacute ruminal acidosis in dairy cows. J Dairy Sci 2004;87(E Suppl):E36–8.
2. Beede DK. Evaluation of water quality and nutrition for dairy cattle. Available at: https://wwwmsuedu/~beede/dairycattlewaterandnutritionpdf. Accessed March 3, 2014.
3. Oetzel GR, Villalba FP, Goodger WJ, et al. Comparison of on-farm methods for estimating the dry matter content of feed ingredients. J Dairy Sci 1993;76(1):293.
4. Oetzel GR. Application of forage particle length determination in dairy practice. Compend Contin Educ Pract Vet 2001;23(3):S30–7.
5. Kononoff PJ, Heinrichs AJ, Buckmaster DR. Modification of the Penn State forage and total mixed ration particle separator and the effects of moisture content on its measurements. J Dairy Sci 2003;86(5):1858–63.
6. Heinrichs J. Evaluating particle size of forages and TMRs using the new Penn State forage particle separator. Penn State Dairy Extension Publication DSE 2013-186. Available at: http://extensionpsuedu/animals/dairy/health/nutrition/forages/forage-quality-physical/separator. Accessed March 3, 2014.
7. Hutjens M, Dann H. Grain processing: it is too coarse or too fine?. Available at: http://c3412693r93cf0rackcdncom/D10181GrainProcessingpdf. Accessed March 3, 2014.
8. Roche JR, Kay JK, Friggens NC, et al. Assessing and managing body condition score for the prevention of metabolic disease in dairy cows. Vet Clin North Am Food Anim Pract 2013;29(2):323–36.
9. Hutjens M. Evaluating manure on the farm. Illini DairyNet Papers. Available at: http://wwwlivestocktraillillinoisedu/dairynet/paperDisplaycfm?ContentID=550. Accessed March 3, 2014.
10. Nordlund KV, Cook NB, Oetzel GR. Investigation strategies for laminitis problem herds. J Dairy Sci 2004;87(E Suppl):E27–35.
11. Oetzel GR. Monitoring and testing dairy herds for metabolic disease. Vet Clin North Am Food Anim Pract 2004;20(3):651–74.
12. Ospina PA, McArt JA, Overton TR, et al. Using nonesterified fatty acids and β-hydroxybutyrate concentrations during the transition period for herd-level monitoring of increased risk of disease and decreased reproductive and milking performance. Vet Clin North Am Food Anim Pract 2013;29(2):387–412.
13. Bertoni G, Trevisi E. Use of the liver activity index and other metabolic variables in the assessment of metabolic health in dairy herds. Vet Clin North Am Food Anim Pract 2013;29(2):413–31.
14. Edmonson AJ, Lean IJ, Weaver LD, et al. A body condition scoring chart for Holstein dairy cows. J Dairy Sci 1989;72(1):68–78.

Index

Note: Page numbers of article titles are in **boldface** type.

Vet Clin Food Anim 30 (2014) 789–804
http://dx.doi.org/10.1016/S0749-0720(14)00071-1
0749-0720/14/$ – see front matter © 2014 Elsevier Inc. All rights reserved.

vetfood.theclinics.com

Moving?

Make sure your subscription moves with you!

To notify us of your new address, find your **Clinics Account Number** (located on your mailing label above your name), and contact customer service at:

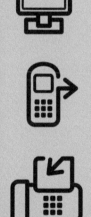

Email: journalscustomerservice-usa@elsevier.com

800-654-2452 (subscribers in the U.S. & Canada)
314-447-8871 (subscribers outside of the U.S. & Canada)

Fax number: 314-447-8029

Elsevier Health Sciences Division
Subscription Customer Service
3251 Riverport Lane
Maryland Heights, MO 63043

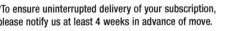

*To ensure uninterrupted delivery of your subscription, please notify us at least 4 weeks in advance of move.

Printed and bound by CPI Group (UK) Ltd, Croydon, CR0 4YY

03/10/2024

01040490-0012